Hansen's Disease

Patrícia D. Deps
Editor

Marcos Cesar Florian
Marcos da Cunha Lopes Virmond
Associated Editors

Hansen's Disease

A Complete Clinical Guide

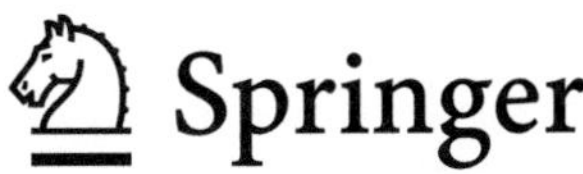 Springer

Editor
Patrícia D. Deps
Social Medicine Department
Universidade Federal do Espírito Santo
Vitória, Brazil

ISBN 978-3-031-30895-6   ISBN 978-3-031-30893-2   (eBook)
https://doi.org/10.1007/978-3-031-30893-2

This Springer imprint is published by the registered company Springer Nature Switzerland AG
The registered company address is: Gewerbestrasse 11, 6330 Cham, Switzerland

Hansen's disease is as ancient as mankind, yet it still poses challenges to science, to people affected by the disease, and to health workers who care for them. We have written this book in the hope that, one day, those challenges will be overcome. Until then, our book is intended to serve as a practical guide for doctors and other professionals who may encounter Hansen's disease in their clinical practice.

Preface

The three editors and reviewers of this book are to be congratulated for bringing together this important collection of chapters on Hansen's Disease (Leprosy). The various chapters use 'Leprosy' and 'Hansen's Disease' interchangeably. The book includes a section on the history of leprosy; it reflects on the important developments that have taken place over recent decades and indicates what research can have an impact on the future. The book has a strong international flavour and represents the work of 42 authors from 10 different countries. It has been edited by three internationally distinguished experts in the field.

The book highlights the key advances that have been influential in the very significant progress that has been made to the field in recent years. These advances include the discovery of *Mycobacterium leprae* as the primary cause of leprosy and the more recent sequencing of the genome of the bacteria. Introduction of effective short course Multidrug Therapy has changed the landscape of the epidemiology of leprosy as well as changing the lives of people affected. The book also recognizes the vital impact made by the UN endorsement of the principles and guidelines for the elimination of discrimination against persons affected by Hansen's disease. The implementation of the guidelines by health care workers can ensure people affected have access to the highest standards of physical and mental health on an equal basis with others. These are important innovations that have had a profound effect on our understanding of the disease and the quality of life of those affected.

The changing epidemiology of leprosy is described as well as the interventions that have an impact on the occurrence of leprosy. The inclusion of leprosy as one of the Neglected Tropical Diseases is seen as an important global strategy to strengthen and sustain leprosy programmes. The COVID-19 pandemic had a substantial impact on the detection and treatment of leprosy during 2020–21 and is still to recover. It is anticipated that new diagnostics tests in combination with new strategies particularly post-exposure prophylaxis will interrupt transmission in the future. There is an intrigued chapter on the existence of both environmental and zoonotic reservoirs of *M. Leprae,* there will be more on this topic, watch this space.

The book also focusses on the innovations that can impact on leprosy in the future. Attention is given to innovations in the detection of disease and diagnosis. There are chapters on both molecular and immunological diagnostic methods as well as the clinical application of existing tools using active case finding approaches and targeted post-exposure prophylaxis. A whole chapter is dedicated to the importance of leprosy in children as an indicator of transmission in the community stressing the critical issue of early diagnosis of leprosy in children. The potential of novel diagnostic imaging is discussed using advanced radiological and ultrasound technologies, and electroneuromyography. The book includes helpful clinical chapters on the differential diagnosis of dermatological and neurological presentations.

The book provides comprehensive coverage of a range of issues in leprosy such as ophthalmic, osteoarticular and otolaryngological complications of the disease. Challenges of immunosuppression and co-infections are dealt with in a dedicated chapter. There is a special focus on psychosocial implications of leprosy, a long-neglected aspect of leprosy work. The frequency of depression and anxiety is now well recognized, and the importance of social support and interventions aimed at improving mental wellbeing. This complements the innovations on elimination of stigma and discrimination and human rights-based approaches.

A strong theme in the book, which is addressed by many of the authors, is reactions, nerve injury and the prevention of disability. This is very important both to health care staff and to people affected. There is a chapter dedicated to reactions, which recognizes the importance of early diagnosis and effective treatment while much of the immunopathogenesis remains to be elucidated. A separate chapter by leading experts explores the mechanism of nerve injury, and another chapter addresses the evaluation, monitoring and prevention of disabilities.

Treatment of leprosy is covered in several chapters, a dominant theme is the importance of early diagnosis, especially in children. The importance of multidrug therapy is emphasized. There is coverage of the issues of drug reactions and drug resistance in multidrug therapy and discussion of alternative regimens. The implications and options in both immune-prophylaxis and chemoprophylaxis are described.

The book identifies the major advances in the past which have changed the course of the history of leprosy. It also provides descriptions of the current priorities in the diagnosis and treatment of leprosy, in the psychosocial interventions and in the changing societal attitudes towards those affected. The authors also identify the issues that could change future approaches to leprosy including the potential for a range of novel diagnostic modalities to change the detection and diagnosis of leprosy. Novel public health strategies can promote early detection and implement approaches of prevention. There is the potential of research described in the book to improve our understanding of the basic pathophysiology of leprosy, particularly the work of the late Milton Ozorio Moraes and his colleagues on the metabolic, genetic and immunological mechanism in susceptibility to leprosy.

The Editors have compiled a fascinating and comprehensive series of chapters on leprosy, past, present and future. They are to be congratulated for this contribution to the literature on leprosy which provides something for everyone, no matter what aspect of leprosy you are interested in or actively involved with, many thanks to the Editors and to the many international authors.

University of Aberdeen   Cairns Smith
Aberdeen, Scotland, UK

Foreword

Between diagnosis and cure of Leprosy or Hansen's disease there are people. There are also families, communities, bacillus, histories, policies, evidence-based knowledge, drugs, technologies, stigma, discrimination, health services, advocacy services, social welfare services, government entities, nongovernmental organizations and organizations of persons affected. Regardless of the order of existence, persons affected by leprosy should be at the centre of the process. This book has been written by 42 persons from 10 different countries, committed to improving the process of care and social inclusion for persons affected by Hansen's disease.

Hansen's disease is a communicable, chronic and curable disease. This statement has become a mantra among the community of scientists and persons affected by the disease. Throughout the twentieth century, the discoveries made in the natural sciences contributed to the understanding of the health-disease process and led to the organization of health care models. A century passed between the identification of *Mycobacterium leprae* by Gerhard Armauer Hansen in 1873 and the combination of antibiotics in multidrug therapy in 1982.

If on the one hand, we remember two World Wars. On the other hand, we forget the daily struggles experienced by those marginalized by society. Among them, people affected by Hansen's disease who were isolated in institutions as a prophylactic measure against the disease. Supported by science and health policies, segregation continued after the discovery of the first antibiotic capable of treating the disease. Compulsory isolation separated thousands of families around the world, perpetuating the stigma related to Hansen's disease and discrimination against those affected by it in the following decades.

The first three chapters of this work introduce us to the historical and technical-scientific aspects of the disease. In the first chapter, the professors and researchers Marcos Florian, Marcos Virmond and Patrícia Deps introduce us to the general aspects of Hansen's disease. In the second chapter, David Scollard discusses the history of scientific advances, from the discovery of the bacillus to the production of a vaccine. In the third chapter, Charlotte A. Roberts, fascinates us by unravelling the mysteries of an almost prehistoric bacillus. Knowledge of the evolutionary and socio-historical processes of Hansen's disease are fundamental to understanding the current situation and envisioning a future of 'zero leprosy'.

At some stage, you will ask yourself: are there still people affected by Hansen's disease? The answer is simple: yes, there are. I am one of them! According to the World Health Organization, the disease is still a public health problem for a group of 23 countries, where high disease burden and discrimination against affected persons and their families persist. Now, you may be asking yourself: why have these countries not eliminated Hansen's disease? Unlike the first one, this answer is complex and traverses the integration of natural and social sciences.

In Chap. 4, Alice Cruz and Patricia Deps discuss a human rights-based approach. For decades, persons affected by the disease and their family members have had their rights violated. In some countries, discriminatory laws still exist. Regardless of history, culture, self-determination of peoples and various forms of colonization, we need to defend the life, equality and dignity of these people in society.

The Covid-19 pandemic reminded everyone of the importance of decisions based on scientific evidence, both for the mistakes and the successes. Hansen's disease as a neglected disease has fewer resources for research. New research on the bacillus, its integration with the environment and its interaction with humans (from transmission to disease development) is needed to understand the disease process, care and prevention.

These topics are addressed in a set of Chaps. 5–10. Renowned researchers, such as Milton Ozório (in memoriam), have dedicated their lives to research and to providing the opportunity to broaden knowledge on the clinical and epidemiological aspects of the disease. This book is a strategy for translating and facilitating access to knowledge for health professionals and people affected by Hansen's disease in places we cannot even imagine.

One of these days, I was approached to guide a family. Initially, the first health professionals did not suspect Hansen's disease, the person was a 5-year-old girl. According to the mother, the first signs and symptoms started when she was 3 years old. Such a small child with Hansen's disease, how is this possible? In Chap. 11, Jerome Leonard and Jessica Fairley teach us about the clinical complexity of these cases. In addition, we need to remember that children and adolescents also suffer discrimination in their living spaces. We must guarantee and preserve the right to education, care, housing, food, and family love. In order to take care of both the physical body and the mental health of our children.

One of the biggest problems of Hansen's disease is physical disability. The physical deformities caused by the disease are among those responsible for stigma and discrimination. Physical disabilities increase the chances of exclusion of affected persons in different areas of life. Strategies to prevent disability need to articulate the biopsychosocial and physical aspects of care. For this, we need to understand the neurological and immunological aspects of the diseases, existing diagnostic technologies, contact prophylaxis, as well as the psychosocial aspects that affect the mental health of these people. These aspects are covered between Chaps. 12 and 25.

Hansen's disease is curable. The discovery and implementation of multidrug therapy has revolutionized the lives of people affected. The last chapter deals with the treatment of the disease. A combination of antibiotics capable of eliminating a bacillus, with appropriate use and within a specified period. The free distribution of the drug and follow-up in primary health care units have allowed more people to be cured and reduced disability. However, the new challenge is to overcome bacterial resistance and research new effective drugs in a shorter treatment time.

Reading this book contributes to expanding knowledge about leprosy so that people affected can be at the centre of the processes and care. Being a person affected by Hansen's disease is not simple since any disease that also affects the soul can upset and transform life. Perhaps the secret is in how and with whom we face this process. However, we also need to remember that guaranteeing rights is a constitutional political duty. So as people affected by Hansen's disease, we need to claim these rights. I thank the editors for this learning opportunity.

Faculty of Nursing, Rio de Janeiro State University   Paula Soares Brandão

Rio de Janeiro, Brazil

Acknowledgements

Andrea Maia Fernandes de Araújo Fonseca from the Health Department of the Municipality of Petrolina, Pernambuco, Brazil.

Chinwe Chika Eze, Nnamdi Azikiwe University/ Nnamdi Azikiwe Teaching Hospital, Nnewi, Anambra State, Nigeria.

Cléverson Teixeira Soares, Lauro de Souza Lima Institute, São Paulo, Brazil.

Dâmaris Versiani Caldeira Gonçalves, Hospital Israelita Albert Einstein, Brazil.

Márcia Helena Oliveira, HC-Universidade Federal de Pernambuco, Brazil.

Marília de Moraes Delgado, HC-Universidade Federal de Pernambuco, Brazil.

Milena de Oliveira Amui Abud, Centro de Controle de Hanseníase in Uberaba, Brazil.

Paula Maria Rodrigues de Barros Corrêa Damázio, HC-Universidade Federal de Pernambuco, Brazil.

Rachel Azevedo Serafim, Secretaria Estadual de Saúde of Espírito Santo, Brazil.

Rafael Maffei Loureiro, Hospital Israelita Albert Einstein, São Paulo, Brazil.

Vânia Azevedo de Souza, Secretaria de Saúde de Serra, Brazil.

Contents

Introduction to Hansen's Disease

Marcos Cesar Florian, Marcos da Cunha Lopes Virmond, and Patrícia D. Deps

Hansen's disease (HD), also called leprosy, has been historically a worldwide problem, including as a major scourge of Europe in the Middle Ages. Nowadays, it is considered to be a 'neglected tropical disease' that most often affect the poorest people living in low- and middle-income countries in the tropical and subtropical regions. Currently, the three countries with the highest number of people affected are India, Brazil, and Indonesia [1].

Increased risk of Hansen's disease has been associated with individual and household factors including older age, male gender, poor sanitary and socioeconomic conditions, lower level of education, and food insecurity. However, there is limited understanding of the roles of infected and asymptomatic people in the transmission of the disease [2]. The complex social, political, environmental, and human health aspects of Hansen's disease present challenges to the implementation of effective public health policies to prevent and control Hansen's disease.

Hansen's disease is a chronic infectious disease that mainly affects peripheral nerves and the skin. It typically starts as a localized disease which, in susceptible individuals, can become generalized. Involvement of the peripheral nerves causes motor and sensory dysfunction leading to disabilities especially in the hands, feet, and eyes.

M. C. Florian
Universidade Federal de São Paulo, São Paulo, Brazil
e-mail: mcflorian@unifesp.br

M. da Cunha Lopes Virmond (✉)
Universidade de São Paulo, Bauru, Brazil
e-mail: mvirmond@usp.br

P. D. Deps
Universidade Federal do Espírito Santo, Vitória, Brazil
e-mail: patricia.deps@ufes.br

Although the World Health Organization (WHO) multidrug therapy (MDT) treatment regimen (dapsone, rifampicin, and clofazimine) has achieved high cure rates and dramatically reduced the number of Hansen's disease cases, a large number of people still develop long-term complications, including impairment of neural function and consequent disabilities and deformities because MDT does not reverse damage [3]. Further, the acute inflammatory responses—Hansen's disease reactions—which can exacerbate neural damage, among other causes can also be triggered by MDT. To control these reactions, anti-inflammatory drugs, usually corticosteroids at high initial doses, are frequently used alongside MDT.

MDT has been used for around 40 years. Second-line drugs include minocycline, clarithromycin, and ofloxacin/levofloxacin/moxifloxacin. Unfortunately, therapeutic failures, relapses, and *Mycobacterium leprae* with resistance to dapsone, rifampicin, or ofloxacin have been reported in several parts of the world [4]. Endemic countries need to increase the investigation of resistance to components of MDT and second-line drugs, while in vitro, in vivo, and in silico research is needed to identify new drugs.

Much of the long-term morbidity experienced by people after treatment is secondary to the irreversible damage caused by Hansen's disease. However, we cannot rule out continuous primary effects of the pathological processes of the disease, especially chronic or recurrent inflammation, causing parenchymal, neuropathic and osteoarticular changes. This reinforces the need for prompt diagnosis and treatment and the importance of specialized long-term care for people affected by Hansen's disease.

Whether Hansen's disease can be eliminated is questionable [5, 6], but WHO recognizes it as one of twenty neglected diseases and has adopted a global strategy for the elimination of Hansen's disease by 2030 (see box below) [1]. The ten challenges to be solved in this time span comprise: (1) delay in diagnosis; (2) decrease in Hansen's disease specialists; (3) meaningful engagement of relevant stakeholders; (4) deep-rooted stigma and discrimination; (5) significant gaps in research; (6) limited access or referral to essential care services; (7) non-existent routine surveillance systems; (8) weak health information systems; (9) expansion of monitoring of antibiotic resistance and adverse effects; (10) zoonotic transmission (in some areas).

WHO global Hansen's disease strategies 2021–2030

120 endemic countries reporting zero new autochthonous cases
70% reduction in the annual number of new cases detected
90% reduction in the rate (per million) of new cases with grade-2 disabilities
90% reduction in the rate (per million children) of new cases in children

---

1 Aetiological Agents

Mycobacterium leprae was the only known etiologic agent of Hansen's disease since its discovery by Armauer Hansen in 1873, until a second apparently causative mycobacterial species was identified in 2008.

This new species was identified by Han et al. initially in a patient from Mexico who died of diffuse lepromatous HD with a severe HD reaction, known as Lucio's phenomenon [7]. Investigation of the aetiologic agent revealed the presence of acid-fast bacilli (AFB) and PCR identified a sequence of the ribosomal RNA (rRNA) gene that differed slightly from *M. leprae*. The new strain, labelled FJ924, was then found in an archived biopsy specimen from a second similar case (also from Mexico). Based on these results, the existence of a new species of mycobacterium that causes Hansen's disease, named *Mycobacterium lepromatosis*, was announced [7].

Since this discovery, cases reports have identified *M. lepromatosis* infection in 19 patients, including four patients with dual *M. leprae/M. lepromatosis* infection, and 10 retrospective specimen surveys have examined 1260 archived biopsy specimens, detecting *M. lepromatosis, M. leprae* or dual infection in, respectively, 106 (15.8%), 798 (84.6%), and 28 (3.0%) of 943 PCR-positive specimens from Mexico, Brazil, Malaysia, Myanmar, the Philippines and the USA [8].

With the development and validation of a primer for performing PCR testing using a single repeating element for *M. lepromatosis* (RLMP, equivalent to RLEP *M. leprae*) [9], a reliable molecular diagnostic method is now available to expand the investigation of this new species as a causative agent of Hansen's disease [10].

2 Natural History and Pathogenesis

Despite advances in biomolecular research, the fact that the etiological agent cannot be cultured in vitro presents a significant challenge to studying the relationship between agents and hosts (human and animal), leaving important gaps in our understanding of epidemiological, pathological, and immunological aspects of Hansen's disease, which need to be filled if efforts to eliminate the disease are to be successful.

3 Transmission Dynamics

The transmission pathways of the causative agents of HD are still not well understood. Direct dissemination is clearly important in the transmission process. However, the possibility of indirect dissemination cannot be ignored [11]. Even in endemic areas, many newly detected cases report no known history of contact with patients, suggesting a role for other transmission pathways.

Untreated multibacillary (MB) cases of Hansen's disease are likely to be the principal source of transmission of *M. leprae*, through infectious aerosols of nasal secretions created by coughing and sneezing [12], but possibly also via skin-to-skin contact through breaks in the continuity of the skin [13, 14].

Household contacts of MB cases have an estimated five to ten times higher risk of developing Hansen's disease than the general population, while paucibacillary (PB) cases also present an increased risk of onward transmission.

More controversially, transmission from people with subclinical infection by nasal shedding of *M. leprae* has been demonstrated. *M. leprae* DNA has been detected in nasal swabs in up to 5% of healthy individuals in endemic areas [12], and the presence of anti-PGL-1 (phenolic-glycolipid-1) and anti-LID-1 (Leprosy IDRI Diagnostic 1) antibodies in asymptomatic persons from endemic areas indicates the importance of studying subclinical infection.

Isolated cases of *M. leprae* found in the placenta [15] and in breast milk [16] have been reported, but risk of transmission via these routes is uncertain. The literature includes reports of cases of Hansen's disease caused by accidental infection with contaminated needles [17, 18], by material used for tattooing [19], after a dog bite [20], and after BCG vaccination [21].

The incubation period of Hansen's disease ranges from 3 months to 40 years [22]. It has been estimated that 70–90% of the population is resistant to *M. leprae* due to innate immunity, in some instances reinforced by vaccination with BCG or by cross-reaction in people who have been exposed to *Mycobacterium tuberculosis* or other mycobacteria.

It has long been known that *M. leprae* is able to survive outside the human body for several months under favourable conditions. The finding of RNA indicating the presence of viable *M. leprae* in environmental soil and water samples in Brazil and India [23, 24], and that amoeba were capable of ingesting and harbouring viable *M. leprae*, provided further evidence for the survival of *M. leprae* outside a mammalian host [25].

Adopting a One Health approach to Hansen's disease, including consideration of environmental reservoirs and zoonotic transmission of *M. leprae* and *M. lepromatosis* at population level, is more recent. Here transmission involves a circular sequence of steps from transmission of the bacillus from the environment through contact with soil, water, or animal hosts to development of the disease in humans and transmission of the agent back into the environment [26].

4 Mitsuda Test

The intradermal reaction or 'Mitsuda' delayed-type hypersensitivity test evaluates a person's cellular immune response to *M. leprae*. The test is performed by intradermal inoculation of a solution of bacilli killed by heat. In cases where the test is positive, it is possible to identify a papule-nodule type reaction that is considered positive if larger than 3 mm in diameter at the inoculation site after 4 weeks. This indicates an intense Th-1 type cellular immune response associated with low risk of developing MB disease at the Virchowian (lepromatous) pole of the Hansen's disease spectrum.

A negative Mitsuda reaction indicates the absence of a cellular immune response against *M. leprae*, indicating a predominantly Th-2 type humoral response and a higher risk of developing Virchowian (lepromatous) Hansen's disease.

Most of the population in an endemic area will have a positive response to inoculation with Mitsuda antigen and, if infected with *M. leprae*, a person will tend to develop a PB of Hansen's disease or remain free from disease. Although the Mitsuda test has recognized value in clinical practice for assessing the cellular immune response against the causative agent of HD, it is not currently available for use in many countries.

5 Vaccines

The BCG vaccine, used to prevent severe forms of tuberculosis, is given routinely to children in many Hansen's disease endemic countries and has also been shown to be effective in reducing risk of the disease [27]. In a country endemic for HD (Brazil), a second dose of BCG is used in contacts of Hansen's disease cases if signs and symptoms of the disease are not detected. Administration of BCG jointly with chemoprophylaxis against Hansen's disease is being evaluated.

Vaccines derived from *Mycobacterium indicus pranii* [28], *Mycobacterium avium intracellulare complex* (LepVax) [29], and anti-tuberculosis vaccines [30] have been studied as possible future options in the prevention of Hansen's disease. One of the WHO's strategic pillars for 2021–2030 includes scaling up prevention and encouraging research into existing and potential new vaccines [1].

One such candidate is a vaccine developed specifically for Hansen's disease comprising a recombinant protein composed of four *M. leprae* antigens with a synthetic TLR4 agonist (GLA-SE) as adjuvant. In phase 1 trial, this was shown to be a safe and effective inducer of durable T-cell responses [31].

6 Diagnostic Tests

Skin smear microscopy and pathological examination of the skin are important diagnostic tools, but the development of new diagnostic tests to aid clinicians in diagnosing early and PB Hansen's disease cases presents a challenge in Hansen's disease research. Such tests are of importance for those who work in non-specialized centres such as in primary care and remote settings without access to laboratories.

Detection of nerve involvement by peripheral nerve ultrasound is being explored as tool for the diagnosis and follow-up of nerve damage in Hansen's disease patients and will be discussed in a specific chapter on this book.

Biomarker tests for Hansen's disease performed on peripheral blood using the ELISA (enzyme-linked immunosorbent assay) technique to detect IgM anti-PGL-1 and anti-LID-1 antibodies are positive in higher titres in MB forms and in lower titres in PB forms. Hence, lateral flow (rapid) tests using blood smears are more likely to be positive in MB Hansen's disease, but negative results do not rule out PB forms and their positive predictive value in endemic areas is questionable [27].

Molecular DNA detection tests such as rtPCR (real-time polymerase chain reaction) have high diagnostic sensitivity and specificity and can be used with a range of sample types including dermal and conjunctival scrapings and skin and nerve biopsy specimens [10]. However, they require specific laboratory and technical apparatus and expertise, which reduces their widespread use.

7 Nerve Damage

If Hansen's disease were only a dermatological condition, it might not have acquired the same degree of social and medical historical significance. Hansen's disease as a major public health challenge arises from its contagiousness and potential for severe peripheral nerve damage.

It is known that *M. leprae* has a tropism to Schwann cells through pathways that are still being elucidated [32]. However, the relationship between the pathogen and each individual is often unpredictable, ranging from the absence of injury to highly destructive immunological reactions. The latter can lead to damage to the peripheral nerves to varying degrees ranging from slightly decreased sensitivity, to paraesthesia, to complete anaesthesia and loss of muscle strength. Disabilities and deformities follow, often accompanied by neuropathic pain [33, 34].

Early detection to mitigate neural damage is a crucial aspect of Hansen's disease programmes. Although the use of reaction markers, nerve ultrasonography, and a better understanding of neurophysiology have aided in the early detection and follow-up of neural damage, it remains a challenge to completely prevent this consequence of Hansen's disease. Measures to train personnel and facilitate access to specialist care are needed and, for people affected by deformities and disabilities arising from nerve damage, physical rehabilitation should be provided as part of the process of recovery and to aid in social reintegration.

References

1. World Health Organization. Global consultation of National Leprosy Programme managers, partners and affected persons on Global Leprosy Strategy 2021–2030. Geneva: World Health Organization; 2020.
2. Britton WJ, Lockwood DNJ. Leprosy. Lancet Lond Engl. 2004;363:1209–19. https://doi.org/10.1016/S0140-6736(04)15952-7.
3. Lockwood DNJ, Suneetha S. Leprosy: too complex a disease for a simple elimination paradigm. Bull World Health Organ. 2005;83:230–5.
4. Scollard DM, Adams LB, Gillis TP, et al. The continuing challenges of leprosy. Clin Microbiol Rev. 2006;19:338–81. https://doi.org/10.1128/CMR.19.2.338-381.2006.

5. Fine PEM. Leprosy: what is being "eliminated"? Bull World Health Organ. 2007;85:2. https://doi.org/10.2471/blt.06.039206.

6. Meima A, Smith WCS, van Oortmarssen GJ, et al. The future incidence of leprosy: a scenario analysis. Bull World Health Organ. 2004;82:373–80.

7. Han XY, Seo Y-H, Sizer KC, et al. A new Mycobacterium species causing diffuse lepromatous leprosy. Am J Clin Pathol. 2008;130:856–64. https://doi.org/10.1309/AJCPP72FJZZRRVMM.

8. Deps P, Collin SM. *Mycobacterium lepromatosis* as a second agent of Hansen's disease. Front Microbiol. 2021;12:698588. https://doi.org/10.3389/fmicb.2021.698588.

9. Sharma R, Singh P, McCoy RC, et al. Isolation of *Mycobacterium lepromatosis* and development of molecular diagnostic assays to distinguish *Mycobacterium leprae* and *M. lepromatosis*. Clin Infect Dis. 2020;71:e262–9. https://doi.org/10.1093/cid/ciz1121.

10. Avanzi C, Singh P, Truman RW, Suffys PN. Molecular epidemiology of leprosy: an update. Infect Genet Evol. 2020;86:104581. https://doi.org/10.1016/j.meegid.2020.104581.

11. Cree IA, Smith WC. Leprosy transmission and mucosal immunity: towards eradication? Lepr Rev. 1998;69:112–21. https://doi.org/10.5935/0305-7518.19980011.

12. Hatta M, van Beers SM, Madjid B, et al. Distribution and persistence of *Mycobacterium leprae* nasal carriage among a population in which leprosy is endemic in Indonesia. Trans R Soc Trop Med Hyg. 1995;89:381–5. https://doi.org/10.1016/0035-9203(95)90018-7.

13. Araujo S, Freitas LO, Goulart LR, Goulart IMB. Molecular evidence for the aerial route of infection of *Mycobacterium leprae* and the role of asymptomatic carriers in the persistence of leprosy. Clin Infect Dis. 2016;63:1412–20. https://doi.org/10.1093/cid/ciw570.

14. Gama RS, Gomides TAR, Gama CFM, et al. High frequency of *M. leprae* DNA detection in asymptomatic household contacts. BMC Infect Dis. 2018;18:153. https://doi.org/10.1186/s12879-018-3056-2.

15. Bryceson ADM. Leprosy. In: Champion RH, Rook GA, Wilkinson DS, Ebling FJG, editors. Textbook of dermatology: in four volumes. 5th ed. Oxford: Blackwell; 1993.

16. Pedley JC. The presence of *M. leprae* in human milk. Lepr Rev. 1967;38:239–42.

17. Marchoux E. Un cas d'inoculation accidentelle du bacille de Hansen en pays non lepreux. Int J Lepr. 1934;2:1–6.

18. Klingmüller V. Ergebnisse der Lepraforschung seit 1930: Ergänzung zum Beitrage "Lepra in" Handbuch der Haut- und Geschlechtskrankheiten Band X/2, 1930. Berlin: Springer; 2013.

19. Porritt RJ, Olsen RE. Two simultaneous cases of leprosy developing in tattoos. Am J Pathol. 1947;23:805–17.

20. Gupta CM, Tutakne MA, Tiwari VD, Chakrabarty N. Inoculation leprosy subsequent to dog bite. A case report. Indian J Lepr. 1984;56:919–20.

21. Stoner GL, Belehu A, Nsibambi J, Warndorff J. Borderline tuberculoid leprosy following BCG vaccination. A case report. Int J Lepr Mycobact Dis. 1981;49:16–20.

22. Rees RJ, McDougall AC. Airborne infection with *Mycobacterium leprae* in mice. J Med Microbiol. 1977;10:63–8. https://doi.org/10.1099/00222615-10-1-63.

23. Mohanty PS, Naaz F, Katara D, et al. Viability of *Mycobacterium leprae* in the environment and its role in leprosy dissemination. Indian J Dermatol Venereol Leprol. 2016;82:23–7. https://doi.org/10.4103/0378-6323.168935.

24. de Holanda MV, Marques LEC, de Macedo MLB, et al. Presence of *Mycobacterium leprae* genotype 4 in environmental waters in Northeast Brazil. Rev Soc Bras Med Trop. 2017;50:216–22. https://doi.org/10.1590/0037-8682-0424-2016.

25. Ploemacher T, Faber WR, Menke H, et al. Reservoirs and transmission routes of leprosy; a systematic review. PLoS Negl Trop Dis. 2020;14:e0008276. https://doi.org/10.1371/journal.pntd.0008276.

26. Deps P, Rosa PS. One health and Hansen's disease in Brazil. PLoS Negl Trop Dis. 2021;15:e0009398. https://doi.org/10.1371/journal.pntd.0009398.

27. World Health Organization. Guidelines for the diagnosis, treatment and prevention of leprosy. Geneva: World Health Organization; 2017.

28. Singh B, Saqib M, Chakraborty A, Bhaskar S. Lipoarabinomannan from *Mycobacterium indicus pranii* shows immunostimulatory activity and induces autophagy in macrophages. PLoS One. 2019;14:e0224239. https://doi.org/10.1371/journal.pone.0224239.
29. Duthie MS, Pena MT, Ebenezer GJ, et al. LepVax, a defined subunit vaccine that provides effective pre-exposure and post-exposure prophylaxis of *M. leprae* infection. NPJ Vaccines. 2018;3:12. https://doi.org/10.1038/s41541-018-0050-z.
30. Coppola M, van den Eeden SJF, Robbins N, et al. Vaccines for leprosy and tuberculosis: opportunities for shared research, development, and application. Front Immunol. 2018;9:308. https://doi.org/10.3389/fimmu.2018.00308.
31. Ali L. Leprosy vaccines—a voyage unfinished. J Skin Sex Transm Dis. 2021;3:40–5. https://doi.org/10.25259/JSSTD_24_2020.
32. Hess S, Rambukkana A. Cell biology of intracellular adaptation of *Mycobacterium leprae* in the peripheral nervous system. Microbiol Spectr. 2019;7:2019. https://doi.org/10.1128/microbiolspec.BAI-0020-2019.
33. Stump PRNAG, Baccarelli R, Marciano LHSC, et al. Neuropathic pain in leprosy patients. Int J Lepr Mycobact Dis. 2004;72:134–8. https://doi.org/10.1489/1544-581X(2004)072<0134:NPILP>2.0.CO;2.
34. Raicher I, Stump PRNAG, Harnik SB, et al. Neuropathic pain in leprosy: symptom profile characterization and comparison with neuropathic pain of other etiologies. Pain Rep. 2018;3:e638. https://doi.org/10.1097/PR9.0000000000000638.

The Journey to a Scientific Understanding of Leprosy: A Brief Outline

David Scollard

1 Introduction

Leprosy is caused by a germ, but recognition of this dates only to the late 1800s. An account of the long history of human struggle with leprosy before that time is beyond the scope of this chapter. The International Leprosy Association's History of Leprosy Project [1] provides details of historical events, and paleopathological studies are reviewed elsewhere [2]. Patients' memoirs (e.g., see IDEA [3]) provide insight into the suffering this disease has caused. This chapter focuses on the development of the scientific understanding of leprosy that began in the 1800s and has expanded rapidly in recent decades.

2 Beginnings

Leprosy was endemic in Norway in the nineteenth century, and in 1847 two distinguished Norwegian dermatologists, Daniel Danielssen and Carl Boeck, published an Atlas of Leprosy [4]. This marks the beginning of the modern understanding of this disease. The Atlas, with color illustrations, provided a definition of what leprosy is—and is not. It was a *tour de* force of clinical dermatology, as they recognized that both individuals shown in Fig. 1 had leprosy although their appearances differ greatly. The young lady's illness they described as "macular" or "neural"; the gentleman's was described as "nodular." All subsequent classifications reflect this basic distinction. These extreme differences, and the wide diversity of clinical

D. Scollard (✉)
National Hansen's Disease Programs, Retired, Baton Rouge, LA, USA

Wilbraham, MA, USA

P. D. Deps (ed.), *Hansen's Disease*, https://doi.org/10.1007/978-3-031-30893-2_2

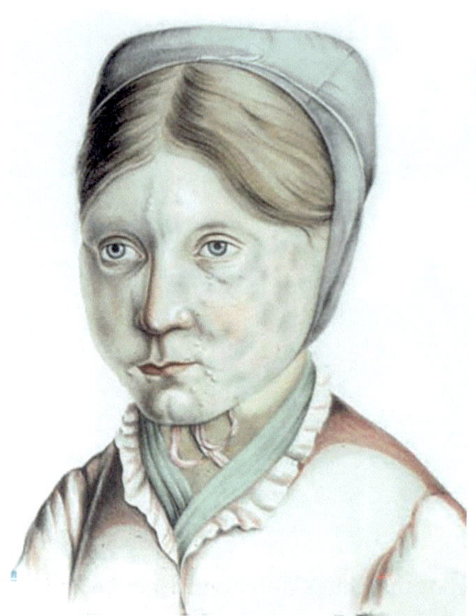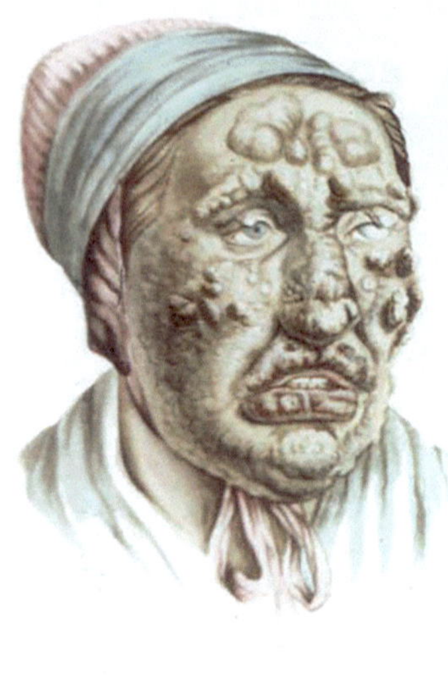

Fig. 1 Two individuals illustrated in the Atlas of Leprosy by Danielssen and Boeck in 1847. The young lady on the left they described as having "macular" or "neural" leprosy; the gentleman on the right they described as "nodular" leprosy. This basic distinction is reflected in the classifications used since that time

lesions between the extremes illustrated in the Atlas, highlighted the conundrum physicians and scientists faced for the next century: How can one disease have so many different appearances? Danielssen and Boeck had no explanation for the etiology of leprosy but, seeing it often occurring within families, they speculated—incorrectly—that it was hereditary.

In the 1870s, another Norwegian doctor, Gerhard Armauer Hansen, was interested in the new scientific reports on germs. On February 28, 1873—exactly 150 years ago—while studying tissue samples under his microscope, he recorded in his notebook that he saw "… small straight rods, which are not destroyed by addition of potash. These are the lepra bacilli" [5]. He published these observations in 1874 [6] (Fig. 2), asserting that the germs he saw caused leprosy. Physicians at that time considered this preposterous because germs were not yet believed to cause human diseases. A few years later, Robert Koch identified and cultured the germ causing tuberculosis. The methods used to stain tubercle bacilli also stained Hansen's bacilli, but Hansen was unable to culture the germ he had discovered. The First International Leprosy Conference in 1887 [7] finally acknowledged that Hansen's bacillus (later designated *Mycobacterium leprae*) caused leprosy. In the 1880s, Rudolph Virchow and others [8, 9] established that *M. leprae* infected nerves. Hansen's discovery was a monumental breakthrough and marks the beginning of modern medical microbiology, but decades would pass before these discoveries benefitted patients.

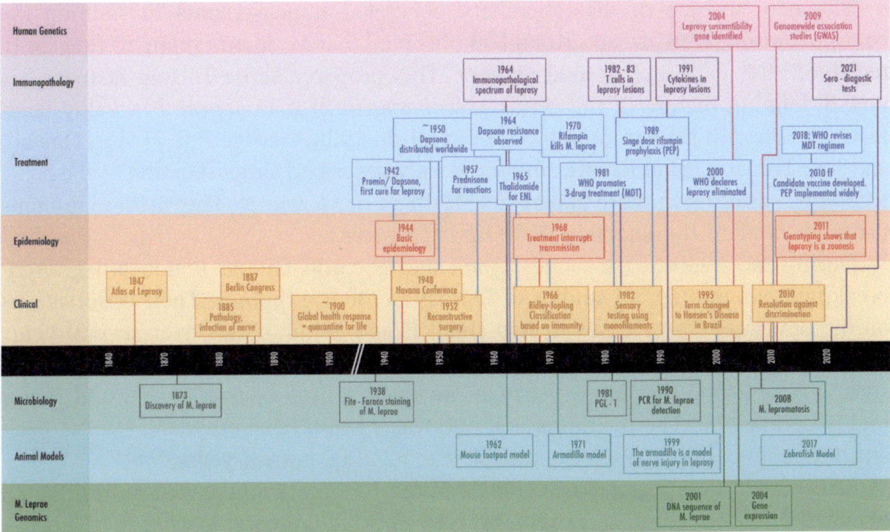

Fig. 2 The expansion of knowledge about leprosy. Major discoveries and landmarks in the development of medical and scientific knowledge about leprosy are indicated on a timeline from 1840–2020. Discoveries related to *M. leprae* and to animal models are shown below the timeline; advances in treatment and understanding of the human host response are shown above the timeline. (Note: The scale of the timeline is not uniform)

During the late 1800s and early 1900s, the realization that germs caused leprosy became part of a global rationale to compel quarantine of patients. This was an egregious distortion of the basic rationale for infectious disease quarantine, i.e., temporary isolation until the incubation period had passed. The incubation period for *M. leprae* was unknown, so quarantine in leprosaria meant quarantine for life. Often this meant severing family relationships, imposing grievous hardship. Hawaiians called it *ma'i ho'oka'awale*, the separating sickness [10].

3   1900–1960: Discoveries and Frustrations

As medical microbiology blossomed in the early 1900s, many other germs were discovered and cultivated, but *M. leprae* remained uncultivable despite diligent efforts. Laboratory testing for antibiotics was impossible. While cures were discovered for other infections, leprosy remained incurable. Scientists sought to demonstrate transmission of *M. leprae* by insects, without success [11, 12]. Others tried inoculating *M. leprae* into a wide range of animals, from frogs to rabbits, without success [13]. Physicians continued to be mystified by the variety of clinical and histological appearances of leprosy, unable to fathom how one germ could cause such diverse lesions.

The new science of histochemistry generated improvements in staining the bacilli. Hansen, Neisser, and Koch had observed that *M. leprae* retained fuchsin (a red dye) after exposure to acid-alcohol. This property, termed "acid-fastness," is now a defining feature of the genus *Mycobacteria*. But *M. leprae* is weakly acid-fast: some bacilli stained poorly or not at all. In 1938, George Fite [14] in Hawaii, and José Faraco [15] in Brazil, simultaneously described a modification of the basic technique resulting in more dependable staining of *M. leprae*. This method remains the gold standard for detecting *M. leprae* in biopsies.

During the 1930s, Drs. James Doull and Ricardo Guinto conducted ground-breaking epidemiological studies of leprosy in the Philippines. Their observations on the development of cases in two small island communities over several years provided the only detailed study of the natural epidemiology of leprosy [16]. These studies established that leprosy has an incubation time of 6–10 *years* and is ***not*** highly contagious. The overall attack rate was <1/1000 person-years, but the peak attack rate, in children 10–14 years old, was >2/1000 person-years.

In 1942, Dr. Guy Faget at Carville conducted a small clinical trial of promin, an injectable sulfone [17] (Fig. 2) and observed slow but dramatic resolution of leprosy lesions. Initially, experts were skeptical, but after seeing the results at the Havana Leprosy Congress in 1948 they were convinced [18]. An oral form of the drug, dapsone, was soon developed [19, 20]. It was effective, safe, and inexpensive. *Leprosy was finally curable.* Dapsone was distributed widely around the world after 1950, following post-war re-establishment of international shipping. Outpatient treatment became possible, and leprosaria began to close.

Although dapsone could cure the infection, leprosy reactions still caused considerable suffering and little treatment was available. The potent anti-inflammatory effects of corticosteroids were discovered in the early 1950s, and in 1957 Jonquieres first reported dramatic benefits of prednisone in treating leprosy reactions [21, 22].

M. leprae infection of nerves may result in anesthesia that often leads to the development of plantar ulcers. Leprosy hospitals commonly had daily foot ulcer clinics. Surgeons performed amputations when necessary, but reconstruction was seldom attempted because the tissues were considered unsuitable for healing. In the 1950s, Dr. Paul Brand challenged this, arguing that these were *pressure ulcers* promoted by insensitivity, and relieving pressure would allow healing. He showed that reconstructive surgery such as tendon transfers (or transpositions) could be performed successfully on hands and feet to restore basic function [23, 24]. These developments launched a new approach to leprosy rehabilitation, probably second only to dapsone treatment in revolutionizing patient care.

4   1960–1999: Rapid Progress

Dapsone worked slowly: some patients were told they must take it for life. It was nevertheless hailed as a miracle drug to cure individual patients, and by the mid-1960s, in a clever home-exposure study, Robert Worth demonstrated that dapsone treatment also interrupted transmission of *M. leprae*. In families in which one or both parents had leprosy, he compared the incidence of leprosy in children born before and after the parent(s) were treated. Among 109 children born before the parent(s) were treated, 10 developed leprosy, while among 35 children born into the same families after the parent(s) were treated, none developed the disease [25].

Meanwhile, *M. leprae* remained uncultivable, impeding laboratory research for new drugs. Physicians could only pursue small clinical trials, usually testing drugs effective against *M. tuberculosis,* since both organisms are mycobacteria. Hypothesizing that *M. leprae* preferred a cooler growth temperature, Charles Shepard, at the United States' CDC, discovered in 1960 that the bacilli would proliferate to a limited extent after injection into mouse foot pads [26]. This was a major breakthrough, enabling scientists to study *M. leprae* in the laboratory.

Antibiotics could now be tested, by feeding them to inoculated mice [27]. But because *M. leprae* grows *very slowly* (dividing only once every 13 days), each test took a year or more to complete. Nevertheless, field isolates began to reveal some dapsone-resistant bacilli after dapsone had been used for only a decade [28]. Seeking new antimicrobials, the efficacy of "B663" (clofazimine) was reported in 1962 [29] and the bactericidal effect of rifampicin in 1970 [30].

In the mid-1960s, scientists had found that *M. leprae* grew abundantly in T-cell deficient mice [31], increasing the quantity of bacilli available for research. However, since the mice were immunocompromised, only limited immunological investigations could be done with this model.

Although leprosy was curable, the wide diversity of lesions remained puzzling. A clinical classification was proposed at the 1953 Leprosy Congress in Madrid [32], identifying two extreme forms (recall the 1847 Atlas), with a "dimorphous" category between them, but the basis for these variations was not understood. In 1964, Olaf Skinsnes, an American pathologist, proposed that this diversity was based on the patient's cellular immune response (CMI). He reasoned that some patients develop granulomatous inflammation in lesions and as a result have few bacilli, indicating strong CMI; others have foamy cells filled with abundant bacilli, i.e., no CMI to *M. leprae*. The broad borderline group displays every degree of CMI between the extremes. He called this the "immunopathological spectrum of leprosy" [33]. Two years later, the English physicians Dennis Ridley and William Jopling published a classification system using clinical and pathological features to position each patient along this immunological spectrum [34]. This classification is still the gold standard for leprosy. Skinsnes' spectrum concept intrigued immunologists and spurred numerous immunological investigations that dominated leprosy research for the rest of the twentieth century. Today, more than 50 years later, the exact mechanisms that regulate CMI to generate this wide spectrum are still not clear and this continues to motivate research.

Prednisone relieved reaction symptoms, including neuropathy, but often required prolonged administration of high doses resulting in serious side effects. In the early 1960s, an Israeli dermatologist, Jacob Sheskin, observed that thalidomide provided rapid relief of *erythema nodosum leprosum* (ENL) [35], a common reaction. By the time this was published in 1965, however, the severe teratogenic effect of thalidomide had been recognized. It was quickly banned worldwide, the only exception being for the treatment of ENL. Having remained in the pharmacopeia *only for ENL*, thalidomide's benefit in some malignancies would be discovered decades later [36].

Since the 1930's, concerns had been raised that the term "leprosy" was a major contributor to the social opprobrium associated with this disease, and suggestions were made that it should instead be called "Hansen's Disease." This cause was championed from the 1960s onward by the Brazilian dermatologist Abrahão Rotberg [37]. After decades, this campaign finally bore fruit:

- 1975—The term Hansen's Disease was mandated by presidential decree in Brazil.
- 1986—The United States' leprosy hospital at Carville was renamed the Gillis W. Long Hansen's Disease Center.
- 1995—The government of Brazil passed a law-making Hansen's Disease the official term for the disease [38].
- The WHO and other entities continue to use both terms interchangeably.

In 1971, researchers at Carville discovered that *M. leprae* proliferated in the nine banded armadillo (*Dasypus novemcinctus*), providing an immunocompetent animal model [39]. However, armadillos were of little interest to other immunologists and no molecular probes, monoclonal antibodies, etc., had been developed for them, so that only limited immunological studies were possible. However, *M. leprae* does grow to considerable numbers in the armadillo, providing very large quantities of bacilli that enabled quantitative biochemical and physiological studies [40]. A century after Hansen discovered *M. leprae*, its physiology could finally be investigated.

In 1982, the World Health Organization recommended multiple drug therapy (MDT) for leprosy, composed of dapsone, rifampin, and clofazimine [41]. This was part of a global initiative that included training of health workers, new metrics— e.g., defining "cure" as completion of MDT, and instructing national programs to remove "cured cases" from registries. Implemented worldwide, it was the greatest anti-leprosy effort in history. Leprosy *prevalence* declined rapidly [42], but it was not clear how much of this was due to cures of new infections vs simply removal of old cases from registries. The program oversimplified a complex disease in ways that were often controversial [43]. By 1990, the WHO, greatly impressed with their apparent success, declared their goal to eliminate leprosy as a public health problem by the year 2000—in one decade [44]. Elimination was defined as a prevalence of less than one case per 10,000 population.

Meanwhile, a 1989 report of trials in the Marquesas islands [45], suggested that a reduction in new cases might be achieved with post-exposure prophylaxis using a single dose of rifampin (SDR-PEP). This prompted renewed studies of prophylaxis against leprosy [46].

As cure of infection advanced, preventing disability became a more urgent goal, requiring earlier detection of nerve involvement. At a leprosy meeting in 1982, nylon monofilaments were proposed as tools for sensory testing in leprosy patients

[47]. The methods were subsequently developed at the Instituto Lauro de Souza Lima in Brazil, and such testing became the global standard of care for leprosy [48].

The discovery of hybridomas in 1975 [49] enabled the development of monoclonal antibodies to identify lymphocyte subsets. Immunostaining using these antibodies revealed that the T-lymphocyte composition in skin lesions across the immuno-pathological spectrum of leprosy [50, 51] correlated well with advancing knowledge about the basic mechanisms of cellular immunity [52]. Discovery of a unique glycolipid (PGL-1) in the cell wall of *M. leprae* in the 1980s [53], and the discovery that some patients make antibodies against this molecule, initiated efforts to develop a serologic test for leprosy. Such a serologic test has still not yet been fully achieved, but the latest developments are very promising [54].

Advances in DNA sequencing in the 1980s and 90s [55] led to the use of polymerase chain reaction (PCR) to detect *M. leprae* DNA [56] and to identify the mutations associated with drug resistance [57]. Similar developments in molecular immunology accelerated leprosy immunology research, for example, correlating T-lymphocyte subsets with cytokine production across the immunologic spectrum [58, 59].

In 1996, researchers observed that nerve involvement in *M. leprae*-infected armadillos closely modeled human nerve injury in leprosy [60]. The immuno-inflammatory processes occurring during *M. leprae* infection of nerves could now be studied under controlled experimental conditions [61, 62].

5   2000–2020

At the 54th World Health Assembly in 2000, the WHO announced that global leprosy prevalence had fallen below their target level [63]. This was widely regarded as a declaration that leprosy had been eliminated. Actually, *surveillance* was eliminated, or widely reduced, and many new cases were still diagnosed in several countries. A later critique suggested that many millions of patients had been missed [64]. In 2018, the WHO revised the recommended treatment [65], an acknowledgment that leprosy had not been eliminated.

After decades of effort to reduce stigma and discrimination, in 2010 the United Nations General assembly adopted Resolution 66/215, *Elimination of discrimination against persons affected by leprosy and their family members* [66]. In 2015, the Human Rights Council adopted this as Resolution 29/5 [67]. These resolutions, together with pressure from patient advocate groups and others, prompted many countries to rescind or revise laws that had sanctioned discrimination based on leprosy.

Since 2000, basic research on *M. leprae* and on host immune responses has been dominated by molecular and genetic techniques. Stewart Cole and colleagues at the Pasteur Institute published the full DNA sequence of *M. leprae* in 2001 [68]. Analysis revealed the absence of several genes for proteins in key metabolic pathways, beginning to explain why *M. leprae* is non-cultivable [40]. Knowledge of the *M. leprae* genome opened up nearly endless possibilities to explore the biology of *M. leprae*. This led to large-scale studies of *M. leprae* function, measured by mRNA transcription of multiple genes using reverse transcription PCR [69]. Studies of the *M. leprae* transcriptome continue to advance knowledge of its metabolism [70].

In the 1800s, Danielssen and Boeck (and others before them) had proposed that leprosy was hereditary [4], but genetic research methods were not sufficient to identify leprosy susceptibility genes until the late 1990s. In 2004, the same year that the full human genome was published, Marcello Mira and colleagues used positional cloning methods to identify a leprosy susceptibility gene on chromosome 6 [71]. Human genetic studies have since flourished and, in 2009, Zhang and colleagues in China published the first leprosy genomewide association study [72].

DNA sequencing technology also enabled Han and colleagues to identify a new organism, dubbed *M. lepromatosis* [73]. Based on a 5% genomic difference from *M. leprae*, *M. lepromatosis* is denoted as a new species. Clinically and histologically it causes the same disease as *M. leprae* [74], but this—and other genetic variants of *M. leprae*—are valuable markers in the new field of molecular epidemiology of leprosy [75].

Research had revealed that *M. leprae* infection had been present in wild armadillos (but never recognized) long before the experimental infections [76]. In 2011, Richard Truman and colleagues demonstrated that *M. leprae* isolated from wild armadillos share the same genotypes as isolates from leprosy patients in the southern United States [77]. Leprosy is thus a zoonosis in this region. Preliminary data indicate that this is also true in Central and South America. Therefore, interruption of human–human transmission of *M. leprae* will not be sufficient to eliminate leprosy from the Western hemisphere, and leprosy control measures must be revised accordingly. Meanwhile, a new zebrafish model was described in 2017 [78] and used to study mechanisms of *M. leprae*-induced nerve injury.

By 2020, several countries had implemented SDR-PEP [79], giving new energy to control programs. Many technical and immunological advances have resulted in the recent development of a candidate leprosy vaccine ready for clinical trials [80]. However, leprosy develops slowly and even with good interventions it declines slowly. It is therefore too early at this writing to know how effective the PEP or vaccine initiatives will be in long-term reduction of new cases.

6 Conclusions

After 150 years of research, we understand a great deal about leprosy. Scientifically, this includes landmark discoveries in microbiology, immunology, and genetics (Table 1) led by advances in technology. Medically, effective treatment and physical rehabilitation have made this an "outpatient" disease. Millions of patients have been cured since 1950 and, as a result, millions more infections have been prevented.

Table 1 Summary of advances in scientific and medical knowledge about leprosy since 1850, and challenges remaining

	Knowledge and capabilities gained	Major gaps remaining
Etiology	Leprosy is caused by *M. leprae*	
	M. leprae is not cultivable It grows very slowly	Metabolism of *M. leprae* not fully understood
	It can infect peripheral nerves	Neurotropism of *M. leprae* is unexplained
	PCR identification is now available	
	Full genome is sequenced	Much is still unknown about *M. leprae* physiology
	Drug-resistance mutations are identified	
Epidemiology	Attack rate is low	Can prophylaxis prevent infection?
	Incubation time is very long	
	Transmission: human–human and zoonotic (armadillo)	Mechanism of transmission is uncertain
Host immune response	Most people have native immunity: some susceptibility genes are identified	Mechanisms of native immunity?
	Extraordinary immunopathological spectrum	Mechanisms/regulation of adaptive immunity?
		Immunology of reactions remain unclear
		Can a vaccine prevent leprosy?
Clinical	Curable–effective antimicrobials are available	Better/shorter drug regimens are needed
	Neuropathy is detectable earlier, treatable with corticosteroids	Better methods are needed to treat/prevent neuritis and reactions
	Nerve injury model (armadillo) is available	Mechanisms of nerve injury remain unclear
	Reconstructive surgery is available	
Social response	International anti-discrimination policies are promulgated	Fear prevails. Stigma and discrimination continue
	Increasingly articulate patient advocacy	

Scores of leprosaria have been closed and the few that remain are specialized treatment centers, not quarantine prisons. But reactions and nerve injury remain challenging, and basic questions such as the means of transmission and the mechanisms of immune regulation remain unexplained. In addition, social and psychological progress has lagged considerably in dispelling fear and ostracism. The knowledge gained has not fully translated into a wide acceptance that this is a natural and curable disease. Instead, fear prevails, and widespread stigma and discrimination remain. This is a different kind of challenge. Possibly, advances in social science research will lead to new approaches to reduce stigma and discrimination; perhaps leprosy research will lead the way.

Acknowledgements Portions of this material were presented at a symposium on the history of the Penikese Island Leprosarium, Oct 21, 2021, sponsored by the Public Health Museum, Tewksbury, Massachusetts (USA) (www.publichealthmuseum.org). I am deeply grateful to Darikka Scollard and Digital Turf (https://digitalturf.net) for expert assistance in the construction of the timeline figure. The author, and all who search the literature for insight into leprosy, owe a profound debt to Dr. Marcos Virmond, distinguished surgeon and leprologist. During his tenure as President of the International Leprosy Association, he was responsible for digitizing all 73 Volumes of the International Journal of Leprosy, making them available at no cost at http://ijl.ilsl. br/. Many of the major developments in leprosy occurred between 1931 and 2005 and are recorded in the pages of the Journal: discoveries, disagreements, and disappointing (but important) dead-ends. The online access to the Journal that Dr. Virmond organized will provide future generations of scientists and historians with invaluable information. I am also grateful to Prof. Patricia Deps, Prof. Magnus Vollset of the University of Bergen, Norway, and Elizabeth Schexnyder of the NHDP Museum, USA, for their assistance and suggestions. For all of its many difficulties, outstanding physicians and scientists from every era have been drawn to the challenge of understanding leprosy. All of their efforts are gratefully acknowledged. Constraints of space required that many excellent and important studies could not be cited in this brief account. Any attempt to define historical landmarks in medical and scientific discovery inevitably depends upon personal judgment. For the most recent decades, this is especially difficult, as we lack sufficient historical perspective. In the future, the significance of these recent discoveries can be judged more objectively.

References

1. https://leprosyhistory.org/. Accessed 10 Jan 2022.
2. Roberts C. Leprosy past and present. Gainesville: University of Florida Press; 2020.
3. https://www.leprosy-information.org/organization/idea-international-association-integration-dignity-and-economic-advancement.
4. Daniellsen DC, Boeck CW. Om Spedalskhed. Oslo: Christiana; 1847.
5. Carter HV. Report on leprosy and leper-asylums in Norway, with references to India. London: G E Eyre and W Spottiswoode; 1974.
6. Hansen GA. (1874) Spedalskhedens Arsager (Causes of Leprosy). Norsk Mag Laegeevidensk 4:36–79. Int J Lepr. 1955;23:307–9.
7. Internationalen Wissenschaftlichen Lepra Conferenz, No. 1, Berlin. 1897.
8. Arning E. Ueber das Vorkommen des bacillus leprae bei Lepra anaesthetica sive nervorum. Archiv Pathol Anat. 1884;97:170–1. https://doi.org/10.1007/BF02563919.
9. Dehio K. 1897. On the lepra anesthetica and the pathogenetical relation of its disease appearances. [article in German] proceedings of the international scientific leprosy conference in Berlin. Translated and reprinted in Lepr. Lepr India. 1952;24:78–83.
10. Bloombaum M, Gugelyk T. The separating sickness, Mai Ho'oka'awale: interviews with exiled leprosy patients at Kalaupapa. Honolulu: Anoai Press; 1996.
11. Anonymous News. Insects as leprosy carriers. Science. 1929;69(1779):1–3. https://doi.org/10.1126/science.69.1779.l.u.
12. Sousa-Araujo HC. Infeccão espontânea e experimental de Hematófogos em leprosos. Possibilidade de serem elas vectores ou transmissores da lepra. [article in Portuguese] (Natural and experimental infection of blood-sucking insects and leeches from leprosy patients.) Mem Inst Oswaldo Cruz 38:447–484. English summary, Int J Lepr. 1943;14:146.
13. Walsh DS. Chapter 10.1. Overview of Animal Models. *In* Scollard DM, & Gillis TP. (Eds.), International Textbook of Leprosy. American Leprosy Missions, Greenville, SC. 2020. https://doi.org/10.1489/itl.10.1.
14. Fite GL. The staining of acid-fast bacilli in paraffin sections. Am J Pathol. 1938;14(4):491–507.

15. Faraco J. Bacillos de Hansen e Cortes de Parafina. Bras J Lepr. 1938;6:177–80.
16. Doull JA, Guinto RS, Rodreguez JN, Bancroft H. Risk of attack in leprosy in relation to age at exposure. Am J Trop Med Hyg. 1945;25:435–9. https://doi.org/10.4269/ajtmh.1945.s1-25.435.
17. Faget GH, Pogge RC, Johansen FA, Dinan JF, Prejean BM, Eccles CG. The promin treatment of leprosy: a progress report. Publ Heath Rep. 1943;65:1147.
18. Wade WA. Report on the Havana congress. Int J Lepr. 1948;16:179–84.
19. de Lima LS. Present status of sulfone therapy at the Padre Bento Sanitorium. Int J Lepr Other Mycobact Dis. 1948;16:127–38.
20. Lowe J. Treatment of leprosy with diamino-diphenyl sulphone by mouth. Lancet. 1950;1(6596):145–50. https://doi.org/10.1016/s0140-6736(50)90257-1.
21. Jonquieres ED. Control of tuberculoid reactions in leprosy with prednisone. Sem Med. 1957;111(7):313–7.
22. Jopling WH, Cochrane RG. The place of cortisone and corticotrophin in the treatment of certain acute phases of leprosy. Lepr Rev. 1957;28:5.
23. Brand PW. Reconstructive surgery of the hand in leprosy. Ann R Coll Surg Engl. 1952;11(6):350–61.
24. Fritschi EP, Brand PW. The place of reconstructive surgery in the prevention of foot ulceration in leprosy. Int J Lepr. 1957;25(1):1–8.
25. Worth RM. Is it safe to treat the lepromatous patient at home? A study of home exposure to leprosy in Hong Kong. Int J Lepr. 1968;36:296–302.
26. Shepard CC. The experimental disease that follows the injection of human leprosy bacilli into footpads of mice. J Exp Med. 1960;112:445–54.
27. Shepard CC, Chang YT. Effect of several anti-leprosy drugs on multiplication of human leprosy bacilli in footpads of mice. Proc Soc Exp Biol Med. 1962;109:636–8.
28. Pettit JH, Rees RJ. Sulfone resistance in leprosy. An experimental and clinical study. Lancet. 1964;2(7361):673–4. https://doi.org/10.1016/s0140-6736(64)92482-1.
29. Browne SG, Hogerzeil LLM. "B 663" in the treatment of leprosy. Preliminary report of a pilot trial. Lepr Rev. 1962;33:6–10.
30. Rees RJ, Pearson JM, Waters MF. Experimental and clinical studies on rifampicin in treatment of leprosy. Br Med J. 1970;1(5688):89–92. https://doi.org/10.1136/bmj.1.5688.89.
31. Lenz S, Collins JH, Lahiri R, Adams LB. Chapter 10.3. Rodent Models in Leprosy Research. *In* Scollard DM, & Gillis TP. (Eds.), International Textbook of Leprosy. American Leprosy Missions, Greenville, SC. 2020. https://doi.org/10.1489/itl.10.3.
32. International Congress of Leprosy. Report of the committee on classification. Int J Lepr. 1953;21:504–16.
33. Skinsnes OK. The immunological spectrum of leprosy. In: Cochrane RG, Davey TF, editors. Leprosy in theory and practice. Baltimore: Williams and Wilkins; 1964. p. 156–62.
34. Ridley DS, Jopling WH. Classification of leprosy according to immunity—a five-group system. Int J Lepr Other Mycobact Dis. 1966;34:255–73.
35. Sheskin J. Thalidomide in the treatment of lepra reactions. Clin Pharmacol Ther. 1965;6:303–6. https://doi.org/10.1002/cpt196563303.
36. Botting J. The history of thalidomide. Drug News Perspect. 2002;15(9):604–11. https://doi.org/10.1358/dnp.2002.15.9.840066.
37. Rotberg S. "Hanseniasis", the new official name of "leprosy" in S. Paulo, Brazil, and its prophylactical results. An Bras Dermatol. 1969;44(3):199–204.
38. Deps P, Cruz A. Why we should stop using the word leprosy. Lancet Infect Dis. 2020;20(4):e75–8. https://doi.org/10.1016/S1473-3099(20)30061-X.
39. Kirchheimer WF, Storrs EE. Attempts to establish the armadillo (*Dasypus novemcinctus* Linn.) as a model for the study of leprosy. I. Report of lepromatoid leprosy in an experimentally infected armadillo. Int J Lepr Other Mycobact Dis. 1971;39(3):693–702.
40. Brennan PJ, Spencer JS. Chapter 5.1. The Physiology of *Mycobacterium leprae*. *In* Scollard DM, & Gillis TP. (Eds.), International Textbook of Leprosy. American Leprosy Missions, Greenville, SC. 2019. https://doi.org/10.1489/itl.5.1.

41. WHO Study Group. Chemotherapy of leprosy for control programmes. Geneva: World Health Organization; 1982.
42. World Health Organization. Leprosy Elimination Project: status report, 2003–2004. Geneva: World Health Organization; 2004.
43. Lockwood DN, Suneetha S. Leprosy: too complex a disease for a simple elimination paradigm. Bull World Health Organ. 2005;83(3):230–5.
44. World Health Assembly. Elimination of leprosy: resolution of the 44th World Health Assembly. Resolution No. WHA 44.9. Geneva: World Health Organization; 1991.
45. Cartel JL, Chanteau S, Boutin JP, Taylor R, Plichart R, Roux J, et al. Implementation of chemoprophylaxis of leprosy in the Southern Marquesas with a single dose of 25 mg per kg rifampin. Int J Lepr Other Mycobact Dis. 1989;57:810–6.
46. Moet FJ, Pahan D, Oskam L, Richardus JH, COLEP Study Group. Effectiveness of single dose rifampicin in preventing leprosy in close contacts of patients with newly diagnosed leprosy: cluster randomized controlled trial. BMJ. 2008;336(7647):761–4. https://doi.org/10.1136/bmj.39500.885752.BE.
47. Pearson JM. The evaluation of nerve damage in leprosy. Lepr Rev. 1982;53:119–30.
48. Lehman LF, Orsini MB, Nicholl AR. The development and adaptation of the Semmes–Weinstein monofilaments in Brazil. J Hand Ther. 1993;6(4):290–7. https://doi.org/10.1016/s0894-1130(12)80330-9.
49. Köhler G, Milstein C. Continuous cultures of fused cells secreting antibody of predefined specificity. J Immunol. 2005;174(5):2453–5.
50. van Voorhis WC, Kaplan G, Sarno EN, Horwitz MA, Steinman RM, Levis WR, et al. The cutaneous infiltrates of leprosy: cellular characteristics and the predominant T-cell phenotypes. N Engl J Med. 1982;307:1593–7.
51. Narayanan RB, Bhutani LK, Sharma AK, Nath I. T cell subsets in leprosy lesions: in situ characterization using monoclonal antibodies. Clin Exp Immunol. 1983;51:421–9.
52. Weiss DI, Do TH, de Andrade Silva BJ, Teles RMB, Andrade PR, Ochoa MT, Modlin RL. Chapter 6.2. Adaptive Immune Response in Leprosy. *In* Scollard DM, & Gillis TP. (Eds.), International Textbook of Leprosy. American Leprosy Missions, Greenville, SC. 2020. https://doi.org/10.1489/itl.6.2.
53. Brennan PJ. *Mycobacterium leprae*—the outer lipoidal surface. J Biosci. 1984;6:685–9.
54. Tió-Coma M, Kiełbasa SM, van den Eeden SJF, Mei H, Roy JC, Wallinga J, et al. Blood RNA signature RISK4LEP predicts leprosy years before clinical onset. EBioMedicine. 2021;68:103379. https://doi.org/10.1016/j.ebiom.2021.103379.
55. Heather JM, Chain B. The sequence of sequencers: the history of sequencing DNA. Genomics. 2016;107(1):1–8. https://doi.org/10.1016/j.ygeno.2015.11.003.
56. Williams DL, et al. The use of a specific DNA probe and polymerase chain reaction for the detection of *M. leprae*. J Infect Dis. 1990;162:193–200.
57. Gillis TP, Booth RJ, Looker D, Watson JD. Simultaneous detection of *Mycobacterium leprae* and its susceptibility to dapsone directly from clinical specimens. J Clin Microbiol. 2001;39:2083–8.
58. Yamamura M, Uyemura K, Deans RJ, Weinberg K, Rea TH, Bloom BR, Modlin RL. Defining protective responses to pathogens: cytokine profiles in leprosy lesions. Science. 1991;254:277–9.
59. Misra N, Murtaza A, Walker B, Narayan NP, Misra RS, Ramesh V, et al. Cytokine profile of circulating T cells of leprosy patients reflects both indiscriminate and polarized T-helper subsets: T-helper phenotype is stable and uninfluenced by related antigens of *Mycobacterium leprae*. Immunology. 1995;86:97–103.
60. Scollard DM, Lathrop G, Truman RW. Infection of distal peripheral nerves by *M. leprae* in infected armadillos: an experimental model of nerve involvement in leprosy. Int J Lepr. 1996;64:146–51.
61. Scollard DM, McCormick GM, Allen J. Localization of *Mycobacterium leprae* to endothelial cells of epineurial and perineurial blood vessels and lymphatics. Am J Pathol. 1999;154:1611–20.

62. Sharma R, Lahiri R, Scollard DM, Pena M, Williams DL, Adams LB, et al. The armadillo: a model for the neuropathy of leprosy and potentially other neurodegenerative diseases. Dis Model Mech. 2013;6:19–24. https://doi.org/10.1242/dmm.010215.
63. World Health Organization. Leprosy-global situation. Wkly Epidemiol Rec. 2002;77:1–8.
64. Smith WC, van Brakel W, Gillis T, Saunderson P, Richardus JH. The missing millions: a threat to the elimination of leprosy. PLoS Negl Trop Dis. 2015;23:e0003658. https://doi.org/10.1371/journal.pntd.0003658.
65. World Health Organization. Guidelines for the diagnosis, treatment, and prevention of leprosy. 2018. ISBN: 978 92 9022 638 362.
66. United Nations General Assembly. Elimination of discrimination against persons affected by leprosy and their family members. Resolution 66/215. 2011.
67. Human Rights Council. Elimination of discrimination against persons affected by leprosy and their family members. Resolution. 29/5. 2015.
68. Cole ST, Eiglmeier K, Parkhill J, James KD, Thomson NR, Wheeler PR, et al. Massive gene decay in the leprosy bacillus. Nature. 2001;409(6823):1007–11.
69. Williams DL, Torrero M, Wheeler PR, Truman RW, Yoder M, Morrison N, et al. Biological implications of *Mycobacterium leprae* gene expression during infection. J Mol Microbiol Biotechnol. 2004;8:58–72. https://doi.org/10.1159/000082081.
70. Ojo O, Williams DL, Adams LB, Lahiri R. *Mycobacterium leprae* transcriptome during in vivo growth and ex vivo stationary phases. Front Cell Infect Microbiol. 2022;11:817221. https://doi.org/10.3389/fcimb.2021.817221.
71. Mira MT, Alcaïs A, Nguyen VT, et al. Susceptibility to leprosy is associated with PARK2 and PACRG. Nature. 2004;427(6975):636–40. https://doi.org/10.1038/nature02326.
72. Zhang FR, Huang W, Chen SM, Sun LD, Liu H, Li Y, et al. Genomewide association study of leprosy. N Engl J Med. 2009;361:2609–18. https://doi.org/10.1056/NEJMoa0903753.
73. Han XY, Seo YH, Sizer KC, Schoberle T, May GS, Spencer JS, et al. A new Mycobacterium species causing diffuse lepromatous leprosy. Am J Clin Pathol. 2008;130:856–64. https://doi.org/10.1309/AJCPP72FJZZRRVMM.
74. Sharma R, Singh P, McCoy RC, Lenz SM, Donovan K, Ochoa MT, et al. Isolation of *Mycobacterium lepromatosis* and development of molecular diagnostic assays to distinguish *Mycobacterium leprae* and *M. lepromatosis*. Clin Infect Dis. 2020;71:e262–9. https://doi.org/10.1093/cid/ciz1121.
75. Avanzi C, Singh P, Truman RW, Suffys PN. Molecular epidemiology of leprosy: an update. Infect Genet Evol. 2020;86:104581. https://doi.org/10.1016/j.meegid.2020.104581.
76. Truman RW, Shannon EJ, Hagstad HV, Hugh-Jones ME, Wolff A, Hastings RC. Evaluation of the origin of *Mycobacterium leprae* infections in the wild armadillo, *Dasypus novemcinctus*. Am J Trop Med Hyg. 1986;35:588–93. https://doi.org/10.4269/ajtmh.1986.35.588.
77. Truman RW, Singh P, Sharma R, Busso P, Rougemont J, Paniz-Mondolfi A, et al. Probable zoonotic leprosy in the southern United States. N Engl J Med. 2011;364:1626–33. https://doi.org/10.1056/NEJMoa1010536.
78. Madigan CA, Cameron J, Ramakrishnan L. A zebrafish model of *Mycobacterium leprae* granulomatous infection. J Infect Dis. 2017;216:776–9. https://doi.org/10.1093/infdis/jix329.
79. Schoenmakers A, Mieras L, Budiawan T, van Brakel WH. The state of affairs in post-exposure leprosy prevention: a descriptive meta-analysis on immuno- and chemo-prophylaxis. Res Rep Trop Med. 2020;11:97–117. https://doi.org/10.2147/RRTM.S190300.
80. Duthie MS, Frevol A, Day T, Coler RN, Vergara J, Rolf T, et al. A phase 1 antigen dose escalation trial to evaluate safety, tolerability and immunogenicity of the leprosy vaccine candidate LepVax (LEP-F1 + GLA-SE) in healthy adults. Vaccine. 2019;38:1700–7. https://doi.org/10.1016/j.vaccine.2019.12.050.

The Origin, Evolution and History of Leprosy Through a Palaeopathological Lens

Charlotte A. Roberts

1 Introduction

While leprosy remains a challenge for management today in certain parts of the world, we should remember that it is an infection that has a long and interesting history. This has been demonstrated by historians interrogating medical historical evidence [1], and by documenting evidence in skeletons from archaeological sites [2, 3]. This evidence can provide a deep time perspective for understanding the disease today [4].

2 Palaeopathology and Leprosy

Palaeopathological study entails the identification of damage to bones that result from different diseases, often using information gleaned from clinical sources [5] with standard accepted methods and bearing in mind its limitations [6, 7], and in an ethical manner [8]. Palaeopathology enables us to view the long history of disease through the remains of people who were affected and link the evidence to major transitions such as from foraging to farming and industrialization [9, 10]. The causative organism of leprosy is *Mycobacterium leprae* (or the more recently discovered *M. lepromatosis*), and leprosy is one such disease that can affect the bones and teeth, but it only affects a person's skeleton in 3–5% of untreated people [11]. Diagnosis can be tricky, especially if a skeleton is not well preserved, which can be the case in archaeological contexts. This is because the distribution of characteristic changes

C. A. Roberts (✉)
Department of Archaeology, Durham University, Durham, UK
e-mail: c.a.roberts@durham.ac.uk

P. D. Deps (ed.), *Hansen's Disease*, https://doi.org/10.1007/978-3-031-30893-2_3

needs to be considered. Further, the disease affects often small and fragile parts of the skeleton which, in particular circumstances, can be damaged postmortem during burial in the ground (often for thousands of years), or in the course of excavation, analysis or during storage for future work.

3 Bone Changes of Leprosy

Leprosy has a broad immune spectrum [12], but palaeopathologists usually recognize the effects of low resistance leprosy in the skeleton, or lepromatous, leprosy, while appreciating that high resistance, or tuberculoid, leprosy is much more challenging to identify [13] (but see Matos 2009 who suggests, from clinical data, that bilateral or unilateral hand and foot bone changes with no rhinomaxillary syndrome are consistent with tuberculoid leprosy). Palaeopathologists of leprosy have benefitted much from the research of two Danish doctors: Vilhelm Møller-Christensen (Fig. 1) who excavated and analysed skeletons from a medieval leprosy hospital site in Denmark [14]; and Johs Andersen, who was a practising leprologist [15]. Leprosy affects the bones of the face, hands and feet and, albeit rarely, can affect the normal development of the tooth roots, particularly of the upper incisors (*leprogenic odontodysplasia*) [16]—Figs. 2 and 3.

Fig. 1 Vilhelm Møller-Christensen, who first described the bone changes of leprosy in archaeological skeletons

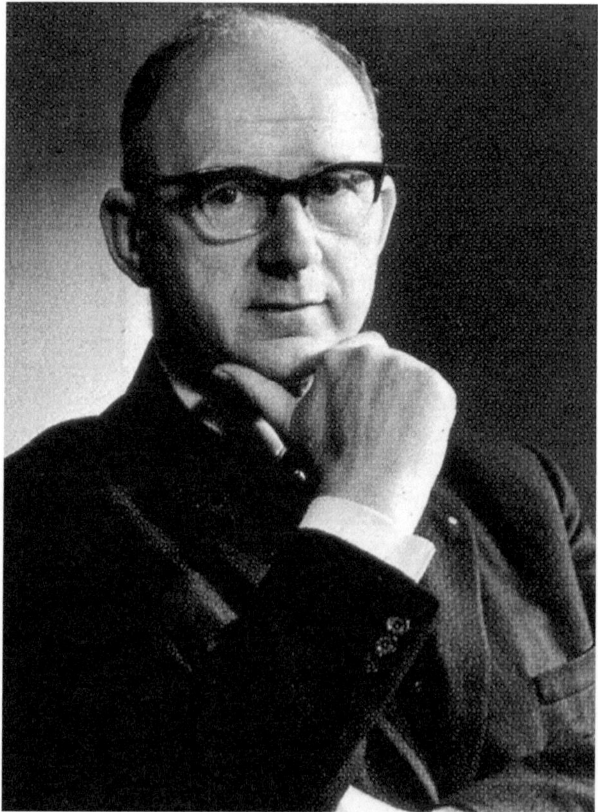

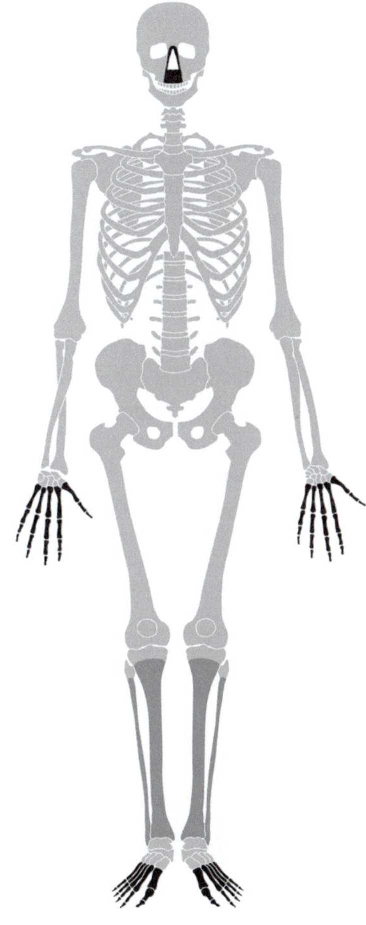

Fig. 2 Distribution of bone changes in leprosy in the skeleton (in black)

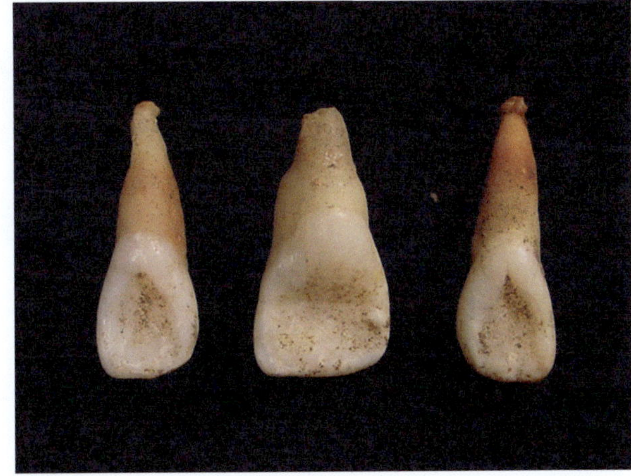

Fig. 3 Leprogenic odontodysplasia affecting the roots of the upper incisors in a medieval skeleton from a leprosy hospital cemetery in Odense, Denmark (courtesy of Vitor Matos)

3.1 Facial Bones and Leprosy

As the leprosy bacteria are inhaled, we must first turn to the facial bones of the skull to appreciate how the bones are damaged (termed "rhinomaxillary syndrome"), and recognize that there are differential diagnoses for these bone changes (e.g. tuberculosis and treponemal disease). The bacteria directly affect the mucous membranes of the mouth and nose of the respiratory system and subsequently the underlying bones, including the turbinate bones and the bony part of the septum. Due to the development of inflammation of the mucous membranes, the nasal bones, anterior nasal spine, and the alveolar process of the maxilla are subject to absorption/loss of bone; and the nasal and oral surface of the palatine bones become pitted, with new bone formation (Figs. 4 and 5). Destructive perforations in the palate can also occur so that there is a connection between the nose and mouth.

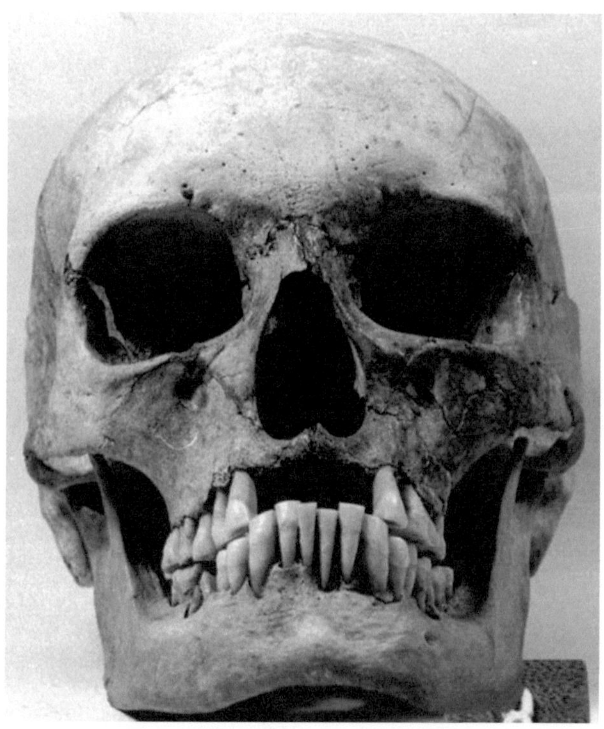

Fig. 4 Rhinomaxillary syndrome affecting the facial bones of a medieval skeleton from Denmark (Naestved leprosy hospital)

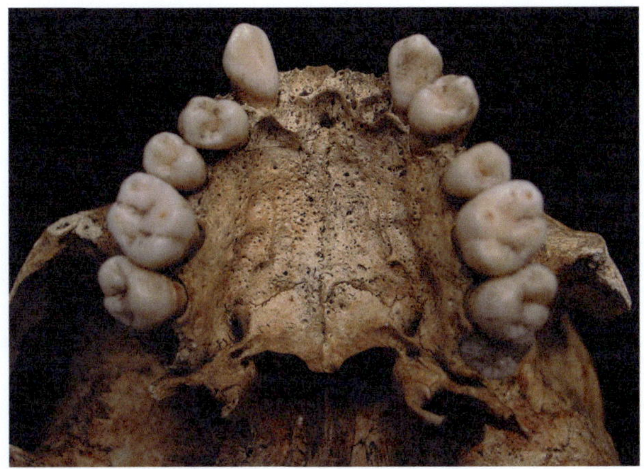

Fig. 5 Porosity of the oral surface of the palate ('holes) affecting a medieval skeleton from a leprosy hospital in Odense, Denmark (courtesy of Vitor Matos)

3.2   Nerve Damage and Bone Changes of Leprosy

The bacteria also affect the sensory, motor and autonomic peripheral nerves, which can indirectly and particularly affect the bones of the hands and the feet (Figs. 6 and 7). The damage to the **sensory nerves** causes a lack of sensation which leads to injury, and ulceration of the fingertips and palms of the hand; if not treated secondary bacterial infection can spread to the bones and joints of the hands and feet. Septic arthritis (infection of the joints that can lead to osteoarthritis) and an inflammatory bone response on the bone surfaces may ensue. Finger-tip absorption and subsequent erosion of the ends of the distal phalanges can occur. The bones subsequently 'shorten' and the skin contracts around the remaining bone ends, with the index and middle (longest) fingers most affected. The carpal bones may also disintegrate, albeit rarely. A similar process occurs in the feet: loss of sensation and ulceration, especially in the forefoot, precedes secondary bacterial infection of the foot bones and joints; the tarsals disintegrate more readily than the carpals. Cup and peg deformities of the joints may also occur. **Motor nerve** involvement can lead to paralysis of muscles, and dislocation and subluxation of interphalangeal joints, with hyperextension of the metacarpophalangeal and metatarsophalangeal joints, and hyperflexion of the interphalangeal joints. The hyperflexion can cause palmar and plantar defects of the phalanges, and lateral popliteal nerve involvement may lead to a drop foot, causing new bone formation on the dorsal surfaces of the tarsal bones caused by stress to the attached ligaments as the foot drops. Damage to the autonomic nervous system leads to concentric diaphyseal remodeling of the metacarpal and metatarsal shafts and proximal/middle phalanges. This may lead to loss of the

Fig. 6 Destruction of
some of the distal ends of
the proximal and
middle hand phalanges of a
medieval skeleton from
Denmark (Naestved
leprosy hospital)

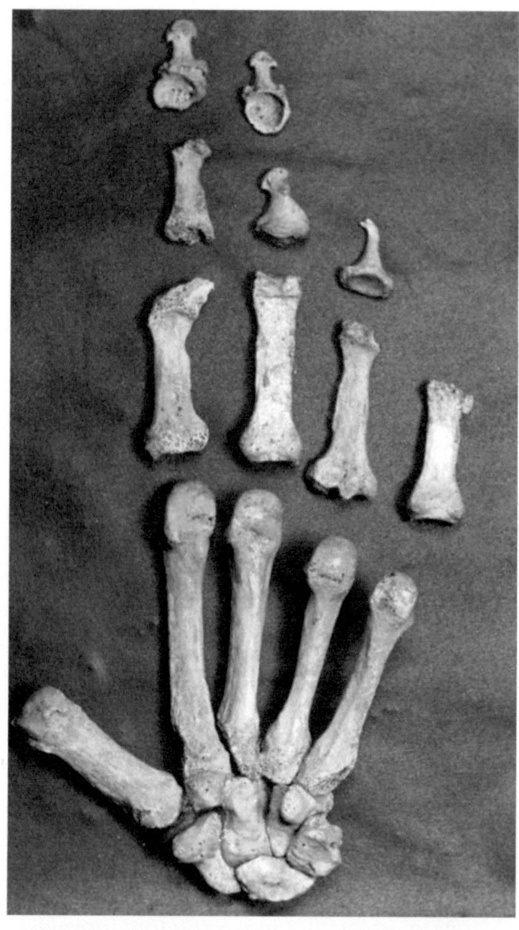

Fig. 7 Loss of the distal
ends of three metatarsals,
diaphyseal concentric
remodelling of two middle
phalanges, and fusion of
middle and distal
phalanges affecting a
medieval skeleton from a
leprosy hospital in
Chichester, England
(courtesy of Don Ortner)

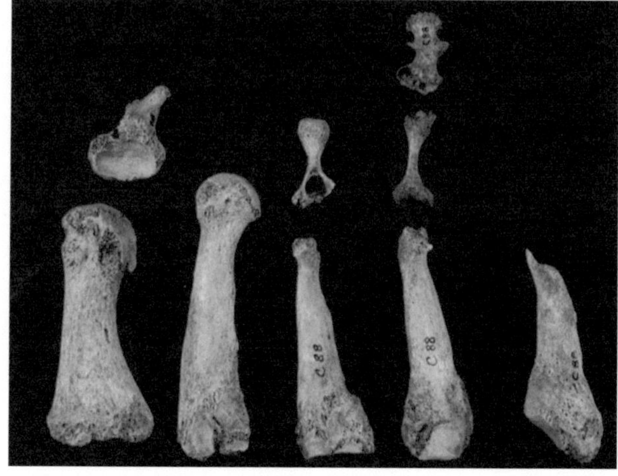

medullary cavity. The metatarsal heads may be destroyed with resulting cup-and-peg deformity at the metatarso-phalangeal joints. New bone formation can occur on long and short tubular bones, and often on the tibial and fibular shafts alongside the described bone changes described above (Fig. 8). In summary, rhinomaxillary syndrome, or rhinomaxillary syndrome and involvement of the hand and foot bones, may be accepted as evidence for lepromatous leprosy. However, we should also note research that has helped researchers to estimate the specificity and sensitivity of lesions of leprosy [17].

At this point, the osteological paradox should be mentioned [7] in relation to diagnosis of leprosy. We have already seen that there is a low percentage of untreated people whose skeleton may be affected and, as this is primarily a soft tissue disease, many people with leprosy whose skeletons are found as part of the archaeological record may not even have developed bone changes prior to death. To a certain extent new methods of analysis in palaeopathology can solve some of the problems.

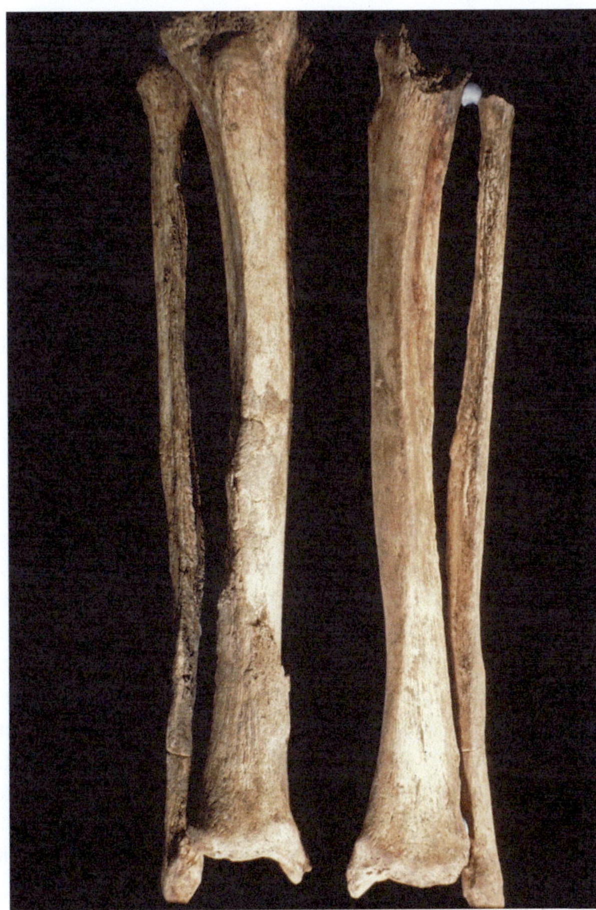

Fig. 8 Inflammatory-related new bone formation on the lower leg bones affecting a medieval skeleton from a leprosy hospital in Chichester, England (courtesy of Don Ortner)

4　Methods of Analysis in Palaeopathology

Over the last 30 years or so, imaging, histological and biomolecular methods have led to advances in diagnosis and new understandings of the origin, evolution and history of leprosy as a human disease. This is notwithstanding that the routine recording of pathologically induced bone changes in each skeleton continue to underpin the use of more advanced diagnostic techniques. Easily the most advances have been seen in ancient DNA analysis.

The first evidence for ancient DNA being preserved in an archaeological human skeleton was reported just over 30 years ago [18], and it was not long before reports of preserved ancient pathogen DNA started to appear. The first was evidence for tuberculosis (1993), but it was closely followed by a paper reporting ancient bacterial DNA of leprosy found in a sample of bone from a metatarsal dated to AD 600 from Israel [19]. By 2001, the modern genome of *M. leprae* had been sequenced [20] while the more recently discovered *M. lepromatosis* had its genome sequenced in 2008 [21]. Schuenemann et al. became the first to sequence an ancient *M. leprae* genome [22]. Most recently, *M. leprae* DNA has been found preserved in dental calculus [23].

The study of leprosy aDNA has been helped by modern *M. leprae* sequencing, including the important work documenting strains/subtypes of *M. leprae* across the globe [24, 25]. This has led to researchers exploring the strains of *M. leprae* affecting the skeletons of people who had the infection in the past [26–30], and in tandem with stable isotope analysis looking at the impact of mobility of people with leprosy on taking their infections (and strains) with them. However, it should be remembered that even if aDNA of leprosy can be extracted from skeletons and analysed, it does not mean that the person experienced the disease. They could have had subclinical leprosy and had no signs or symptoms of the infection.

5　Skeletal Evidence for Leprosy

When considering the evidence for leprosy in the archaeological record, our direct evidence is from skeletons (or mummies), although we should not forget that leprosaria were prominent institutions in medieval Europe in particular. However, very few have been excavated and even fewer have seen attention paid to their associated cemeteries. Some exceptions include those in Chichester and Winchester in England [31, 32] and Naestved in Denmark [33]. Skeletons with signs of leprosy have been excavated on four continents, to date and remain absent from the archaeological record in the Americas, Antarctica and Australasia. Asia, the Pacific region, and the Middle East have revealed very little evidence. The evidence is very much dependent on what excavations take place, and most importantly who is available and well versed with the bone changes of leprosy to be able to identify skeletons with those bone changes. Some parts of the world have few palaeopathologists working in them. Most evidence comes from medieval cemeteries in Europe (12th–16th centuries AD), and especially Britain, Denmark, Hungary and Sweden; in fact, Northern Europe as a whole has the most evidence. However, a general decline in leprosy in Europe is noted from the fourteenth century AD onwards, overtaken by a rise in tuberculosis, likely due to a cross immunity between the two infections [34]. This perhaps reflects extensive palaeopathological "activity", but it appears to corroborate historical evidence for leprosy in this period. The earliest evidence is from Hungary (3700–3600 BC), India (2500–2000 BC), Iran (6200–5700 BC), Pakistan (2550–2030 BC), Sudan (2300 BC), and Turkey (2700–2300 BC). Of particular interest, and relevant to challenging the myth that people with leprosy were all stigmatized and ostracized, "The majority of the skeletons with bone changes of leprosy around the world have been found in non-leprosy hospital cemeteries and were buried normally for their communities in those regions and time periods" [16]. This strongly suggests that people with leprosy were much more accepted within their communities than is/has been thought. As stigma in relation to leprosy remains a challenge to manage today, revisiting and reinterpreting the myth of stigma in the past is important.

While no evidence has been forthcoming in the Americas, more recent documentary data and modern DNA studies indicate that leprosy affected people in the Americas as a result of the slave trade and colonialism [24, 25]. The modern DNA studies also suggested that leprosy originated in East Africa or the Near East and spread east along northern (Silk Road) and southern routes to Asia, and west to Europe and west Africa with migrating populations, and finally to the Americas over the last 500 years. These hypotheses are now being tested using ancient DNA analysis using well-dated skeletal remains with leprosy that are geberating ancient DNA strain data, according to modern geographic location, to explore the global distribution of different ancient strains. Research to date on skeletons seems to be supporting these hypotheses. Some really fascinating research is also combining stable isotope analysis for dietary and mobility history from individual skeletons with DNA data. For example, a young male skeleton from an 11th–12th century leprosy hospital cemetery in Winchester, England was buried with a scallop shell (medieval pilgrim "badge") [35]. Isotope data showed he was not locally raised in the region where he was buried, and he harboured the 2F strain of *M. leprae* which is common in Central Asia and the Middle East today. This suggests he had been a pilgrim who had travelled around and was eventually buried in England [26]. A skeleton at the same site also had a European strain of leprosy that is also found in Europe today, and in the southern United States (including in nine banded armadillos), the latter supporting evidence that leprosy was taken to the Americas and then affected humans and other animals. A final strand of the interpretation further noted that red squirrels on Brownsea Island, off the south coast of England, and very close to Winchester, have been identified with the same strain as that found at the Winchester site. Of course, in recent years red squirrels in Britain and Ireland have been discovered to be affected by leprosy [36].

References

1. Rawcliffe C. Leprosy in medieval England. Woodbridge: Boydell Press; 2006.
2. Roberts CA, Manchester K. The archaeology of disease. 3rd ed. Gloucester: Sutton Publishing; 2005.
3. Buikstra JE. Ortner's identification of pathological conditions in human skeletal remains. London: Academic Press; 2019a.
4. Roberts CA, Scollard DM, Fava VM. The origin, evolution of tuberculosis from clinical, genetic and palaeopathological perspectives. In: Plomp K, Roberts CA, Elton S, Bentley G, editors. Palaeopathology and evolutionary medicine: an integrated approach. Oxford: Oxford University Press; 2022.
5. Resnick D, editor. Diagnosis of bone and joint disorders. London: W.B. Saunders; 2002.
6. Buikstra JE. A brief history and 21st century challenges. In: Buikstra JE, editor. Ortner's identification of pathological conditions in human skeletal remains. London: Academic Press; 2019b. p. 11–9.
7. Wood JW, Milner GR, Harpending HC, Weiss KM. The osteological paradox: problems of inferring prehistoric health from skeletal samples. Curr Anthropol. 1992;33:343–70.
8. Lambert PM. Ethics and issues in the use of skeletal remains in paleopathology. In: Grauer AL, editor. A companion to paleopathology. Cambridge: Cambridge University Press; 2012. p. 17–33.
9. Cohen M, Armelagos G, editors. Palaeopathology at the origins of agriculture. Academic Press: London; 1984.
10. Newman SL, Gowland RL, Caffell AC. North and south: a comprehensive analysis of non-adult growth and health in the industrial revolution (AD 18th–19th C), England. Am J Biol Anthropol. 2019;169(1):104–21. https://doi.org/10.1002/ajpa.23817.
11. Paterson DE, Rad M. Bone changes of leprosy: their incidence, progress, prevention and arrest. Int J Lepr Other Mycobact Dis. 1961;29:393–422.
12. Ridley DS, Jopling WH. Classification of leprosy according to immunity: a five-group system. Int J Lepr Other Mycobact Dis. 1966;34:255–73.
13. Matos VMJ. The retrospective diagnosis of leprosy: clinical and paleopathological complementarities in the medical files from the Rovisco Pais Hospital-Colony (20th Century, Tocha, Portugal) and in the skeletal collection from the medieval leprosarium of St. Jorgen's (Odense, Denmark). Coimbra: Universidade de Coimbra; 2009.
14. Møller-Christensen V. Bone changes in leprosy. Copenhagen: Munksgaard; 1961.
15. Andersen JG. Studies in the mediaeval diagnosis of leprosy in Denmark. Copenhagen: Costers Bogtrykkeri; 1969.
16. Roberts CA. Leprosy. Past and present. Gainesville: University of Florida Press; 2020.
17. Boldsen JL. Epidemiological approach to the paleopathological diagnosis of leprosy. Am J Phys Anthropol. 2001;115(4):380–7.
18. Hagelberg E, Sykes B, Hedges R. Ancient bone DNA amplified. Nature. 1989;342:485.
19. Rafi A, Spigelman M, Stanford J, Lemma E, Donoghue H, Zias J. DNA of *Mycobacterium leprae* detected by PCR in ancient bone. Int J Osteoarchaeol. 1994;4:287–90.
20. Cole ST, Eiglmeier K, Parkhill J, James KD, Thomson NR, Wheeler PR, Honor N, Garnier T, Churcher C, Harris D, et al. Massive gene decay in leprosy bacillus. Nature. 2001;409:1007–11.
21. Singh P, Benjak A, Schuenemann VJ, Herbig A, Avanzi C, Busso P, Nieselt K, Krause J, Vera-Cabrera L, Cole ST. Insight into the evolution and origin of leprosy bacilli from the genome sequence of *Mycobacterium lepromatosis*. Proc Natl Acad Sci USA. 2015;112:4459–64.
22. Schuenemann VJ, Singh P, Mendum TA, Krause-Kyora B, Jager G, Bos KI, Herbig A, Economou C, Benjak A, Busso P, et al. Genome-wide comparison of medieval and modern *Mycobacterium leprae*. Science. 2013;341:179–83.
23. Fotakis AK, Denham SD, Mackie M, Orbegozo MI, Mylopotamitaki D, Gopalakrishnan S, Sicheritz-Pontén T, Olsen JV, Cappellini E, Zhang G, Christophersen A, Gilbert MTP, Vågene

AJ. Multi-omic detection of *Mycobacterium leprae* in archaeological human dental calculus. Philos Trans R Soc B. 2020;375:20190584.

24. Monot M, Honor N, Garnier MT, Arao R, Copp J-Y, Lacroix C, Sow S, Spencer JS, Truman RW, Williams DL, et al. On the origin of leprosy. Science. 2005;308(5724):1040–2.

25. Monot M, Honor N, Garnier MT, Zidane N, Sherafi D, Paniz-Mondolfi A, Matsuoka M, Taylor GM, Donoghue HD, Bouwman A, et al. Comparative genomic and phylogeographic analysis of *Mycobacterium leprae*. Nat Genet. 2009;41:1282–9.

26. Taylor GM, Tucker K, Butler R, Pike AW, Lewis J, Roffey S, Marter P, Lee O-Y, Wu HH, Minnikin DE, Besra GS, et al. Detection and strain typing of ancient *Mycobacterium leprae* from a medieval leprosy hospital. PLoS One. 2013;8(4):e62406. https://doi.org/10.1371/journal.pone.0062406.

27. Economou C, Kjellstrom A, Lidén K, Panagopoulos I. Ancient-DNA reveals an Asian type of *Mycobacterium leprae* in medieval Scandinavia. J Archaeol Sci. 2013;40:465–70.

28. Donoghue HD, Taylor GM, Marcsik A, Molnár E, Pálfi G, Pap I, Teschler-Nicola M, Pinhasi R, Erdal YS, Velemínsky P, et al. A migration-driven model for the historical spread of leprosy in medieval eastern and Central Europe. Infect Genet Evol. 2015;31:250–6.

29. Schuenemann VJ, Avanzi C, Krause-Kyora B, Seitz A, Herbig A, Inskip S, Bonazzi M, Reiter E, Urban C, Pedersen DD, et al. Ancient genomes reveal a high diversity of *Mycobacterium leprae* in medieval Europe. PLoS Pathog. 2018;14(5):e1006997.

30. Pfrengle S, Neukamm J, Guellil M, Keller M, Molak M, Avanzi C, Kushniarevich A, Montes N, Neumann G, Tukhbatova RI, Berezina NY, Buzhilova AP, Sergeevich KD, Hamre SS, Matos V, Ferreira MT, González-Garrido L, Wasterlain SN, Lopes C, Santos AL, Antunes-Ferreira N, Duarte V, Silva AM, Melo L, Sarkic N, Saag L, Tambets K, Reiter E, Busso P, Cole ST, Roberts CA, Sheridan A, Cessford C, Robb J, Krause J, Scheib CL, Inskip SA, Schuenemann VJ. *Mycobacterium leprae* diversity and population dynamics in medieval Europe from novel ancient genomes. BMC Biol. 2021;19:220. https://doi.org/10.1186/s12915-021-01120-2.

31. Magilton J, Lee F, Boylston A, editors. 'Lepers outside the gate'. Excavations at the cemetery of the Hospital of St James and St Mary Magdalene, Chichester, 1986–1987 and 1993. York: Council for British Archaeology Research Report 158/Chichester Excavations 10; 2008.

32. Roffey S, Tucker K. A contextual study of the medieval hospital and cemetery of St Mary Magdalen, Winchester, England. Int J Paleopathol. 2012;2:170–80.

33. Møller-Christensen V. Changes in the maxillary bone with leprosy. Int J Lepr Other Mycobact Dis. 1953;21:616–7.

34. Manchester K. Tuberculosis and leprosy in antiquity: an interpretation. Med Hist. 1984;28:162–73.

35. Roffey S, Tucker K, Filipek-Ogden K, Montgomery J, Cameron J, O'Connell T, Evans J, Marter P, Taylor GM. Investigation of a medieval pilgrim burial excavated from the leprosarium of St Mary Magdalen Winchester, UK. PLoS Negl Trop Dis. 2017;11(1):e0005186. https://doi.org/10.1371/journal.pntd.0005186.

36. Avanzi C, Del-Pozo J, Benjak A, Stevenson K, Simpson VR, Busso P, McLuckie J, Loiseau C, Lawton C, Schoening J, et al. Red squirrels in the British Isles are infected with leprosy bacilli. Science. 2016;354(6313):744–7.

Hansen's Disease and Human Rights

Alice Cruz and Patrícia D. Deps

1 Introduction

Medical practice is intrinsically related to maintaining or restoring people's health. WHO defines health as *a state of complete physical, mental and social wellbeing and not merely the absence of disease or infirmity.* This broad concept of health has given rise to the paradigm of humanized medicine, biopsychosocial practice, or person-centered medicine. In this context, it can be argued that physicians and other healthcare workers need to engage actively in promoting equality, dignity, and social justice and, in the case of Hansen's disease, with tackling and eliminating stereotyping, stigmatization, and discrimination against persons affected by the disease.

Stigmatization related to Hansen's disease, and its consequences, were discussed in the previous chapter. In particular, how stigmatization can damage the well-being of persons affected by Hansen's disease. In 2021, stigma was identified by WHO as an obstacle to the elimination of Hansen's disease, classified into four types:

(a) Individual stigma—sometimes referred to as *self-stigmatization,* although the authors agree with others that this classification blames the victim and would propose the alternative concept of *internalized stigma*, placing society and not the individual as the source.
(b) Stigmatization by healthcare workers.
(c) Institutionalized stigma, such as when clinics and hospitals fail to provide care.

A. Cruz (✉)
Office of the United Nations High Commissioner for Human Rights, Geneva, Switzerland

P. D. Deps
Universidade Federal do Espírito Santo, Vitória, Brazil
e-mail: patricia.deps@ufes.br

© The Author(s), under exclusive license to Springer Nature Switzerland AG 2023
P. D. Deps (ed.), *Hansen's Disease*, https://doi.org/10.1007/978-3-031-30893-2_4

(d) Structural stigma—stigmatization at the level of officialdom, through policies that lead to insufficient resourcing, lack of innovation in health technology such as diagnostic and therapeutic methods, inadequate mental healthcare, and lack of support for research and rehabilitation.

Disease-related stigma carries a destructive potential that is sometimes underestimated by public health policy-makers. Hansen's disease has a long history of stigmatization, discrimination, and violation of human rights, destroying countless lives over thousands of years [1]. Yet, formal recognition of stigmatization as a violation of human rights is a relatively recent development.

The second decade of the twenty-first century was marked by an acknowledgment that the medicalization of stigma and discrimination namely, the idea that providing medical treatment and disseminating medical understanding and scientific knowledge of a disease would remove stigma and discrimination, was not enough. Discrimination encompasses much more than the interpersonal stigmatization which occurs at the level of the community, and which has been the primary focus of most stigma reduction strategies. Discrimination can be direct and indirect, leading to stigmatization, loss of opportunities, material deprivation, structural disadvantage, and limited access to public services and state benefits.

Adopting a human rights-based approach, the essence of which is full recognition of the rights of persons affected by Hansen's disease, is necessary to move public and private interventions in Hansen's disease stigmatization beyond the predominant medical and charitable models. Attention needs to be paid to the "looping effect" between biology and culture [2]. For instance, it is widely known that the gender of the healthcare workforce can act as a barrier in the access of women to diagnosis and treatment of Hansen's disease in endemic regions, and that the physically demanding labor which is the daily reality for many persons affected can aggravate physical impairments related to nerve damage caused by Hansen's disease.

In the present day, persons affected by Hansen's disease are still subjected to stereotyping and to interpersonal, institutional, and structural violence, manifesting ultimately in the most dehumanizing form of stigmatization—internalized stigma [3]. More than 100 laws that discriminate directly against persons affected by Hansen's disease persist in 30 countries, while indirect discrimination through the discriminatory application of laws that appear neutral at face value has also been reported [4].

Stigmatization and discrimination are major obstacles to the elimination of Hansen's disease. In recognition of this, the United Nations General Assembly adopted, in 2010, resolution 65/215 on the elimination of discrimination against persons affected by Hansen's disease and their family members, documented in principles and guidelines named after the resolution. These constitute a non-legally binding human rights instrument that interprets and translates legally binding norms in relation to the conditions and needs of persons affected by Hansen's disease and their family members. They provide countries with a road map to enforce

Table 1 Principles and guidelines for the elimination of discrimination against persons affected by leprosy and their family members

Principles	
Persons affected by leprosy and their family members	
1	Should be treated as people with dignity and are entitled, on an equal basis with others, to all the human rights and fundamental freedoms proclaimed in the Universal Declaration of Human Rights, as well as in other relevant international human rights instruments to which their respective States are parties, including the International Covenant on Economic, Social and Cultural Rights, the International Covenant on Civil and Political Rights, and the Convention on the Rights of Persons with Disabilities
2	Should not be discriminated against on the grounds of having or having had Hansen's disease
3	Should have the same rights as everyone else with respect to marriage, family, and parenthood. To this end: (a) no one should be denied the right to marry on the grounds of Hansen's disease; (b) Hansen's disease should not constitute a ground for divorce; (c) A child should not be separated from his or her parents on the grounds of Hansen's disease
4	Should have the same rights as everyone else in relation to full citizenship and obtaining identity documents
5	Should have the right to serve the public, on an equal basis with others, including the right to stand for elections and to hold office at all levels of government
6	Should have the right to work in an environment that is inclusive and to be treated on an equal basis with others in all policies and processes related to recruitment, hiring, promotion, salary, the continuance of employment, and career advancement
7	Should not be denied admission to or be expelled from schools or training programs on the grounds of Hansen's disease
8	Are entitled to develop their human potential to the fullest extent and to fully realize their dignity and self-worth. Persons affected by Hansen's disease and their family members who have been empowered and who have had the opportunity to develop their abilities can be powerful agents of social change
9	Have the right to be, and should be, actively involved in decision-making processes regarding policies and programs that directly concern their lives

Source: UN General Assembly "Principles and guidelines for the elimination of discrimination against persons affected by leprosy and their family members" A/HRC/15/30 pp. 3–7

international human rights law in the specific case of persons affected by Hansen's disease and their family members (Table 1).

Discrimination related to Hansen's disease often intersects with other identity labels connected with oppression, marginalization, exclusion, and violence. Most common among these social conditions and identities are gender, ethnicity and/or race, age, disability, migration, and poverty [5]. In practice, this means that Hansen's disease discrimination affects in different ways a person according to his or her social status and capital. Women and children are particularly vulnerable. In many parts of the world, women's access to healthcare services is dependent on permission from a third party, while children affected by Hansen's disease are subjected to bullying and can even be prohibited from attending school. The life course effects of the multifaceted stigmatization experienced by adults who were diagnosed with Hansen's disease in childhood can end in attempts by people to end their lives [3].

2 Issues Related to Treatment

Multidrug therapy was created by the WHO in the 1980s, combining three drugs to prevent drug resistance. The component drugs were also cheap, which was important in achieving and sustaining mass distribution [6]. Economic factors have always been at play against the right to the highest attainable standard of health for persons affected by Hansen's disease. This is illustrated by decisions about the dosage of the more powerful component of the multidrug regimen—rifampicin—being based mainly on cost criteria [7]. Similarly, many Hansen's disease experts disagree with global guidance regarding the duration of multidrug therapy. According to the WHO, almost all new cases can now be cured within 6–12 months. In reality, longer treatment is often needed. Patients who have a weaker immune response to Hansen's disease may experience extremely severe, disabling and painful episodes and even relapse after many years. Some Hansen's disease experts also believe that centralized decisions about treatment might increase transmission, while others disagree with guidance about the drugs themselves. In practice, patients with more purchasing power may opt for drugs that have fewer side effects, such as alternatives to clofazimine, a component of WHO multidrug therapy that causes darkening of the skin which in turn reinforces stigmatization.

Hansen's disease reactions are one of the biggest challenges in managing the disease, and they can cause much physical and mental suffering. Reactions frequently occur during and after anti-mycobacterial treatment. They are associated with the nerve damage which is the main cause of physical impairment. Hansen's disease reactions may require prolonged treatment, sometimes for several years [8]. The mechanisms of reactions are poorly understood, and treatment is largely empirical. Unlike multidrug therapy, most of the drugs used for treating Hansen's disease reactions are not provided to countries free of charge. These include steroids and thalidomide—both of which can cause problematic side effects. As is well known, thalidomide during pregnancy can harm the fetus and cause malformation of the limbs, while steroids can cause dependence and dramatic bodily changes.

Hansen's disease treatment and management of reactions both rely on obsolete and cheap drugs that can cause major side effects. The commodification of health and lack of interest of the pharmaceutical industry in neglected tropical diseases, together with the low priority that governments give to Hansen's disease, explain why persons affected by Hansen's disease are offered such low-quality medical treatment.

Despite being curable with multidrug therapy, if not detected and treated promptly, Hansen's disease can become a chronic disease that demands a continuum of medical and psychosocial care including rehabilitation, reconstructive surgery, the provision of assistive devices, and psychosocial support. Such care should be fully addressed by effective referral within national healthcare systems. However, the harsh reality of healthcare for persons affected by Hansen's disease has been the progressive dismantlement of Hansen's disease services and infrastructure, such as laboratories, and a gradual loss of expertise [9]. These factors aggravate systemic barriers to access to diagnosis and treatment widely faced by persons affected by Hansen's disease in both endemic and non-endemic countries. Another issue of great concern is that access to quality healthcare services after bacteriological cure is extremely limited for persons affected by Hansen's disease, despite this being critical for preventing physical impairments. This inequity in provision of care is another manifestation of discrimination against persons affected by Hansen's disease within healthcare systems [10].

3   Roles and Responsibilities of Healthcare Professionals

As already mentioned, healthcare workers play an important role in eliminating stigmatization and discrimination, including through the services that they provide. However, here it is important to mention the role of intersectoral policy-making. Elimination of discrimination cannot be expected to be undertaken through National Hansen's Disease Programs alone. This societal task needs to be mainstreamed into government bodies other than the Ministry of Health, including those governing education, employment, and justice, and also through agencies responsible for protecting the rights of vulnerable groups such as women, children, the elderly, and people with disabilities.

Health systems should be people-centric and resourced to ensure the following for persons affected by Hansen's disease: (1) availability and physical and economic accessibility of services; (2) active and informed participation of service-users; (3) gender-sensitive and culturally sensitive strategies; (4) child-friendly services; (5) accountability of healthcare professionals, using indicators to facilitate monitoring. Healthcare systems should enable and encourage community engagement and participation, by providing social support and individual and family psychosocial counselling, linking with self-care and self-help groups, and peer support and peer health promoters, establishing channels for patient-provider communication, and conducting outreach activities in partnership with organizations for persons affected by Hansen's disease. A holistic strategy needs to include a rights-based approach to mental health, which should be ethically respectful, culturally appropriate, gender-sensitive and empowering to individuals, making use of peer support an integral part of recovery-based services.

Persons affected by Hansen's disease require follow-up after being discharged from treatment and should not be disconnected from healthcare services after apparent cure. A continuum of care is essential to guarantee the right of persons affected to the highest attainable standard of physical and mental health. This care should be multidisciplinary, encompassing early diagnosis of reactions, prompt and appropriate use of drugs, individual and group therapies including physiotherapy and occupational therapy, and provision of wound care, surgery, orthotics, and prosthetics according to patient need. For persons affected by Hansen's disease who have impairments or disabilities, provision of assistive devices is important in maintaining quality of life.

It is incumbent on healthcare professionals to support campaigns and assist programs that aim to guarantee a high standard of care by providing well-trained medical professionals, counselling, outreach and other allied services, and access to new and better treatments, particularly for managing Hansen's disease reactions. Clinicians need to be up-to-date with alternative treatments, such as substitutes for clofazimine which can cause dyschromia, a side-effect linked to stigmatization. Healthcare professionals are responsible for preventing and reporting violations of the rights of persons affected by Hansen's disease. These include those summarized in Table 2, with specific actions that health professionals can take, and as illustrated in the two case studies at the end of this chapter.

To support healthcare professionals in these matters, clinical education and training should be extended to foster an in-depth understanding of the root causes of

Table 2 Levels at which human rights violations can occur and actions that healthcare professionals can take

Level	Violation	Action
Society	Prohibition to marry, work (including public and elected posts), live, and study in certain areas and schools, have a normal social life, use public transport and public offices, attend churches, and move to another place	Combat practices that directly discriminate against persons affected by Hansen's disease including segregation and legal prohibitions
Workplace	Dismissal, removal, or segregation of any nature	Identify physical limitations and restrictions, guiding employers to promote adaptation or temporary change of tasks or posts, avoiding dismissal
School	Children and adolescents bullied at or banned from schools	Guarantee the reception of young people in schools and promote the inclusion of students in all appropriate activities
Healthcare	Discrimination at this level is often imperceptible and perpetrated by healthcare professionals in their work routine. It includes stereotyping persons affected by Hansen's disease and making prejudiced assumptions, disregard for physical and mental suffering, failing to facilitate access to hospitals and clinics, and separating persons affected by Hansen's disease from other patients	Building the patient–physician relationship provides an opportunity for inclusivity. The healthcare professional should recognize physical and mental suffering, ensure equal access to facilities and services, and counter and correct misinformation such as risk of transmission. Healthcare services should ensure participation of persons affected by Hansen's disease, their families and support groups, and organizations
All	Structural discrimination and denials of rights	Formal and substantive recognition of persons affected by Hansen's disease and their family members as holding equal rights. Meaningful participation of persons affected in policy-making, monitoring, and evaluation. Implementation of affirmative measures and provision of accessible mechanisms for filing complaints on the violation of rights

discrimination and pathways to the emotional distress experienced by patients. The final two aspects of providing care for persons affected by Hansen's disease in a way that respects rights and counters stigma and discrimination are the fundamental importance of the act of caring itself, by which we mean a compassionate patient–physician relationship built on trust and understanding (important in any context) [11], and participation, in the sense of meaningful inclusion (not as a mere formality) of affected persons and their family members to ensure that their rights are protected.

4   Monitoring and Evaluation

To measure progress towards elimination of discrimination related to Hansen's disease, collection of monitoring data requires significant improvement, for which we make the following recommendations:

- Clearly-defined targets, indicators, and benchmark measures need to be established routine data collection should include disaggregation not only by demographic variables but also by other identities recognized in human rights law as basis for discrimination, such as race/ethnicity and disability data collection, processing, and dissemination must respect the principles of consent to participate (or opt out), data protection, and the right to privacy.
- Monitoring and evaluation should be supported by mechanisms to ensure accountability and transparency, including sharing information with stakeholders such as patient support groups and organizations for persons affected by Hansen's disease.
- An accessible mechanism should be provided for registering complaints or concerns regarding violations of rights—these should be appropriate to the local and national context and be developed, implemented, and maintained with the participation of organizations for persons affected by Hansen's disease.

5   Case Study 1: Rights-Based Counselling

Stigmatization and discrimination are multifaceted, demanding contextual and multisectoral approaches and interventions. In Indonesia, a Rights-Based Counselling Module (RBCM) based on Cognitive Behavioural Therapy (CBT) raised awareness of human rights in general and rights related to healthcare specifically [12]. The module was offered to individuals, families, and groups. One interesting outcome was that people who had experienced stigma then became counsellors, thereby fulfilling Principle No. 8 of the principles and guidelines for the elimination of discrimination which states that *persons affected by Hansen's disease and their family members who have been empowered and who have had the opportunity to develop their abilities can be powerful agents of social change.*

6 Case Study 2: Eliminating "Leprosy"

Principle No. 9 of the principles and guidelines provides for the active involvement of persons affected by Hansen's disease in decision-making processes regarding policies and programs that directly concern their lives. Recorded complaints of stigmatization related to use of the word "leprosy" and requests to change it date back to 1931, when Hansen's disease patients in the USA reported that "leprosy" and its derivatives (leper, leprous) brought humiliation and made life impossible in their communities. In 1976, by presidential decree, Brazil adopted the term "hanseníase," with use of the old term in official and professional practice prohibited by law in 1995. Besides being the preference of persons affected by Hansen's disease [13], the change distances Hansen's disease from "leprosy," a disease associated in the popular imagination with "biblical leprosy" and its strong negative connotations (sin, uncleanliness, and contagion). Although officially only Brazil has effected the name change by law, use of the term Hansen's disease is increasingly widespread either instead of or alongside leprosy, and we believe that this is an important step towards eliminating stigma and discrimination [14].

References

1. Deps P. The day I changed my name: Hansen's disease and stigma = O dia em que mudei de Nome: Hanseniase e estigma. Paris: Éditions de Boccard; 2019.
2. Hacking I. The looping effects of human kinds. In: Sperber D, Premack D, Premack AJ, editors. Causal cognition: a multidisciplinary debate. Oxford: Oxford University Press; 1995.
3. Cruz A. Stigmatization as dehumanization: wrongful stereotyping and structural violence against women and children affected by leprosy. In: Office of the United Nations High Commissioner for Human Rights (OHCHR). Geneva: World Health Organization; 2019.
4. Cruz A. An unfinished business: discrimination in law against persons affected by leprosy and their family members. In: Office of the United Nations High Commissioner for Human Rights (OHCHR). Geneva: World Health Organization; 2021.
5. Cruz A. Office of the United Nations High Commissioner for Human Rights (OHCHR). Geneva: World Health Organization; 2018.
6. WHO Study Group on Chemotherapy of Leprosy for Control Programmes, World Health Organization. Chemotherapy of leprosy for control programmes: report of a WHO study group [meeting held in Geneva from 12 to 16 October 1981]. Geneva: World Health Organization; 1982.
7. Sansarricq H, UNDP/World Bank/WHO Special Programme for Research and Training in Tropical Diseases. Multidrug therapy against leprosy: development and implementation over the past 25 years. Geneva: World Health Organization; 2004.
8. Lockwood DNJ, Lambert S, Srikantam A, et al. Three drugs are unnecessary for treating paucibacillary leprosy—a critique of the WHO guidelines. PLoS Negl Trop Dis. 2019;13:e0007671. https://doi.org/10.1371/journal.pntd.0007671.
9. Costa LG, Cortela D, Soares RCFR, Ignotti E. Factors associated with the worsening of the disability grade during leprosy treatment in Brazil. Lepr Rev. 2015;86:265–72.
10. de Cury MRCO, Paschoal VD, Nardi SMT, et al. Spatial analysis of leprosy incidence and associated socioeconomic factors. Rev Saude Publica. 2012;46:110–8. https://doi.org/10.1590/s0034-89102011005000086.

11. Deps P, Charlier P. Medical approach to refugees: importance of the caring physician. Ann Glob Health. 2020;86:41. https://doi.org/10.5334/aogh.2779.
12. Lusli M, Peters R, van Brakel W, et al. The impact of a rights-based counselling intervention to reduce stigma in people affected by leprosy in Indonesia. PLoS Negl Trop Dis. 2016;10:e0005088. https://doi.org/10.1371/journal.pntd.0005088.
13. Delboni L, Deps P. Consensus in Brazil on the renaming of leprosy to Hansen's disease. Trans R Soc Trop Med Hyg. 2021;115:1086–7. https://doi.org/10.1093/trstmh/trab115.
14. Deps P, Cruz A. Why we should stop using the word leprosy. Lancet Infect Dis. 2020;20:e75–8. https://doi.org/10.1016/S1473-3099(20)30061-X.

Leprosy Agents and Principal Methods of Detection, Identification, and Characterization of the Leprosy Agents

Sofie Marijke Braet ⓘ, Patrícia Sammarco Rosa ⓘ, John Stewart Spencer ⓘ, and Charlotte Avanzi ⓘ

1 Characteristics of the Leprosy Agents

Leprosy is a neglected tropical disease caused by two acid-fast rod-shaped Gram-positive mycobacteria, *Mycobacterium leprae* and *Mycobacterium lepromatosis*. The genome of *M. leprae* and *M. lepromatosis* (3.26 Mbp [1] and 3.27 Mbp [2], respectively) are extremely reduced and show a large proportion of pseudogenes. A consequence is the complete dependency of both bacilli to host machinery and thus on intracellular growth. This observation also explains the lack of success in growing these bacteria on axenic media. Alternatively, the leprosy bacilli can

S. M. Braet
Institute of Tropical Medicine, Antwerp, Belgium

University of Antwerp, Antwerp, Belgium

Research Foundation Flanders, Brussels, Belgium
e-mail: sbraet@itg.be

P. S. Rosa
Division of Research and Education, Instituto Lauro de Souza Lima, Bauru, São Paulo, Brazil
e-mail: prosa@ilsl.br

J. S. Spencer
Department of Microbiology, Immunology and Pathology, Colorado State University,
Fort Collins, CO, USA
e-mail: john.spencer@colostate.edu

C. Avanzi (✉)
Mycobacteria Research Laboratories, Department of Microbiology,
Immunology and Pathology, Colorado State University, Fort Collins, CO, USA

Swiss Tropical and Public Health Institute, Basel, Switzerland

University of Basel, Basel, Switzerland
e-mail: charlotte.avanzi@colostate.edu

P. D. Deps (ed.), *Hansen's Disease*, https://doi.org/10.1007/978-3-031-30893-2_5

successfully be maintained for short periods in cell culture such as macrophages or cultivated in laboratory models such as mouse footpad (MFP) and armadillos [3]. Growth of the leprosy bacilli in an animal model, requiring a high number of bacilli to inoculate, takes several months because of the pathogen's doubling time of 12 days [3]. These are expensive and technically challenging techniques that only a handful of laboratories have the expertise worldwide.[1]

Both bacilli trigger the full spectrum of leprosy symptoms in humans, except for *M. lepromatosis*, for which tuberculoid forms have not yet been described [4]. *M. leprae* infection in humans are found worldwide while *M. lepromatosis* cases are mainly located in Mexico, the Caribbean region and in Central and South America with sporadic cases in Asia [4, 5]. In Mexico, pure *M. lepromatosis* infections as well as co-infections with *M. leprae* [4] are reported, whereas outside Mexico, *M. lepromatosis* is mostly reported under the form of co-infection[2] with *M. leprae* [4]. *M. leprae* naturally infects a wide range of animal reservoirs such as armadillos [7], red squirrels [8], and chimpanzees [9]. *M. lepromatosis* was identified in the red squirrel in the British Isles but no animal reservoir has been identified in the Americas yet [8]. In the USA, leprosy is recognized as a zoonosis with sporadic cases in the south-eastern part of the country while in other endemic countries, human-to-human transmission is regarded as the main route of infection [5, 10, 11].

2 Methods of Identification of the Leprosy Causative Agents

Leprosy diagnosis relies on three cardinal signs: (1) definite loss of sensation in a pale (hypopigmented) or reddish skin patch; (2) thickened or enlarged peripheral nerve with loss of sensation and/or weakness of the muscles supplied by that nerve; or (3) presence of acid-fast bacilli in a slit-skin smear (SSS), as defined by the World Health Organization (WHO) guidelines [12]. The leprosy bacilli are mainly detected in skin and nerve tissue (Table 1) with various sensitivity depending on the disease's form [26]. Multibacillary (MB) patients (>5 skin lesions) will harbor a high number of bacteria in skin lesions while few or no leprosy bacilli are expected in paucibacillary (PB) patients (≤5 skin lesions). Diagnosis of PB patients will often require several samplings (including nerve sampling in case of pure neural leprosy) and methods to confirm the diagnosis microbiologically. SSSs and nasal swabs are less invasive than skin biopsies and often preferred by patients, but fewer bacilli are usually observed, decreasing the sensitivity of detection especially for PB patients. Moreover, healthy household contacts of leprosy patients or healthy individuals from endemic countries may harbor bacilli in these samples, representing a

---

[1]National Hansen Disease Program, Baton Rouge, Louisiana, USA; Instituto Lauro de Souza Lima, Bauru, Brazil; Centre National de Référence des mycobactéries, Paris, France; Schieffelin Institute of Health, Karigari, India; National Institute of Infectious Diseases: Leprosy Research Center, Tokyo, Japan.

[2]Except one case of pure *M. lepromatosis* case reported in Dominican Republic [6].

Table 1 Methods available for the detection, identification, and viability measurement of the leprosy bacilli in various clinical samples

Purpose of the detection	Preferred sample type	Principle	Methods	Commercially available	References
Identification of leprosy bacilli					
Qualitative					
Immunodiagnostics	Venous blood or fingerstick blood	Antigen-based detection Cellular immunity	ELISA Lateral flow test Lateral flow test	Yes	[13–15]
Quantitative					
Microscopy	SSS[b] Skin biopsies	Bacterial coloration	Bacillary index (ZN) Bacillary index (FF)	No	[16–18]
Molecular methods	SSS[b] Skin biopsies	Quantification of *M. leprae* and *M. lepromatosis*-specific target from DNA samples	qPCR RLEP (*M. leprae*) RLPM (*M. lepromatosis*)	Yes (RLEP)	[4, 19, 20]
Viability of the leprosy bacilli					
Microscopy	SSS[b] Skin biopsies	Assessment of bacterial integrity (solid *vs.* fragmented bacilli)	Morphology index	No	[21]
In vivo	–	Inoculation from fresh skin biopsies in the footpad of immunocompetent mice	Shepard method	No	[22]
Molecular methods	Skin biopsies	Quantification of *M. leprae* transcripts in RNA extracts, measured on a defined number of *M. leprae* calculated by RLEP PCR	qPCR[a] *hsp18* and *esxA* 16S rRNA	No	[23–25]

[a]There is no viability assay developed for *M. lepromatosis* [b] *Slit Skin Smear*

prognostic marker rather than a confirmatory diagnostic marker [27]. The edges of active skin lesions are the areas where the highest quantity of bacilli is found. Therefore, for diagnostic purposes, a skin biopsy (4 mm) at the edge of an active lesion is preferred for downstream molecular applications (detection, genotyping, and drug susceptibility) as well as for inoculation in mouse footpad. Nevertheless,

SSS is often used for monitoring bacterial load during treatment because it is less invasive than skin biopsies. Given the tropism for skin and nerve cells, leprosy bacilli are rarely found in the systemic circulation, only in patients with high level of infection. Blood samples are thus less relevant for bacterial identification but can be used for serological or immunological diagnosis.

2.1 Identification and Quantification of Leprosy Bacilli in Skin Lesion by Microscopy

The most common method of identifying leprosy bacilli in tissue is microscopy on SSS, biopsy of a skin lesion and in rare cases on a nerve biopsy. Ziehl Neelsen (ZN) staining is the standard coloration for acid-fast bacilli (AFB). However, since *M. leprae* and *M. lepromatosis* are weakly acid-fast [28, 29], the ZN procedure is performed with a shorter discoloration time [16]. The adapted ZN method named Fite-Faraco staining is recommended for skin biopsies preserved in formalin and paraffin (Fig. 1) [17, 31, 32]. After staining, the rod-shaped bacilli turn uniformly pink and can be identified as isolated or grouped in globi, which is characteristic for a leprosy infection.

Subsequently to staining, the number of bacilli or bacillary index (BI) is counted based on a semi-logarithmic scale from +1 to +6 (Table 2). A patient's BI usually represents the mean of BIs calculated from SSS collected from the ear lobe, elbow, and knee. This measure is performed before and at different time points during treatment. An increase of BI during treatment must be considered as treatment inefficiency or failure.

In parallel, the type of leprosy is can be characterized by specific histopathologic changes in the lesions following the well-described classification of Ridley and Jopling from lepromatous to tuberculoid forms [18, 33–35]. Alternatively, in

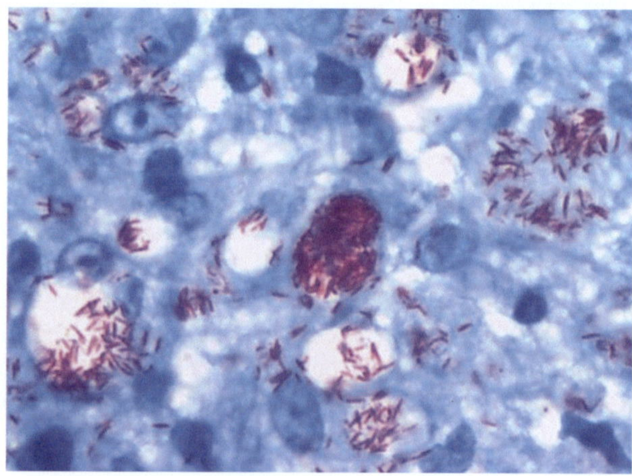

Fig. 1 Bacilloscopy varying from 4+ to 6+. Presence of bacilli in neural branches, macrophages, interstitial cells, in perivascular and periadnexal inflammatory infiltrates and occasionally in the walls of vessels and endothelium. In the center macrophages with intracytoplasmic vacuoles filled with numerous bacilli (globi) (Fite-Faraco ×100). Figure and caption adapted from [30]

Table 2 Bacillary index

Negative (0)—no bacilli per 100 high-power field
Positive (1+)—1 to 10 bacilli per 100 high-power field
Positive (2+)—1 to 10 bacilli per 10 high-power field
Positive (3+)—1 to 10 bacilli per high-power field
Positive (4+)—10 to 100 bacilli per high-power field
Positive (5+)—100 to 1000 bacilli per high-power field
Positive (6+)—More than 1000 bacilli per high-power field

absence of microscopy, the WHO recommends the classification of leprosy solely based on the number of skin lesions (MB *vs.* PB) patients for treatment purposes [12]. MB usually includes lepromatous forms while PB includes tuberculoid forms [36].

2.2 Molecular Methods

Molecular assay is currently the only method able to differentiate between *M. leprae* and *M. lepromatosis* infection. The analysis of both genomes [1, 2] has revealed genetic differences and singularities exploited to develop sensitive and specific molecular assay to differentiate both pathogens.

The genome of *M. leprae* contains four families of dispersed repetitive elements including one, RLEP, present in 37 copies [37]. The molecular amplification of the conserved core region of this element is highly specific to *M. leprae* [38] and sensitive with a limit of detection down to three bacilli using TaqMan quantitative PCR (Table 3) [19, 43, 44]. In case of waning clinical acumen or suspected early leprosy or PB patients, which are difficult to detect clinically or histologically, molecular detection using the RLEP target is the method of choice, provided that good practice and control of the qPCR conditions are applied.

Two tests based on RLEP detection are commercially available. The GenoType LepraeDR from Hain LifeScience (Germany) is a reverse hybridization DNA strip that also allows detection of drug resistance, which requires a thermocycler and an automated washing and shaking device [45]. The second test is a loop-mediated isothermal amplification, the RLEP LAMP assay soon to be commercialized by Amplex Diagnostics (Germany) [20]. The LAMP assay uses six primers and a Bst DNA polymerase and can be executed at one single temperature, circumventing the need for a (q)PCR machine.

There is no commercial test available yet for molecular detection of *M. lepromatosis* but infection by *M. leprae* or *M. lepromatosis* can be distinguished on the basis of their 16S rRNA sequence being only 98% identical [46]. The method requires sequencing of the amplicon. Similarly, the pathogens can be differentiated based on a 45 bp insertion in the *M. lepromatosis rpoT* sequence and the difference can be observed on agarose gel [40]. However, in case of co-infection with *M. leprae*, 16S rRNA, and *rpoT* amplification can be difficult to interpret. Singh and colleagues

Table 3 List of primers and probes to perform identification, quantification, and viability assay for the leprosy bacilli

Purpose of assays	Target gene	Primer/probe sequences (5′–3′)	References
Quantification of *M. leprae*	RLEP	Fw: GCAGCAGTATCGTGTTAGTGAA Rv: CGCTAGAAGGTTGCCGTAT P: CGCCGACGGCCGGATCATCGA	[39]
Quantification of *M. lepromatosis*	RLPM	Fw: TTGGTGATCGGGGTCGGCTGG Rv: CCCCACCGGACACCACCAACC P: AAGTGACGCGGGCGTGGATT	[40]
Drug resistance rifampicin[a]	*rpoB*	Fw: GTCGAGGCGATCACGCCGC Rv: CGACAATGAACCGATCAGAC	[41]
Drug resistance dapsone[a]	*folP1*	Fw: CCTGACGATGCTGTCCAGC Rv: CACCAGACACATCGTTGACG	[41]
Drug resistance ofloxacin[a]	*gyrA*	Fw: GATGGTCTCAAACCGGTACATC Rv: ACCCGGCGAACCGAAATTG	[41]
Viability *M. leprae*	*hsp18* *esxA*	Fw: CGATCGGGAAATGCTTGC Rv: CGAGAACCAGCTGACGATTG P: ACACCGCGTGGCCGCTCG Fw: CCGAGGGAATAAACCATGCA Rv: CGTTTCAGCCGAGTGATTGA P: TGCTTGCACCAGGTCGCCCA	[39]
Viability *M. leprae*	16S rRNA	Fw: GCATGTCTTGTGGTGGAAAGC Rv: CACCCCACCAACAAGCTGAT P: CATCCTGCACCGCA	[23]

Fw forward, *Rv* reverse
[a]Mutations conferring drug resistance and validated in mouse footpad are described by Aubry and colleagues [42]

developed a specific 244 bp PCR amplification assay targeting *hemN,* a gene absent in the genome of *M. leprae* due to reductive evolution [2, 6], but this gene is present in other mycobacteria making the assay not specific. Recently, Sharma et al. developed a qPCR targeting the *M. lepromatosis* repetitive element RLPM [4], occurring 5–6 times in the *M. lepromatosis* genome and being highly specific. The RLPM qPCR assay is currently the most sensitive and specific assay available to detect the presence of *M. lepromatosis* in DNA samples. [47].

2.3 *Immunodiagnostics*

Molecular methods are highly specific but lack sensitivity at early stages of disease progression when symptoms are rare or to measure exposure and assess risk of disease progression in healthy contacts [48]. This is where host biomarkers can be complementary. However, due to the spectral variability in the immune response in leprosy patients, specific tests measuring antibody response (MB) and cell-mediated immunity (PB) are necessary to cover the full leprosy spectrum [48]. Several antigens are shown to mount a strong antibody response and include the native phenolic glycolipid I (PGL-I) or its mimotope, the natural disaccharide octyl bovine serum albumin (ND-O-BSA)[3] that is part of the cell wall of *M. leprae* and *M. lepromatosis* (IgM response), and the leprosy IDRI diagnostic 1 (LID-1), which is a fusion protein of two known *M. leprae* antigens, ML0405 and ML2331 (IgG response) [49]. However, their sensitivity remains low especially for PB patients [49]. Additionally, when performed in an endemic country, healthy contacts can also have positive antibody response to these antigens, but the vast majority of these individuals will not progress toward the disease [48]. The qualitative tests in a lateral flow test format are commercially available in Brazil for both NDO-LID and PGL-I antigens [13, 50]. A qualitative test (ML Flow test) assessing the antibody response to PGL-I is commercialized by Bioclin (Brazil) and a recently developed quantitative test is commercially available in The Netherlands, the UCP-LFA [51] for quantification of anti-PGL-I response.

To cover the full spectrum of leprosy forms, a lateral flow test measuring multiple host proteins was recently developed and is currently being tested in several endemic countries [14]. This multi-biomarker test includes six previously identified host biomarkers able to diagnose all leprosy forms as well as differentiate between MB and PB cases. The test is performed on fingerstick blood and is minimally invasive [14].

3   Monitoring Treatment Efficacy

Leprosy is curable using multidrug therapy, combining rifampicin, dapsone, and clofazimine for all forms of leprosy, for 6 (PB) to 12 months (MB). Drugs are administered by supervised dose (monthly), taken at the health center, associated with self-administered doses (daily) at home. The patient is discharged after full completion of the number of doses recommended by the therapeutic scheme and following to the results of the dermato-neurological examination [12]. MDT can be pursued if clinical signs persist at the end of the recommended treatment period (treatment inefficiency) up to 24 months. After this period, persistence of symptoms is considered treatment failure [52]. A handful of laboratory methods are available to support clinical assessment and are described below.

---

[3]Antigens available through BEI Resources (pure PGL-I: NR-19342; ND-O-BSA: NR-19346). LID-1 is not available from BEI Resources.

3.1   *Bacterial Index and Morphology Index by Microscopy*

BI determination can be performed before and at different time points during treatment to monitor the evolution of the bacterial load. BI determination is not a measure of viability, as a slow decrease in AFB is commonly observed during treatment (one log/year). In contrast, the morphology index (MI) is measured of bacterial viability based on cell integrity. Solid bacilli are considered viable while fragmented or granular bacilli are non-viable (Fig. 2) [21]. This method relies on previous observation that morphological changes of the leprosy bacillus correlate with effective treatment of lepromatous patients [35]. It is expressed as a percentage of viability measured on 200 bacilli [35]. The MI in untreated MB leprosy usually ranges between 25 and 75 and should decline to 0 after 6 months of effective chemotherapy. This method might reduce the variation seen with acid-fast staining and can be done subsequently to the BI measurement. However, it is considered to be an imperfect measure of viability since it is variable depending on the operator and requires a high number of bacilli in sample.

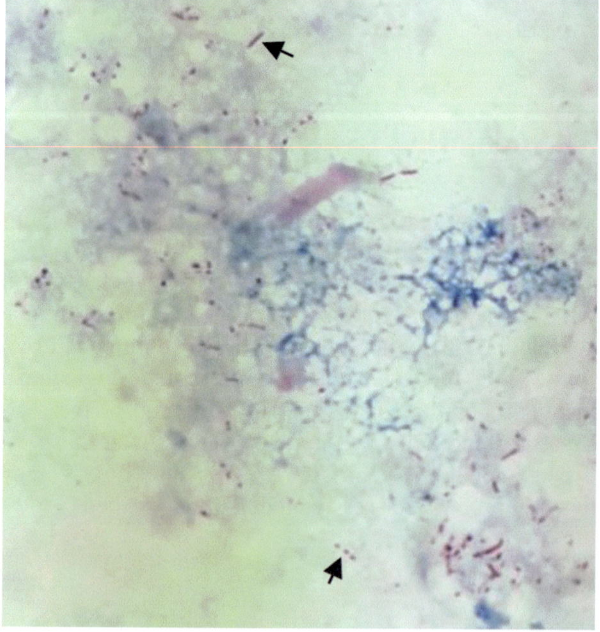

Fig. 2 Morphology assessment of bacilli in microscopy—the arrow in the upper part represents a solid bacillus considered viable while the arrow in the lower part of the figure shows a fragmented non-viable bacillus (× 1000). Figure provided by Suzana M. Diório

3.2 In Vivo Inoculation

Alternatively, bacterial viability in clinical samples can be assessed by inoculation of bacteria from human skin biopsies to MFPs in immunocompromised nude mice followed by the microscopic evaluation of bacterial replication 6–12 months later [24]. However, this method requires bacterial isolation to be performed from the skin biopsies freshly collected (maximum 4 days after collection) and only few laboratories in the world have the capacity to perform such experiments [16, 24].

3.3 RNA-Based Approaches

The current validated molecular viability assays (Tables 1 and 3) are based on the quantification of transcripts, *hsp18* and *esxA*, or 16S rRNA measured on a defined number of *M. leprae* calculated by RLEP PCR [25, 39]. Both assays determine absolute viability at the time of harvest and do not rely on a paired "pretreatment" sample [3]. Nevertheless, since patients' response to treatment is variable from one individual to another and because of the slow growth of the pathogen, longitudinal viability testing should be performed to properly measure the impact of the drugs on bacterial viability [25]. RNA-based methods represents currently the fastest way to assess drug efficacy and strongly correlates with the MFP assay. They were also validated on samples from infected mice and clinical isolates [23, 25].

4 Methods to Monitor Drug Resistance

The main cause of treatment inefficacy is the development of drug-resistant bacteria. Systematic monitoring of drug susceptibility in leprosy is very important since clinical signs of therapeutic inefficiency are seldom present before 12 months of standard MDT treatment. In addition, resistance to dapsone may be hidden by the bactericidal action of rifampicin, and most likely, dapsone-resistant patients will relapse late after the end of treatment [53]. Therefore, drug susceptibility testing should be performed in all cases prior to treatment initiation to detect infection with drug-resistant strains and when treatment insufficiency and relapse is suspected.

Drug resistance in *M. leprae* is most often attributable to mutations in specific part of chromosomal genes encoding drug targets, known as drug-resistant determining regions (DRDR) [54], rather than horizontal gene transfer [55]. Patients with the highest BI (lepromatous patients harboring 10^{11}–10^{12} *M. leprae* bacilli per gram of tissue) are more likely at risk of selecting drug-resistant mutants [54]. Empirically, the gold standard method for drug susceptibility testing is the Shepard method [22]. Briefly, the method relies on the isolation of at least 10^4 viable bacilli from lesions of MB patients and inoculation within about 3 days following collection of the clinical specimen into the footpads of immunocompetent mice. The bacilli are recovered from the inoculated footpads after 6–10 months of treatment, compared to untreated group and recovery of $\geq 1 \times 10^5$ bacilli per foot pad is considered positive growth. Because of the 12-days doubling time of *M. leprae* results may only be available after the end of the treatment of the patient [3]. This method is only applicable to patients with a high bacillary load. Alternatively, molecular methods targeting the DRDR of specific targets have been validated and implemented in all endemic countries as part of the WHO drug resistance surveillance network [56]. The validated targets include *folP1* (dapsone), *rpoB* (rifampicin), and *gyrA* (ofloxacin) by identification of mutations in the DRDRs of these targets using specific primers (Table 3). Recommended methods include a polymerase chain reaction (PCR) step coupled with Sanger sequencing [41], the commercial DNA strip test GenoType LepraeDR [45], or whole-genome sequencing [55]. There is currently no validated targets for the leprosy drugs clofazimine, minocycline, and clarithromycin [42].

Treatment of *M. lepromatosis* infection is empirically similar to the one administered for MB cases of *M. leprae* infection [6]. While it is likely that rifampicin is active against *M. lepromatosis*, it is not yet clear whether the bacterium is susceptible to dapsone or clofazimine [42]. There is currently no molecular test available to amplify the drug resistant determining regions of *rpoB, folP1,* and *gyrA* for *M. lepromatosis* and drug susceptibility testing in mice has not yet been performed.

Contributions
SMB, PSR, JSS, CA wrote the manuscript. All authors reviewed the last version of the manuscript.

Funding CA is supported by the Heiser Program of the New York Community Trust for Research in Leprosy grant number P21-000127, the European Union's Horizon 2020 research and innovation program under the Marie Sklodowska-Curie grant No. 845479. JSS is supported by a Fulbright Scholar to Brazil grant, 2019–2022. CA and PSR would like to thank the Raoul Follereau Foundation for the support given to the fight against leprosy, and particularly for the annual support given to the work conducted in their respective laboratories. SMB is supported by the Fonds Wetenschappelijk Onderzoek (FWO, grants 1189219N and V408322N, https://www.fwo.be/) and European and Developing Countries Clinical Trials program (EDCTP2) supported by the European Union (grant number RIA2017NIM-1847-PEOPLE, https://www.edctp.org/#).

Declarations of Interest None.

References

1. Cole ST, Eiglmeier K, Parkhill J, James KD, Thomson NR, Wheeler PR, et al. Massive gene decay in the leprosy bacillus. Nature. 2001;409(6823):1007–11.
2. Singh P, Benjak A, Schuenemann VJ, Herbig A, Avanzi C, Busso P, et al. Insight into the evolution and origin of leprosy bacilli from the genome sequence of *Mycobacterium lepromatosis*. Proc Natl Acad Sci U S A. 2015;112(14):4459–64. https://doi.org/10.1128/spectrum.01692-21.
3. Adams LB. Susceptibility and resistance in leprosy: studies in the mouse model. Immunol Rev. 2021;301(1):157–74.
4. Sharma R, Singh P, McCoy RC, Lenz SM, Donovan K, Ochoa MT, et al. Isolation of *Mycobacterium lepromatosis* and development of molecular diagnostic assays to distinguish *Mycobacterium leprae* and *M. lepromatosis*. Clin Infect Dis. 2020;71(8):e262–9.
5. Deps P, Collin SM. *Mycobacterium lepromatosis* as a second agent of Hansen's disease. Front Microbiol. 2022;12:698588. https://doi.org/10.3389/fmicb.2021.698588.
6. Fernández JDP, Pou-Soarez V, Arenas R, Juárez-Duran ER, Luna-Rojas SL, Xicohtencatl-Cortes J, et al. *Mycobacterium leprae* and *Mycobacterium lepromatosis* infection. A report of six multibacillary cases of leprosy in Dominican Republic. Jpn J Infect Dis. 2022;75(4):427–30.
7. Ploemacher T, Faber WR, Menke H, Rutten V, Pieters T. Reservoirs and transmission routes of leprosy; a systematic review. PLoS Negl Trop Dis. 2020;14(4):e0008276.
8. Avanzi C, Del-Pozo J, Benjak A, Stevenson K, Simpson VR, Busso P, et al. Red squirrels in the British Isles are infected with leprosy bacilli. Science. 2016;354(6313):744–7.
9. Hockings KJ, Mubemba B, Avanzi C, Pleh K, Düx A, Bersacola E, et al. Leprosy in wild chimpanzees. Nature. 2021;598(7882):652–6.
10. da Silva MB, Portela JM, Li W, Jackson M, Gonzalez-Juarrero M, Hidalgo AS, et al. Evidence of zoonotic leprosy in Pará, Brazilian Amazon, and risks associated with human contact or consumption of armadillos. PLoS Negl Trop Dis. 2018;12(6):e0006532.
11. Vera-Cabrera L, Ramos-Cavazos CJ, Youssef NA, Pearce CM, Molina-Torres CA, Avalos-Ramirez R, et al. *Mycobacterium leprae* infection in a wild nine-banded armadillo, Nuevo León, Mexico. Emerg Infect Dis. 2022;28(3):747–9.
12. World Health Organization. Regional Office for South-East Asia. Guidelines for the diagnosis, treatment and prevention of leprosy. 2018. https://apps.who.int/iris/handle/10665/274127. Accessed 24 Jan 2022.
13. Teles SF, Silva EA, de Souza RM, Tomimori J, Florian MC, Souza RO, et al. Association between NDO-LID and PGL-1 for leprosy and class I and II human leukocyte antigen alleles in an indigenous community in Southwest Amazon. Braz J Infect Dis. 2020;24(4):296–303.
14. van Hooij A, Fat EMTK, de Jong D, Khatun M, Soren S, Chowdhury AS, et al. Prototype multi-biomarker test for point-of-care leprosy diagnostics. iScience. 2021;24(1):102006. https://www.cell.com/iscience/abstract/S2589-0042(20)31203-7
15. Buhrer-Sekula S, Smits HL, Gussenhoven GC, van Leeuwen J, Amador S, Fujiwara T, et al. Simple and fast lateral flow test for classification of leprosy patients and identification of contacts with high risk of developing leprosy. J Clin Microbiol. 2003;41(5):1991–5.
16. Trombone APF, Pedrini SCB, Diório SM, de Belone AFF, Fachin LRV, do Nascimento DC, et al. Optimized protocols for *Mycobacterium leprae* strain management: frozen stock preservation and maintenance in athymic nude mice. J Vis Exp. 2014;85:50620.
17. Fite GL. The staining of acid-fast bacilli in paraffin sections. Am J Pathol. 1938;14(4):491–507.
18. Scollard DM. Histopathological diagnosis of leprosy. Lepr Rev. 2022;93(1):92–3.
19. Truman RW, Andrews PK, Robbins NY, Adams LB, Krahenbuhl JL, Gillis TP. Enumeration of *Mycobacterium leprae* using real-time PCR. PLoS Negl Trop Dis. 2008;2(11):e328.
20. Saar M, Beissner M, Gültekin F, Maman I, Herbinger KH, Bretzel G. RLEP LAMP for the laboratory confirmation of leprosy: towards a point-of-care test. BMC Infect Dis. 2021;21(1):1186.
21. Ridley DS. The SFG (solid, fragmented, granular) index for bacterial morphology. Lepr Rev. 1971;42(2):96–7.

22. Shepard CC. The experimental disease that follows the injection of human leprosy bacilli into foot-pads of mice. J Exp Med. 1960;112(3):445–54.
23. Davis GL, Ray NA, Lahiri R, Gillis TP, Krahenbuhl JL, Williams DL, et al. Molecular assays for determining *Mycobacterium leprae* viability in tissues of experimentally infected mice. PLoS Negl Trop Dis. 2013;7(8):e2404. https://doi.org/10.3389/fitd.2022.967351.
24. Adams LB, Lahiri R. Cultivation and viability determination of *Mycobacterium leprae*. In: Scollard DM, Gillis TP, editors. The international textbook of leprosy; 2016.
25. Martinez AN, Lahiri R, Pittman TL, Scollard D, Truman R, Moraes MO, et al. Molecular determination of *Mycobacterium leprae* viability by use of real-time PCR. J Clin Microbiol. 2009;47(7):2124–30. https://doi.org/10.47276/lr.94.1.7.
26. Frade MAC, de Rosa DJF, Bernardes Filho F, Spencer JS, Foss NT. Semmes–Weinstein monofilament: a tool to quantify skin sensation in macular lesions for leprosy diagnosis. Indian J Dermatol Venereol Leprol. 2021;87(6):807–15.
27. da Silva MB, Li W, Bouth RC, Gobbo AR, Messias ACC, Moraes TMP, et al. Latent leprosy infection identified by dual RLEP and anti-PGL-I positivity: implications for new control strategies. PLoS One. 2021;16(5):e0251631.
28. Brennan PJ, Spencer JS. The physiology of *Mycobacterium leprae*. In: International textbook of leprosy. Berlin: Springer; 2016. https://internationaltextbookofleprosy.org/chapter/mycobacterium-leprae.
29. Romano LA, Klosterhoff MC, de Medeiros AFF, Pedrosa VF. Comparative study of Ziehl–Neelsen's technique and the Fite–Faraco technique in the histopathological diagnosis of Mycobacteriosis in fish. Asian J Res Anim Vet Sci. 2020;27:27–34.
30. Deps PD, Rosa PS. Agentes Etiologicos e principal metodos pae detecçao do *M. leprae*. In: Hanseníase na prática clínica. São Paulo: Editora dos editores; 2022. https://www.barnesandnoble.com/w/hansen-ase-na-pr-tica-cl-nica-patr-cia-deps/1141330656?ean=9786586098655.
31. Fontes AB, Cruz O, Flavio I, Lara A, Santos AR, et al. Pathogen detection. In: International textbook of leprosy. Berlin: Springer; 2017.
32. Girma S, Avanzi C, Bobosha K, Desta K, Idriss MH, Busso P, et al. Evaluation of Auramine O staining and conventional PCR for leprosy diagnosis: a comparative cross-sectional study from Ethiopia. PLoS Negl Trop Dis. 2018;12(9):e0006706.
33. Ridley DS, Jopling WH. Classification of leprosy according to immunity. A five-group system. Int J Lepr Other Mycobact Dis. 1966 Sep;34(3):255–73.
34. Worobec SM. Current approaches and future directions in the treatment of leprosy. Res Rep Trop Med. 2012;3:79–91.
35. World Health Organization. Leprosy unit. Laboratory techniques for leprosy. Geneva: World Health Organization; 1986. https://apps.who.int/iris/handle/10665/61778
36. Britton WJ, Lockwood DN. Leprosy. Lancet. 2004;363(9416):1209–19.
37. Cole ST, Supply P, Honoré N. Repetitive sequences in *Mycobacterium leprae* and their impact on genome plasticity. Lepr Rev. 2001;72(4):449–61.
38. Braet S, Vandelannoote K, Meehan CJ, Fontes ANB, Hasker E, Rosa PS, et al. The repetitive element RLEP is a highly specific target for detection of *Mycobacterium leprae*. J Clin Microbiol. 2018;56(3):e01924–17.
39. Collins JH, Lenz SM, Ray NA, Balagon MF, Hagge DA, Lahiri R, et al. A sensitive and quantitative assay to enumerate and measure *Mycobacterium leprae* viability in clinical and experimental specimens. Curr Protoc. 2022;2(2):e359.
40. Dwivedi P, Sharma M, Patel P, Singh P. Simultaneous detection and differentiation between *Mycobacterium leprae* and *Mycobacterium lepromatosis* using novel polymerase chain reaction primers. J Dermatol. 2021;48(12):1936–9.
41. World Health Organization. A guide for surveillance of antimicrobial resistance in leprosy: 2017. New Delhi: World Health Organization, Regional Office for South-East Asia, 2017. https://www.who.int/publications/i/item/9789290225492. Accessed 24 Jan 2022.
42. Aubry A, Rosa PS, Chauffour A, Fletcher ML, Cambau E, Avanzi C. Drug resistance in leprosy: update following 70 years of chemotherapy. Infect Dis Now. 2022;52(5):243–51.

43. Beissner M, Woestemeier A, Saar M, Badziklou K, Maman I, Amedifou C, et al. Development of a combined RLEP/16S rRNA (RT) qPCR assay for the detection of viable *M. leprae* from nasal swab samples. BMC Infect Dis. 2019;19(1):753.

44. de Manta FSN, Jacomasso T, de Rampazzo RCP, Moreira SJM, Zahra NM, Cole ST, et al. Development and validation of a multiplex real-time qPCR assay using GMP-grade reagents for leprosy diagnosis. PLoS Negl Trop Dis. 2022;16(2):e0009850.

45. Cambau E, Chauffour-Nevejans A, Tejmar-Kolar L, Matsuoka M, Jarlier V. Detection of antibiotic resistance in leprosy using GenoType LepraeDR, a novel ready-to-use molecular test. PLoS Negl Trop Dis. 2012;6(7):e1739.

46. Han XY, Sizer KC, Thompson EJ, Kabanja J, Li J, Hu P, et al. Comparative sequence analysis of *Mycobacterium leprae* and the new leprosy-causing *Mycobacterium lepromatosis*. J Bacteriol. 2009;191(19):6067–74.

47. Martinez AN, Talhari C, Moraes MO, Talhari S. PCR-based techniques for leprosy diagnosis: from the laboratory to the clinic. PLoS Negl Trop Dis. 2014;8(4):e2655.

48. van Hooij A, Geluk A. Immunodiagnostics for leprosy. In: International textbook of leprosy. Berlin: Springer; 2016. https://internationaltextbookofleprosy.org/chapter/immunodiagnostics-leprosy.

49. Espinosa OA, Benevides Ferreira SM, Longhi Palacio FG, da Cortela DCB, Ignotti E. Accuracy of enzyme-linked immunosorbent assays (ELISAs) in detecting antibodies against *Mycobacterium leprae* in leprosy patients: a systematic review and meta-analysis. Can J Infect Dis Med Microbiol. 2018;2018:e9828023.

50. Duthie MS, Goto W, Ireton GC, Reece ST, Cardoso LPV, Martelli CMT, et al. Use of protein antigens for early serological diagnosis of leprosy. Clin Vaccine Immunol. 2007;14(11):1400–8.

51. Zhou Z, Pena M, van Hooij A, Pierneef L, de Jong D, Stevenson R, et al. Detection and monitoring of *Mycobacterium leprae* infection in nine banded armadillos (*Dasypus novemcinctus*) using a quantitative rapid test. Front Microbiol. 2021;12:763289. https://doi.org/10.3389/fmicb.2021.763289.

52. de Neto FBA, Buarque Feitosa RD, da Soares Silva M. Daily moxifloxacin, clarithromycin, minocycline, and clofazimine in nonresponsiveness leprosy cases to recommended treatment regimen. Int J Trop Dis. 2020;3(2):35.

53. Gonçalves FG, de Belone AFF, Rosa PS, Laporta GZ. Underlying mechanisms of leprosy recurrence in the Western Amazon: a retrospective cohort study. BMC Infect Dis. 2019;19(1):460.

54. Williams DL, Gillis TP. Drug-resistant leprosy: monitoring and current status. Lepr Rev. 2012;83(3):269–81.

55. Benjak A, Avanzi C, Singh P, Loiseau C, Girma S, Busso P, et al. Phylogenomics and antimicrobial resistance of the leprosy bacillus *Mycobacterium leprae*. Nat Commun. 2018;9(1):352.

56. Cambau E, Saunderson P, Matsuoka M, Cole ST, Kai M, Suffys P, et al. Antimicrobial resistance in leprosy: results of the first prospective open survey conducted by a WHO surveillance network for the period 2009–2015. Clin Microbiol Infect. 2018;24(12):1305–10.

Epidemiology of Hansen's Disease

Eliane Ignotti ⓘ and Peter Steinmann ⓘ

Hansen's disease (HD) is classified as a neglected tropical disease (NTD) amenable to elimination. The epidemiology of this curable infectious disease is strongly associated with social determinants, such as malnutrition, unfavorable living conditions and poverty [1]. Besides *Mycobacterium leprae*, also *M. lepromatosis* causes a closely related clinical picture [2].

The diagnosis of HD is mainly based on clinical signs and symptoms. HD cases are operationally classified as paucibacillary (PB) or multibacillary (MB), with implications for the treatment which is based on multidrug therapy (MDT) over 6 and 12 months, respectively [3]. Upon completion of treatment, HD cases are considered cured. However, many treated people depend on further medical and social assistance due to disabilities and/or impairments that developed prior to diagnosis or during treatment [4].

HD is likely transmitted directly and via droplets, from the nose and mouth, during close and frequent contact with untreated cases. In endemic communities, person-to-person spread is the main mode of transmission, but other pathways have also been described [5]. Characteristic for HD is the very long incubation period of up to several decades but more commonly around 2–7 years on average, and that many exposed individuals never develop disease [6]. Healthy but infected individuals potentially contribute to transmission [7], but it is known that *M. leprae* is shed in large numbers from the skin, mouth, and nose of untreated MB patients [8]. Close

E. Ignotti (✉)
Universidade do Estado de Mato Grosso, Cáceres, Brazil

Universidade Federal de Mato Grosso, Cuiabá, Brazil
e-mail: eliane.ignotti@unemat.br

P. Steinmann
Swiss Tropical and Public Health Institute, Allschwil, Switzerland

University of Basel, Basel, Switzerland
e-mail: peter.steinmann@swisstph.ch

P. D. Deps (ed.), *Hansen's Disease*, https://doi.org/10.1007/978-3-031-30893-2_6

contacts of index patients—understood as the first documented case in a group—are the most vulnerable population, with domestic, neighbor, and social contacts having an elevated but decreasing risk which is further modulated by physical proximity, contact duration, blood relationship, and HD type of the index patient [9].

There is consensus that *M. leprae* also circulates in the environment. Indeed, HD is considered a zoonosis in the USA where cases can be clearly linked to direct and indirect contact with armadillos which are a known reservoir of the bacillus and the only available animal model [10, 11].

The current HD burden varies between countries. While cases are reported from over 100 countries, most cases occur in poor developing countries in the tropical climate zone. India, Brazil, and Indonesia report more than 70% of the roughly 200,000 new cases notified every year (74% in 2020). Many developed countries have interrupted local transmission but still report cases related to migration or patients diagnosed long after transmission ceased. The registered prevalence of HD (the number of cases on treatment) was 129,192 at the end of 2020, with a rate of 16.6 per million population. Globally, the number of reported cases was 127,396 for a new case detection rate (NCDR) of 16.4 per million population (WHO) in 2020 [12]. Illustrating the start differences, Brazil reported 132,021 new cases per million inhabitants in 2019 while the Philippines and Portugal presented 19,627 and 0.587, respectively [13].

Only 127 countries (of 221) provided data to the World Health Organization (WHO) in 2020; the reduction in 2020 reflected operational factors related to the Covid-19 pandemic rather than an underlying epidemiological shift or progress in leprosy control. Prior to the advent of COVID-19, the NCDR was following a steady decline of around 3% per year while the pace suddenly accelerated to more than 37.1% between 2019 and 2020 [12]. The figures for 2021 were comparable but it is conceivable that numbers will again increase after the cessation of COVID-19 barrier measures and the resumption of normal-intensity primary health care services (https://www.who.int/news-room/fact-sheets/detail/leprosy).

The epidemiology of HD is characterized by the clinical form of the case, aspects of transmission, the clinical evolution, completeness of treatment, relapse after treatment completion, and surveillance among cases and contacts including for antibiotic resistance. As a transmissible disease that is potentially disabling, we highlight the need to interpret trends cautiously, especially variables that may suggest a delay in diagnosis. The reduced number of cases in some countries or localities may mean that primary health personnel is unfamiliar with the clinical picture. A lack of awareness among the population, stigma as well as limited financial support for HD programs govern access to diagnosis. For these reasons, in the last 5 years at least 7% of the new cases were diagnosed with physical disabilities or impairments defined as new cases with grade-2 disability (G2D)—or "visible disabilities" [12, 13]. The delayed detection, often due to a lack of awareness in the community of the early signs of HD, impact on care seeking while limited capacity of the health system hinders to recognize symptoms early [13].

The epidemiological status of the disease in a country or area is described by standardized indicators of the burden of disease—incidence, prevalence, relapse—combined with indicators related to operational aspects. The latter describe the quality of the health services relevant for the HD program—including the proportion of cases evaluated and diagnosed with disabilities, the proportion cured, and the number of patients abandoning treatment. Cases with worsening disabilities during and after MDT, misdiagnosis, and death due to HD are also relevant for the quality of the program [4, 14].

There are no sudden leprosy outbreaks due to the long incubation period and the slow evolution of the disease. Consequently, changes in the trend of incidence indicators are slow except for the effects of operational factors. HD presents an asymptomatic infection period with slow evolution, and it will regress without any manifestation of the disease for the majority of those infected. Taken together, this means that the patients diagnosed today were infected several years ago, and that the effects of interventions to limit transmission only become apparent after several years. Currently, the NCDR is the best proxy for the incidence indicator—representing the risk of illness in a locality and over a defined time. The NCDR can be disaggregated by age group and gender or by other variables like ethnicity, education level, and professional activity. For the general population and those younger than 15 years old, there are parameters defined by WHO to facilitate the comprehensive reporting of the endemicity level. Trends in the reduction of this indicator for the general population but not followed by a reduction of the rates for children, signal continued transmission in the community, particularly in the domiciliary environment where children are commonly infected.

Differences in the detection rates or in terms of severity of the cases at the time of diagnosis between gender indicate differences in the risk of illness between these groups. In some countries, the disease is often more advanced in males at the time of diagnosis, while elsewhere it is in females, indicating mainly differences in the access to diagnosis for cultural or religious reasons [12, 13]. Nonetheless, biological aspects also influence these differences in the evolution of the disease until diagnosis between gender and age groups [15].

The prevalence of HD indicates the number of people under treatment. Usually, the rates are calculated as a point prevalence to facilitate temporal comparisons among localities. As the prevalence is influenced by the duration of treatment, it is important to consider changes in the therapeutic protocols when analyzing historical series. The quality of the registries of cases under treatment also influences the prevalence rates. Not all countries have updated databases including healing of previous cases post completion of MDT. Considering the long duration and chronic nature of certain symptoms of HD, information systems must be more complex when compared to the information system for acute infectious diseases. Usually, the prevalence rate for HD has been calculated per 10,000 population, the new case detection rate per 100,000 population and the rate of G2D per million population. Globally, all these indicators are currently calculated per million population using the standard population projections of the United Nations (https://population.un.org/wpp/Download/Standard/Population/). A customized data collection tool was developed within District Health Information System version 2 (DHIS2), which is an open-source software. This way, the data can be verified easily by all interested stakeholders (https://www.who.int/data/gho/data/themes/topics/leprosy-hansens-disease).

                                                                              E. Ignotti and P. Steinmann

Indicators related to new cases, G2D and MB cases at the time of diagnosis help in the interpretation of epidemiological trends in terms of delay of diagnosis, because G2D and MB are related to advance of the disease before diagnosis. For this reason, data from areas presenting an increase of the proportion of cases with G2D and/or MB while reporting a reduction of new cases overall should be interpreted cautiously. However, the proportion of MB cases typically increases with progress towards interruption of transmission. In such situations, only sporadic child cases would be expected.

Under a scenario of low and very low endemicity overall, it is expected that HD cases would be living in isolated areas, and, therefore, they have a higher risk of presenting G2D, and most of them would be MB cases. The declining awareness and capacity of health workers to identify signs and symptoms of the disease become major issues in such situations. The transmission occurring in low-prevalence areas does not represent the same challenges as in high endemicity areas, with most new cases occurring among very close (family) contacts of known index patients [16]. On the other hand, sites with high endemicity commonly observe less than 10% G2D. In both epidemiological situations, it is imperative to fully assess the responsiveness of the health system and the burden of HD since the interpretation of the epidemiological profile depends on the local endemicity combined with the capacity and infrastructure of the health system, and the level of integration of the HD program into primary health care services.

There is an extensive literature speculating about thousands (or millions) of HD cases left undiagnosed, maintaining the chain of transmission globally [17]. Indeed, more intensive case finding activities in an area routinely identify leprosy cases that were previously missed. Taking into count the number of cases prior to the COVID-19 pandemic without diagnosis and adding those not diagnosed during the pandemic period suggest the risk of an increase in transmission and of some of these people developing disabilities which may reverse the trend of a slow and gradual decline of HD observed during the last decade. Some of the undiagnosed cases are relapses, but some were not cured even after completion of MDT. These relapses influence partially the prevalence rate, but more than this, are important to evaluate the quality of the HD program and follow-up of former patients. Although the case characteristics have been shown to change during periods of declining incidence, relapses do not represent a large ongoing source of human-to-human transmission [18].

Concomitantly to the COVID-19 pandemic and its economic and social impact on leprosy control, WHO and its Global Leprosy Program published two important documents, as follows: the "Road Map for NTDs 2021–2030" (https://www.who.int/publications/i/item/9789240010352) and the "Global Leprosy Strategy (2021–2030)" (https://www.who.int/publications/i/item/9789290228509). Both lay out the main tools, approaches, and goals for the elimination of the disease. The main strategy is focused on breaking the chain of transmission, mainly through active case detection in both high- and low-burden settings. Innovative interventions such as post-exposure prophylaxis are recommended as well as integration of activities into primary health services. These plans are coherent with wider NTD elimination strategies, and for HD are focusing on three main targets: zero autochthonous cases in 120 countries; reduction of new cases by 70%, and reduction in child and G2D case rates by 90%.

The base for the future interruption of transmission is provided by the introduction of new diagnostic tests in combination with the existing tools for active case detection including contact-tracing, and the scaling up of leprosy prevention with post-exposure prophylaxis [3, 13, 19].

References

1. Pan American Health Organization/World Health Organization. Policy on research for health. Document CD49/10 of the 49th Directing Council, 61st Session of the regional committee of WHO for the Americas. PAHO/WHO. 2009. http://www.paho.org/hq/dmdocuments/2009/CD49-10-e.pdf.
2. Han XY, Sizer KC, Velarde-Félix JS, Frias-Castro LO, Vargas-Ocampo F. The leprosy agents *Mycobacterium lepromatosis* and *Mycobacterium leprae* in Mexico. Int J Dermatol. 2012;51(8):952–9. https://doi.org/10.1111/j.1365-4632.2011.05414.x.
3. World Health Organization. Regional Office for South-East Asia. Guidelines for the diagnosis, treatment and prevention of leprosy. World Health Organization. Regional Office for South-East Asia. 2018. https://apps.who.int/iris/handle/10665/274127.
4. dos Santos AR, Silva PR, Steinmann P, et al. Disability progression among leprosy patients released from treatment: a survival analysis. Infect Dis Poverty. 2020;9:53. https://doi.org/10.1186/s40249-020-00669-4.
5. Bratschi MW, Steinmann P, Wickenden A, Gillis TP. Current knowledge on *Mycobacterium leprae* transmission: a systematic literature review. Lepr Rev. 2015;86(2):142–55. https://doi.org/10.47276/lr.86.2.142.
6. Richardus JH, Ignotti E, Smith WCS. Chapter 1.1: Epidemiology of leprosy. In: Scollard DM, Gillis TP, editors. International textbook of leprosy. Berlin: Springer; 2016. www.internationaltextbookofleprosy.org.
7. Araújo S, Lobato J, Reis ÉDM, Souza DO, Gonçalves MA, et al. Unveiling healthy carriers and subclinical infections among household contacts of leprosy patients who play potential roles in the disease chain of transmission. Mem Inst Oswaldo Cruz. 2012;107:55–9.
8. Job CK, Jayakumar J, Kearney M, Gillis TP. Transmission of leprosy: a study of skin and nasal secretions of household contacts of leprosy patients using PCR. Am J Trop Med Hyg. 2008;78:518–21.
9. Moet FJ, Pahan D, Schuring RP, Oskam L, Richardus JH. Physical distance, genetic relationship, age, and leprosy classification are independent risk factors for leprosy in contacts of patients with leprosy. Int J Infect Dis. 2006;93(3):346–53. https://doi.org/10.1086/499278.
10. Ploemacher T, Faber WR, Menke H, Rutten V, Pieters T. Reservoirs and transmission routes of leprosy; a systematic review. PLoS Negl Trop Dis. 2020;14(4):e0008276. https://doi.org/10.1371/journal.pntd.0008276.
11. Deps P, Rosa PS. One health and Hansen's disease in Brazil. PLoS Negl Trop Dis. 2021;15(5):e0009398. https://doi.org/10.1371/journal.pntd.0009398.
12. World Health Organization. Global leprosy (Hansen disease) update, 2020: impact of COVID-19 on global leprosy control. Wkly Epidemiol Rec No 36, 2021, 96, 421–444. http://www.who.int/wer.
13. World Health Organization. Global leprosy (Hansen disease) update, 2019: time to step-up prevention initiatives. Wkly Epidemiol Rec No 36, 2020, 95, 417–440. http://www.who.int/wer.

14. Neves KVRN, Nobre ML, Machado LMG, Steinmann P, Ignotti E. Misdiagnosis of leprosy in Brazil in the period 2003–2017: spatial pattern and associated factors. Acta Trop. 2021;215:105791. https://doi.org/10.1016/j.actatropica.2020.105791.
15. Rocha MCN, Nobre ML, Garcia LP. Temporal trend of leprosy among the elderly in Brazil, 2001–2018. Rev Panam Salud Publica. 2020;44:e12. https://doi.org/10.26633/RPSP.2020.12.
16. World Health Organization. Global Leprosy Program. Report of the final meeting: Task Force on definitions, criteria and indicators for interruption of transmission and elimination of leprosy. Chengalpattu, India. 2021. https://www.who.int/publications/i/item/SEA-GLP-6.
17. Smith WC, Van Brakel W, Gillis T, Saunderson P. The missing millions: a threat to the elimination of leprosy. PLoS Negl Trop Dis. 2015;9(4):e0003658. https://doi.org/10.1371/journal.pntd.0003658.
18. Hambridge T, Nanjan Chandran SL, Geluk A, Saunderson P, Richardus JH. *Mycobacterium leprae* transmission characteristics during the declining stages of leprosy incidence: a systematic review. PLoS Negl Trop Dis. 2021;15(5):e0009436. https://doi.org/10.1371/journal.pntd.0009436.
19. Steinmann P, Reed SG, Mirza F, Hollingsworth TD, Richardus JH. Innovative tools and approaches to end the transmission of *Mycobacterium leprae*. Lancet Infect Dis. 2017;17(9):e298–305. https://doi.org/10.1016/S1473-3099(17)30314-6.

Hansen's Disease and One Health

Simon M. Collin, Christina Pettan-Brewer, Peter R. Rabinowitz, and Patrícia D. Deps

One Health is the concept that links human health with animal health, plants, and the environment: *One Health is an integrated, unifying approach that aims to sustainably balance and optimize the health of people, animals and ecosystems. It recognizes that the health of humans, domestic and wild animals, plants, and the wider environment (including ecosystems) are closely linked and interdependent* [1].

This idea has origins in ancient civilizations and indigenous wisdom, while its relatively recent reintroduction is rooted in comparative pathology and the writings of William Osler, Rudolf Virchow, Calvin Schwabe, and others, with a focus on "one medicine" [2]. One Health recognizes that many aspects of human health and wellbeing cannot be addressed in isolation but are intrinsically related with other living beings and with the environment [3]. This relationship has come under immense pressure from human population growth and globalization, climate change, wildlife trade and associated health risks, and irreversible ecological damage [4].

S. M. Collin (✉)
Bristol Medical School, University of Bristol, Bristol, UK
e-mail: simon.collin@bristol.ac.uk

C. Pettan-Brewer
Department of Comparative Medicine, School of Medicine, University of Washington, Seattle, WA, USA

Center for One Health Research (COHR), School of Public Health, University of Washington, Seattle, WA, USA
e-mail: kcpb@uw.edu

P. R. Rabinowitz
Center for One Health Research, University of Washington, Seattle, WA, USA
e-mail: peterr7@uw.edu

P. D. Deps
Universidade Federal do Espírito Santo, Vitória, Brazil
e-mail: patricia.deps@ufes.br

1 Animal Hosts and Zoonotic Transmission

Researchers in the USA reported in 1971 that Hansen's disease could be reproduced in armadillos inoculated experimentally with *Mycobacterium leprae* [5]. In 1977, naturally infected armadillos of the species *Dasypus novemcinctus* were identified in the southeastern USA [6]. Subsequently, autochthonous human cases of Hansen's disease from armadillo contact in the absence of other risk factors were reported [7], and the disease in the USA is now considered primarily zoonotic [8–10].

In Brazil, persons affected by Hansen's disease often report no known contact with an index case as source of their infection. A study in the southeast of the country found that 55% of a series of 506 patients had no known contact with an infected individual [11], but 68% of cases (and 48% of a control group without Hansen's disease) reported direct contact with armadillos [12]. Testing of specimens from armadillos in the same region (Espírito Santo state) detected *M. leprae* in 53% (19/36) animals, and a meta-analysis including this and seven similar studies reported a pooled prevalence equivalent to one in ten animals in Brazil being infected [13].

People who have direct contact with armadillos (including hunting, meat preparation, and eating) in Brazil have been found to have approximately double the odds of developing Hansen's disease compared with people who report no contact; in the USA, direct contact is associated with four times higher odds [14].

In Brazil, where hunting and consumption of armadillos is illegal but commonplace, the fraction of Hansen's disease in the population that is attributable to contact with armadillos will depend on multiple factors, including: the risk of infection associated with different types of contact; how prevalent these practices are in the population; the role of human-to-human transmission; and the immunological susceptibility of people in exposed groups. The proportion of all cases of Hansen's disease in an endemic community attributable to contact with armadillos has been estimated to be 3% if 10% of people have direct contact, 10% if one-third have direct contact, and 15% if half the people in the community have direct contact [15].

In Hansen's disease endemic communities where person-to-person spread is the main mode of transmission, the additional risk of zoonotic transmission was evident in a study which reported a higher median anti-PGL-1 titer in people who consumed armadillo meat more than once per month compared with those who did not consume any armadillo [16]. Similarly, a study among child and adolescent household contacts of Hansen's disease cases reported higher anti-NDO-LID antibody levels in those who had consumed armadillo meat compared to those who had not [17].

Other than in armadillos, natural infection of wild animals with *M. leprae* has been reported for only two other non-human species: red squirrels (*Sciurus vulgaris*) in England [18] and chimpanzees in West Africa [19]. The recently discovered second causal agent of Hansen's disease, *M. lepromatosis*, has also been detected in red squirrels in the British Isles [18, 20, 21] but not in armadillos in the Americas [22]. Other than in relation to possible zoonotic cases of Hansen's disease during the Middle Ages, when direct human–squirrel contact was common (through trade in fur and meat), these other animal hosts are unlikely to be of concern for human health today [15, 22].

2 Environmental Reservoirs and Insect Vectors

Viable *M. leprae* (but not *M. lepromatosis*) bacilli have been found in plants, soil, and water sampled in non-endemic and endemic countries [22, 23], including *M. leprae* detected in soil near the homes of persons affected by Hansen's disease in India [24]. However, any apparent associations of increased Hansen's disease risk with such sources are as likely to be reverse causation (affected persons in areas of high endemicity shedding *M. leprae* into environmental sources) as indicative of transmission from environmental reservoirs to people.

Studies investigating possible transmission of *M. leprae* to humans via arthropod vectors are mostly outdated and unreplicated [23]. Recent experiments with the hematophagous triatomine bug (*Rhodnius prolixus*) [25] and tick species (*Amblyomma* spp.) and tick cell lines [26, 27] have revived interest in whether some insect species might serve as vectors for Hansen's disease, but the question remains unanswered.

3 Implications for Policy and Practice

That Hansen's disease in the Americas must be viewed from a One Health perspective (Fig. 1) is incontrovertible. Recognition of Hansen's disease as a zoonosis in the USA, a non-endemic country where few people have close contact with wild armadillos, but not in Brazil, an endemic country where contact with armadillos is more common, is an anomaly that must be challenged by raising awareness among

Fig. 1 One Health and Hansen's disease in the Americas: presence of *M. leprae* in soil, water, armadillos, and humans. [Source: Deps V & Deps P (2022)]

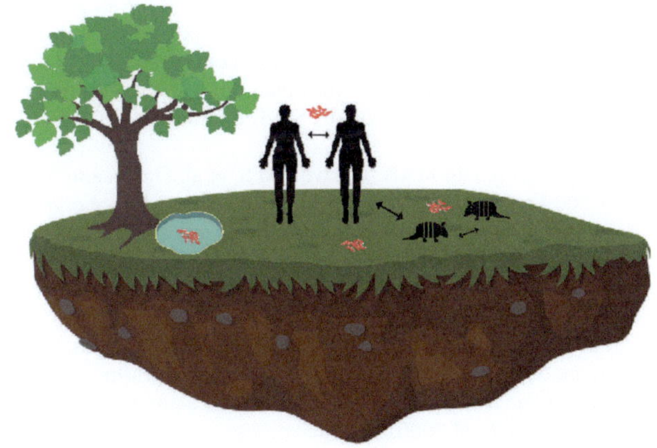

clinicians, public health agencies, and communities, and by conducting further research to build an evidence base for public health interventions.

Although person-to-person transmission is believed to be the main driver in sustaining Hansen's disease endemicity, strategies that aim to achieve elimination must consider animal hosts and environmental reservoirs. This was acknowledged in the WHO Global Hansen's Disease Strategy 2021–2030, which stated that *eradication of [Hansen's disease] is not feasible at this point of time due to presence of a zoonotic reservoir in some areas* and *Studies to understand the mode of zoonotic transmission and its overall epidemiological significance will be needed* [28]. A better understanding of pathways to infection that are not person-to-person could also contribute to destigmatizing Hansen's disease by reducing fears of contagion.

Other important One Health aspects include the ecosystem role of armadillo species, including pest control, seed dispersal, and nutrient cycling, which ultimately benefit rural communities, and the risk of other zoonotic infections through contact with armadillos which are known to host a range of bacterial, fungal, protozoal, and other parasitic agents including members of the genera *Histoplasma, Coccidioides, Trypanosoma, Toxoplasma, Sarcocystis, Leptospira, Sporothrix, Leishmania,* and *Paracoccidioides* [29, 30].

In clinical practice, patients and communities in endemic areas need to be informed of the risk of *M. leprae* infection through contact with armadillos. Newly detected cases of Hansen's disease could be asked about their own and their family members' contact with armadillos as part of tracing procedures to minimize risk of infection within households and to increase awareness.

References

1. Tripartite and UNEP support OHHLEP's definition of "One Health." https://www.who.int/news/item/01-12-2021-tripartite-and-unep-support-ohhlep-s-definition-of-one-health. Accessed 22 Mar 2022.
2. Pettan-Brewer C, Martins AF, de Abreu DPB, et al. From the approach to the concept: one health in Latin America-experiences and perspectives in Brazil, Chile, and Colombia. Front Public Health. 2021;9:687110. https://doi.org/10.3389/fpubh.2021.687110.
3. Gruetzmacher K, Karesh WB, Amuasi JH, et al. The Berlin principles on one health—bridging global health and conservation. Sci Total Environ. 2020;764:142919. https://doi.org/10.1016/j.scitotenv.2020.142919.
4. Laing G, Vigilato MAN, Cleaveland S, et al. One health for neglected tropical diseases. Trans R Soc Trop Med Hyg. 2020;115(2):182–4. https://doi.org/10.1093/trstmh/traa117.
5. Storrs EE. The nine-banded armadillo: a model for leprosy and other biomedical research. Int J Lepr Other Mycobact Dis. 1971;39:703–14.
6. Kirchheimer WF. Occurrence of *Mycobacterium leprae* in nature. Lepr India. 1977;49:44–7.
7. Walsh GP, Meyers WM, Binford CH, et al. Leprosy—a zoonosis. Lepr Rev. 1981;52(Suppl 1):77–83. https://doi.org/10.5935/0305-7518.19810060.
8. Bruce S, Schroeder TL, Ellner K, et al. Armadillo exposure and Hansen's disease: an epidemiologic survey in southern Texas. J Am Acad Dermatol. 2000;43:223–8. https://doi.org/10.1067/mjd.2000.106368.

9. Truman RW, Singh P, Sharma R, et al. Probable zoonotic leprosy in the southern United States. N Engl J Med. 2011;364:1626–33. https://doi.org/10.1056/NEJMoa1010536.

10. Sharma R, Singh P, Loughry WJ, et al. Zoonotic leprosy in the Southeastern United States. Emerg Infect Dis. 2015;21:2127–34. https://doi.org/10.3201/eid2112.150501.

11. Deps PD, Guedes BVS, Bucker Filho J, et al. Characteristics of known leprosy contact in a high endemic area in Brazil. Lepr Rev. 2006;77:34–40.

12. Deps PD, Alves BL, Gripp CG, et al. Contact with armadillos increases the risk of leprosy in Brazil: a case control study. Indian J Dermatol Venereol Leprol. 2008;74:338–42. https://doi.org/10.4103/0378-6323.42897.

13. Deps P, Antunes JM, Santos AR, Collin SM. Prevalence of *Mycobacterium leprae* in armadillos in Brazil: a systematic review and meta-analysis. PLoS Negl Trop Dis. 2020;14:e0008127. https://doi.org/10.1371/journal.pntd.0008127.

14. Deps P, de Antunes JMAP, Collin SM. Zoonotic risk of Hansen's disease from community contact with wild armadillos: a systematic review and meta-analysis. Zoonoses Public Health. 2020;68(2):153–64. https://doi.org/10.1111/zph.12783.

15. Deps P, Rosa PS. One health and Hansen's disease in Brazil. PLoS Negl Trop Dis. 2021;15:e0009398. https://doi.org/10.1371/journal.pntd.0009398.

16. da Silva MB, Portela JM, Li W, et al. Evidence of zoonotic leprosy in Para, Brazilian Amazon, and risks associated with human contact or consumption of armadillos. PLoS Negl Trop Dis. 2018;12:e0006532. https://doi.org/10.1371/journal.pntd.0006532.

17. Serrano-Coll H, Mora HR, Beltran JC, et al. Social and environmental conditions related to *Mycobacterium leprae* infection in children and adolescents from three leprosy endemic regions of Colombia. BMC Infect Dis. 2019;19:520. https://doi.org/10.1186/s12879-019-4120-2.

18. Avanzi C, Del-Pozo J, Benjak A, et al. Red squirrels in the British Isles are infected with leprosy bacilli. Science. 2016;354:744–7. https://doi.org/10.1126/science.aah3783.

19. Hockings KJ, Mubemba B, Avanzi C, et al. Leprosy in wild chimpanzees. Nature. 2021;598:652–6. https://doi.org/10.1038/s41586-021-03968-4.

20. Butler HM, Stevenson K, McLuckie J, Simpson V. Further evidence of leprosy in isle of Wight red squirrels. Vet Rec. 2017;180:407.

21. Simpson V, Hargreaves J, Butler H, et al. Leprosy in red squirrels on the Isle of Wight and Brownsea Island. Vet Rec. 2015;177(8):206–7.

22. Deps P, Collin SM. *Mycobacterium lepromatosis* as a second agent of Hansen's disease. Front Microbiol. 2021;12:698588. https://doi.org/10.3389/fmicb.2021.698588.

23. Ploemacher T, Faber WR, Menke H, et al. Reservoirs and transmission routes of leprosy; a systematic review. PLoS Negl Trop Dis. 2020;14:e0008276. https://doi.org/10.1371/journal.pntd.0008276.

24. Singh V, Turankar RP, Goel A. Real-time PCR-based quantitation of viable *Mycobacterium leprae* strain from clinical samples and environmental sources and its genotype in multi-case leprosy families of India. Eur J Clin Microbiol Infect Dis. 2020;39:2045–55. https://doi.org/10.1007/s10096-020-03958-w.

25. da Neumann AS, de Dias FA, da Ferreira JS, et al. Experimental infection of *Rhodnius prolixus* (Hemiptera, Triatominae) with *Mycobacterium leprae* indicates potential for leprosy transmission. PLoS One. 2016;11:e0156037. https://doi.org/10.1371/journal.pone.0156037.

26. Tongluan N, Shelton LT, Collins JH, et al. *Mycobacterium leprae* infection in ticks and tick-derived cells. Front Microbiol. 2021;12:761420. https://doi.org/10.3389/fmicb.2021.761420.

27. da Ferreira JS, Souza Oliveira DA, Santos JP, et al. Ticks as potential vectors of *Mycobacterium leprae*: use of tick cell lines to culture the bacilli and generate transgenic strains. PLoS Negl Trop Dis. 2018;12:e0007001. https://doi.org/10.1371/journal.pntd.0007001.

28. World Health Organization. Global consultation of National Leprosy Programme managers, partners and affected persons on Global Leprosy Strategy 2021–2030: report of the virtual meeting 26–30 October 2020. World Health Organization Regional Office for South-East Asia. Geneva: World Health Organization; 2020.

29. Richini-Pereira VB, Bosco SMG, Theodoro RC, et al. Importance of xenarthrans in the eco-epidemiology of *Paracoccidioides brasiliensis*. BMC Res Notes. 2009;2:228. https://doi.org/10.1186/1756-0500-2-228.
30. Kluyber D, Desbiez ALJ, Attias N, et al. Zoonotic parasites infecting free-living armadillos from Brazil. Transbound Emerg Dis. 2020;68(3):1639–51. https://doi.org/10.1111/tbed.13839.

Metabolic, Genetic and Immunological Mechanisms in Susceptibility to Leprosy

Milton Ozório Moraes, Roberta Olmo Pinheiro, and Annemieke Geluk

1 Immune Activation in Disease Progression

After *M. leprae* exposure, only a minority of all individuals develop leprosy: the disease is the result of an individual's environmental (e.g., socio-economic conditions, geographic location, vaccination and nutritional status, vitamin D shortage) and genetic factors. Therefore, resistance or susceptibility to infection can vary widely between different ethnic groups and within populations.

Concerning environmental factors, it is noteworthy that leprosy affects the most vulnerable populations in poorer regions of low- and middle-income countries (LMICs). In a cohort of 100 million Brazilians, it was shown that social conditions significantly affected leprosy occurrence, whereas income, education, and sanitation were associated with infection outcomes [1].

Leprosy is not a genetic disease. Instead, exposure intensity and frequency are major risk factors for leprosy. Thus, household- and social contacts of multibacillary (MB) patients have the highest risk of contracting the disease [2]. This is exemplified in follow-up studies of contacts of leprosy patients in Brazil [3] and Bangladesh [4] in which 3.2% and 2% of the contacts, respectively, developed leprosy. Unraveling the immune response induced by the BCG vaccine provided as immunoprophylactic therapy to contacts, showed a protective effect induced by trained immunity-associated genes leading to increased S100A12 and decreased CCL4 levels in healthy contacts [5].

M. O. Moraes · R. O. Pinheiro
Fundação Oswaldo Cruz (FIOCRUZ), Rio de Janeiro, Brazil
e-mail: rolmo@ioc.fiocruz.br

A. Geluk (✉)
Department of Infectious Diseases, Leiden University Medical Center, Leiden, The Netherlands
e-mail: a.geluk@lumc.nl

P. D. Deps (ed.), *Hansen's Disease*, https://doi.org/10.1007/978-3-031-30893-2_8

Nevertheless, in a unique study conducted in an isolated former leprosy colony in the heart of the Amazon region with a high rate of endogamy, even 3–5% of the contacts progressed to disease [6]. This suggests that consanguinity and, consequently, genetics represent an additional risk factor for leprosy outcome which is in line with findings in Bangladesh [2].

A clear demonstration that human genetic variations can favor or block mycobacterial growth and are likely to affect leprosy as well, is *TYK2*, a gene that controls the activation of different pathways involved in viral or bacterial responses funneling to a protective response. In another mycobacterial disease, tuberculosis (TB), a single nucleotide polymorphism (SNP) in *TYK2* causes reduced TYK2 expression [7] leading to decreased production of microbicidal cytokines such as IFNγ and, consequently, to dampening of protective immunity. In general, disruptions of the IFNγ/IL-12 axis (by truncated gene mutations that severely impair IFNγ secretion) favor a phenotype in which avirulent and sometimes attenuated vaccine strains, such as BCG cause disseminated mycobacterial diseases.

For diseases, such as leprosy, it is not expected that the complete abrogation of the activity of a certain gene is solely responsible for disease development. Instead, it is plausible that the combination of partial or moderate effects of several genes underlies disease progression such that human genetic variation (along with environmental factors) results in the plethora of phenotypes observed in the leprosy spectrum.

Human-pathogen co-evolution generated an intricate interaction of checks and balances. Complex and intertwined layers of immune surveillance attempt to eliminate the pathogen, while in turn bacilli have refined escape and hiding strategies to create a safe niche to survive. The bacilli can only reach a successful infection in hosts, who present a combination of genetic and environmental factors advantageous to disease. Innate immunity plays a relevant role in maintaining homeostasis. In fact, in most individuals, innate immune responses clear mycobacteria without induction of adaptive immunity. To this end, macrophages and dendritic cells recognize and phagocytose *M. leprae*, activate autophagy and produce microbicidal peptides to eliminate mycobacteria. Subsequently, these antigen-presenting cells interact with regulatory T-cells that organize robust adaptive responses with secretion of microbicidal cytokines such as IFNγ and TNF and activates cytotoxic T-cells providing a strong and long-term response. Altering the ability to direct the phagocytosed bacteria to autophagy disrupts bacterial clearance as demonstrated by the association between susceptibility to leprosy and SNPs in genes regulating autophagy (*NOD2, LRRK2, PRKN, LACC1*), metabolism (*APOE, HIF1A, LACC1*), or effector pathways (*TNF, IFNG, HLA*) [8].

Nevertheless, *M. leprae* has evolved highly adapted strategies to avoid hostile environments, such as autophagosomes from macrophages and Schwann cells by altering host's metabolism and unbalancing host immunity. These pro-pathogen mechanisms favor maintenance, growth and, eventually, spread of *M. leprae*.

2 Control of Metabolic and Immune Regulation Towards Susceptibility to Infection

2.1 Activation of Autophagy in Resistance and Susceptibility

Resistance to *M. leprae* relies on the host's ability to maintain intracellular homeostasis through autophagy. The process of autophagy controls cellular metabolism by sensing nutrients as well as organelles such as aged mitochondria that are marked to mitophagy. The autophagy process is triggered when there is, for example, nutrient restriction or the need to recycle organelles or process pathogens (xenophagy). Through xenophagy, bacteria (and other pathogens) are phagocytosed and degraded; the pathway, therefore, is central for the direct elimination of bacteria, as well as for the activation of lymphocytes from the presentation of antigens resulting from this processing. Autophagy occurs in all cell types and the activation mechanisms involve several proteins. The process of xenophagy includes phagocytic cells, such as macrophages, as central in organizing the response that eliminates microorganisms. Given the central role of xenophagy in controlling the entry of pathogens into cells, any genetic variation that alters the formation or function of autophagic complex can alter the correct activation of the process and, consequently, favor the escape of the pathogen. Ultimately, xenophagy is responsible for the formation of phagolysosomes that degrade and eliminate the pathogen, which further activates lymphocytes to processing and presenting antigens. Deregulation of this process can progress to the clinical presentation of leprosy and other infectious diseases.

Bacterial survival and decrease in autophagy are also mediated by SNPs in *NOD2*, and *PRKN*. In 2004, a genomic screen in Vietnamese population described the association of leprosy with variants of the PRKN gene that encodes parkin protein a protein of the ubiquitin pathway, which tags bacteria, by ubiquitination, directing them for degradation through xenophagy [9]. Ten years later, functional studies, demonstrated that parkin is critical in the control *M. tuberculosis* infection as well.

The role of the *NOD2* gene was highlighted in the first GWAS in leprosy, carried out in a Chinese population sample in 2010. *NOD2* encodes a pattern recognition receptor that identifies mycobacterial cell wall components, which is one of the first steps in the signaling process for the formation of the autophagic complex. Lower levels of parkin or NOD2 fail to activate the autophagic flux blocking mycobacterial killing. This failed response impairs the activation of T-cells.

3 Subversion Mechanisms

M. leprae tries to control numerous pathways such as nutritional immunity, type I IFN pathway, [10] and glucose metabolism to trick the immune surveillance in order to grant a safe niche for their replication and dissemination in the host. On the other hand, cells try to counteract and contain the bacterial onslaught. The success of the infection is associated with a combination of subtle changes that impair autophagy leading to bacterial survival.

3.1 Type I IFN Pathway

An interesting strategy is an activation of the type I IFN (IFNα and IFNβ) pathway, which is a typical immune response against viral infections. After being engulfed by macrophages and delivered to phagosomes, *M. leprae* induces the rupture of the vesicle membrane allowing the leakage of pathogen DNA into the host cell cytoplasm. This process leads to an activation of type I IFNs that hamper IFNγ production [11]. As a result, there is a reduction in the synthesis of microbicidal peptides. Therefore, it is as if the bacteria assumed the role of "wolf in sheep's clothing," using viral-like behavior as disguise to favor infection. Corroborating this pattern clinical case reports demonstrate that prolonged treatment with IFNα in chronic hepatitis C patients can lead to leprosy [12].

3.2 Nutritional Immunity, Tryptophan Metabolism, IDO, and Kynurenines

IDO-1 mRNA upregulation in skin lesions is a marker of leprosy as compared to other skin diseases irrespective of the clinical form with potential for diagnostics. Although *M. leprae* infection triggers an innate defense mechanism to exhaust tryptophan (trp) trying to block pathogen growth, the tryptophan catabolism generates kynurenine metabolites that are not only microbicidal but can also contribute to peripheral nerve damage. In order to survive, *M. leprae* induces a feedback mechanism caused by high levels of IDO-1 associated with tolerance and immunosuppression of IFNγ-mediated microbicidal responses.

3.3 Metabolism Rewiring a Warburg-Like Effect and Lipid Biogenesis

Besides *M. leprae*-induced pathways, constitutive biochemical pathways also participate in the process of controlling the *M. leprae* infection. Access to energy sources is critical for growth of intracellular pathogens. Indeed, pathogens normally induce metabolic changes that favor their survival. One of these processes is associated with increased glucose uptake towards the pentose pathway in a Warburg-like effect improving glycolysis with decreased mitochondrial respiration. In this way, bacteria activate glucose-6-dehydrogenase whose main function is to produce NADPH that might help obtain nucleotides for its replication and guarantee the supply of energy for their growth by lipid biogenesis.

In a longitudinal, transcriptomic study involving 5352 contacts of leprosy patients, other genes involved in mitochondrial metabolism such as MT-ND2 (mitochondrially encoded NADH dehydrogenase 2) showed potential for prediction of leprosy as it was downregulated in those contacts who later developed PB leprosy [13]. *MT-ND2* together with *MT-ND6* are essential for formation of the mitochondrial membrane respiratory chain NADH dehydrogenase which plays a critical role in oxidative phosphorylation. One of the functions of mitochondrial reactive oxygen species resulting from oxidative phosphorylation is to regulate immunity. *MT-ND2* is under-expressed in leprosy progressors, hence presenting a disadvantage to successful elimination of *M. leprae.*

Other genes associated with mitochondrial respiration are also modulated and overall indicate the shutdown of mitochondrial function and mitophagy [11, 14]. Again, this rewires the metabolism directing it to lipid production [14].

In this context, it is of note that the role of genes such as *APOE*, known for its association with Alzheimer's disease, has been associated with leprosy [15]. Furthermore, SNPs in genes that link processes such as autophagy and energy metabolism (*HIF1A* and *LACC1*) have been convincingly demonstrated to contribute to leprosy susceptibility. A profile of increased activation of lipid metabolism is associated with multibacillary leprosy. The use of statins that reduce intracellular lipids combined with chemotherapy accelerated the elimination of *M. leprae* in experimental models [16].

4 Extreme Phenotypes: Leprosy Paradigm

In contrast to *M. tuberculosis*, *M. leprae* has tropism for Schwann cells or macrophages. It has been described in one study that after infection of Schwann cells, metabolic changes are drastically reshaping cellular phenotype heading to a less differentiated stem-like phenotype [17]. *M. leprae* is the only bacterium capable of initiating this mechanism. This triggers the skin to reprogram host cells to lipid-loaded foamy macrophages, which are highly permissive to bacterial replication and a signature of the lepromatous pole (LL) [18]. Additionally, *M. leprae* induces lipid droplets, which cover its surface antigens and work as a nutrition supply for the pathogen. This cellular phenotype transition is an example of an epithelial–mesenchymal program observed in Schwann cells and likely in keratinocytes. Microarray analysis displayed downregulated genes in LL patients clustered around pathways like "epithelial cell differentiation," "epidermis development," "keratinocyte differentiation," and "cornification" pathways further supporting the mechanisms *M. leprae* uses to evade host immunity [19].

5 Inactivation of Adaptive Immunity

Initial immunological studies provided evidence of the central role of immune response proteins and mediators in leprosy progression and immunopathology [20]. The microenvironment of keratinocytes, endothelial cells, and fibroblast also participates along with macrophages and Schwann cells. Proteins that directly control lymphocyte activation are systematically associated with leprosy, prominently illustrated by HLA: genes and specific alleles in different HLA genes, HLA-A, HLA-B, HLA-DQ, and HLA-DR have been consistently associated since the 1980s and later confirmed in GWAS. Overall, HLA alleles are associated with protection against leprosy, T-cell differentiation towards a protective Th1 pattern, which is correlated with increased production of IFNγ, IL-12, TNF, and IL-17. Genetic variants that increase IFNγ production have been associated with resistance to leprosy. Clinical studies demonstrated that long-term treatment with TNF inhibitors (anti-TNF or TNF receptors) used for autoimmune diseases can trigger the progression of leprosy in *M. leprae*-infected individuals. Therefore, patients undergoing treatment for psoriatic arthritis with "biologicals" such as anti-TNF should be screened for anti-*M. leprae* antibodies before treatment as wells for leprosy lesions during/after treatment. On the contrary, variants that increase TNF production may increase resistance to leprosy outcomes. TNF at optimal doses is capable of inducing microbicidal responses, leading to the elimination of the pathogen.

5.1 Granuloma Formation: Friend or Foe

Paucibacillary (PB) leprosy is an exemplary granulomatous disease. It is likely that the process of granulomatous formation begins with macrophage activation that differentiates into epithelioid cells. These modifications lead to the synthesis of chemoattractant mediators that lead to the migration of lymphocytes that initiate the highly organized structure called a granuloma.

Granuloma formation and the orchestration of this process by cytokines such as IFN-gamma and TNF has been considered a central process in the resistance and susceptibility to *M. leprae* infection. The process of granuloma formation leads to the isolation of the pathogen and eventually its elimination, resulting in spontaneous healing. However, if this process is exacerbated, it can lead to tissue damage, with the appearance of lesions due to exaggerated activation of Th1 immunity, which is observed in PB leprosy.

Transcriptomic studies have shown that granulomatous diseases of the skin, and even other granulomatous-based inflammatory diseases, such as Crohn's disease and juvenile arthritis, exacerbate the activation of pathways that jointly regulate the cellular immune responses. Some pathways are predominant, such as macrophage and lymphocyte activation, and mTOR which controls cellular metabolism, among others. Therefore, the progression to granulomatous diseases with infectious triggers such as *M. leprae*, involves hyperactivation of immunity culminating in granulomatogenesis. In other skin diseases similar to PB leprosy such as granuloma annulare or sarcoidosis, the inhibition of cytokines using to facitinib blocks JAK/STAT activation and suspends communication between macrophages and lymphocytes leading to a "relaxation" of the immune responses. Consequently, there is a disruption of the flow of mediators that maintain the granulomatous structure, which is associated with clinical improvement. Hyperactivation of the mTOR complex (mTORC1), another main player involved in granuloma formation can induce spontaneous sarcoidosis in mice. In this context, the use of everolimus, a known mTORC1 inhibitor, is capable of overturning the formation of granulomas.

6 Conclusion

Currently, we have a clearer, although probably still incomplete, picture of the genes and pathways that participate in the process of susceptibility or resistance to leprosy, which also contributes to better understand the pathogenesis in other chronic inflammatory diseases (Fig. 1).

It should be emphasized that patterns of unregulated excessive inflammation, in part due variation in genes that encode cytokines and proteins, involve granuloma formation mostly in PB patients. Potentially, personalized and adjuvanted treatments could be tailored for this clinical form using drugs that block granuloma formation. On the other hand, for multibacillary leprosy, where lipid accumulates in foamy macrophages statins could be applied as adjuvant therapy. The time is ripe

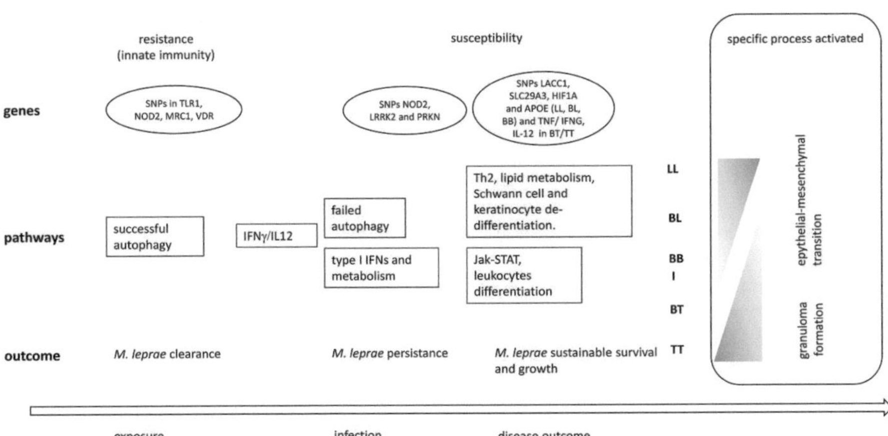

Fig. 1 Schematic flowchart of leprosy progression. The main genes and pathways involved in each stage of the disease (exposure, infection, and outcome) are presented: including the programs involved in granuloma formation in paucibacillary patients and an epithelial-mesenchymal transition in multibacillary patients. Environmental factors such as BCG vaccination and nutrients (food, vitamins) are involved in innate immunity and contribute to disease progression

for the application of integrative biological and genetic knowledge to redefine clinical studies aimed at incorporating new pharmaceuticals into the available resource, improving clinical management, and enabling control of this neglected disease.

References

1. Nery JS, Ramond A, Pescarini JM, Alves A, Strina A, Ichihara MY, et al. Socioeconomic determinants of leprosy new case detection in the 100 million Brazilian cohort: a population-based linkage study. Lancet Glob Health. 2019;7:e1226–36. https://doi.org/10.1016/S2214-109X(19)30260-8.
2. Moet FJ, Meima A, Oskam L, Richardus JH. Risk factors for the development of clinical leprosy among contacts, and their relevance for targeted interventions. Lepr Rev. 2004;75:310–26. https://doi.org/10.47276/lr.75.4.310.
3. Hacker MA, Maria Sales A, Cristina Duppre N, Nunes Sarno E, Ozório Moraes M. Leprosy incidence and risk estimates in a 33-year contact cohort of leprosy patients. Sci Rep. 2021;11:1947. https://doi.org/10.1038/s41598-021-81643-4.
4. Richardus R, Alam K, Kundu K, Chandra Roy J, Zafar T, Chowdhury AS, et al. Effectiveness of single-dose rifampicin after BCG vaccination to prevent leprosy in close contacts of patients with newly diagnosed leprosy: a cluster randomized controlled trial. Int J Infect Dis. 2019;88:65–72. https://doi.org/10.1016/j.ijid.2019.08.035.
5. van Hooij A, van den Eeden SJF, Khatun M, Soren S, Franken KLMC, Chandra Roy J, et al. BCG-induced immunity profiles in household contacts of leprosy patients differentiate between protection and disease. Vaccine. 2021;39:7230–7. https://doi.org/10.1016/j.vaccine.2021.10.027.
6. Lázaro FP, Werneck RI, Mackert CCO, Cobat A, Prevedello FC, Pimentel RP, et al. A major gene controls leprosy susceptibility in a hyperendemic isolated population from north of Brazil. J Infect Dis. 2010;201:1598–605. https://doi.org/10.1086/652007.
7. Boisson-Dupuis S, Ramirez-Alejo N, Li Z, Patin E, Rao G, Kerner G, et al. Tuberculosis and impaired IL-23-dependent IFN-γ immunity in humans homozygous for a common TYK2 missense variant. Sci Immunol. 2018;3(30):eaau8714.
8. Fava VM, Dallmann-Sauer M, Schurr E. Genetics of leprosy: today and beyond. Hum Genet. 2020;139(6–7):835–46. https://doi.org/10.1007/s00439-019-02087-5.
9. Behr MA, Schurr E. A table for two. Nature. 2013;501:498–9. https://doi.org/10.1038/nature12555.
10. Teles RMB, Lu J, Tió-Coma M, Goulart IMB, Banu S, Hagge D, et al. Identification of a systemic interferon-γ inducible antimicrobial gene signature in leprosy patients undergoing reversal reaction. PLoS Negl Trop Dis. 2019;13:e0007764. https://doi.org/10.1371/journal.pntd.0007764.
11. Toledo Pinto TG, Batista-Silva LR, Medeiros RCA, Lara FA, Moraes MO. Type I interferons, autophagy and host metabolism in leprosy. Front Immunol. 2019;9:806. https://doi.org/10.3389/fimmu.2018.00806.
12. Santos M, dos Franco ES, da Ferreira PLC, Braga WSM. Borderline tuberculoid leprosy and type 1 leprosy reaction in a hepatitis C patient during treatment with interferon and ribavirin. An Bras Dermatol. 2013;88:109–12. https://doi.org/10.1590/abd1806-4841.20131986.
13. Tió-Coma M, Kiełbasa SM, van den Eeden SJF, Mei H, Roy JC, Wallinga J, et al. Blood RNA signature RISK4LEP predicts leprosy years before clinical onset. EBioMedicine. 2021;68:103379. https://doi.org/10.1016/j.ebiom.2021.103379.
14. Oliveira MF, Medeiros RCA, Mietto BS, Calvo TL, Mendonça APM, Rosa TLSA, et al. Reduction of host cell mitochondrial activity as *Mycobacterium leprae*'s strategy to evade host innate immunity. Immunol Rev. 2021;301:193–208. https://doi.org/10.1111/imr.12962.

15. Wang D, Zhang D-F, Li G-D, Bi R, Fan Y, Wu Y, et al. A pleiotropic effect of the APOE gene: association of APOE polymorphisms with multibacillary leprosy in Han Chinese from Southwest China. Br J Dermatol. 2018;178:931–9. https://doi.org/10.1111/bjd.16020.
16. Lobato LS, Rosa PS, Da Silva FJ, Da Silva NA, Da Silva MG, Nascimento DC, et al. Statins increase rifampin mycobactericidal effect. Antimicrob Agents Chemother. 2014;58(10):5766–74. https://doi.org/10.1128/C01826.13.
17. Masaki T, Qu J, Cholewa-Waclaw J, Burr K, Raaum R, Rambukkana A. Reprogramming adult Schwann cells to stem cell-like cells by leprosy bacilli promotes dissemination of infection. Cell. 2013;152:51–67. https://doi.org/10.1016/j.cell.2012.12.014.
18. Leal-Calvo T, Avanzi C, Mendes MA, Benjak A, Busso P, Pinheiro RO, et al. A new paradigm for leprosy diagnosis based on host gene expression. PLoS Pathog. 2021;17:e1009972. https://doi.org/10.1371/journal.ppat.1009972.
19. Leal-Calvo T, Moraes MO. Reanalysis and integration of public microarray datasets reveals novel host genes modulated in leprosy. Mol Gen Genom. 2020;295:1355–68. https://doi.org/10.1007/s00438-020-01705-6.
20. Hooij A, Geluk A. In search of biomarkers for leprosy by unraveling the host immune response to *Mycobacterium leprae*. Immunol Rev. 2021;301:175–92. https://doi.org/10.1111/imr.12966.

Clinical Aspects and Classification of Hansen's Disease

Marcos Cesar Florian, Nkechi Anne Enechukwu, and Patrícia D. Deps

Hansen's disease is mainly characterized by peripheral neurological involvement with possible diverse skin lesions. The skin lesions of Hansen's disease (HD) can occur in any area of the body and may be single or numerous, varying widely in shape, presentation, and colour. The margins of the lesions also vary and can be poorly or well defined.

Depending on the individual's ability to react to *M. leprae* infection and the type of immune response that sets in, the disease will develop as tuberculoid (T) HD, the localized form of the disease that is considered less infectious, or as Virchowian (V)/lepromatous (L) HD, which is the generalized, infectious form (we adopt the term Virchowian instead of lepromatous). Between these two poles are clinical and immunological variations comprising the borderline forms (B) of HD with varying potential for transmissibility.

In an attempt to facilitate diagnosis in an endemic country or area, the World Health Organization has established simple criteria by which a diagnosis of HD can be made if a person has one or more of the following [1, 2]:

(a) Definite loss of sensation in a pale (hypopigmented) or reddish skin patch.
(b) Thickened or enlarged peripheral nerve with loss of sensation and/or weakness of the muscles supplied by that nerve.
(c) Presence of visible deformities.
(d) Presence of acid-fast bacilli (AFB) in a slit skin smear (SSS).

M. C. Florian (✉)
Universidade Federal de São Paulo, São Paulo, Brazil
e-mail: mcflorian@unifesp.br

N. A. Enechukwu
Nnamdi Azikiwe University/Nnamdi Azikiwe Teaching Hospital, Nnewi, Anambra Nigeria

P. D. Deps
Universidade Federal do Espírito Santo, Vitória, Brazil
e-mail: patricia.deps@ufes.br

P. D. Deps (ed.), *Hansen's Disease*, https://doi.org/10.1007/978-3-031-30893-2_9

Numbness or tingling in hands and feet, painful sensitivity in nerves, swelling or nodules on face or ears, and painless excoriations or burns on hands or feet should also raise clinical suspicion of HD.

1 Classification of Hansen's Disease

HD has four classifications based on the clinical features of the skin lesions and the bacteriological, histological, and immunological characteristics of the disease process.

Two classifications are operational, the other two are more informative and are widely used by HD specialists and dermatologists. They consider histopathological, immunological, and clinical features of the skin lesions such as type of lesion, number, extension, distribution, the definition of margins and the degree of symmetry of the lesions.

The Madrid Classification from 1952 defines the polar groups, tuberculoid (T) and Virchowian (V), and the interpolar borderline (B) form that encompasses unstable and intermediate pictures of HD. There is also an indeterminate form (I) comprising individuals in the early clinical stage of HD.

The Ridley–Jopling classification was introduced in 1966 [3]. Initially employed in scientific research, it is used in clinical practice in many parts of the world. The Ridley–Jopling system classifies HD as an immune-mediated disease with the tuberculoid form at one end of the spectrum and the Virchowian form at the other. The tuberculoid form (TT) correlates immunologically with cell-mediated immunity capable of forming granulomas and phagocytosing the bacilli, while the Virchowian form (VV) correlates with an inability of cell-mediated immunity to contain bacillary multiplication. Between these two extremes lies the clinically unstable borderline spectrum, subdivided into borderline-tuberculoid (BT), borderline-borderline (BB), and borderline-Virchowian (BV).

In 1981, the World Health Organization (WHO) developed an Operational classification, used in HD control programs, which takes into account the number of skin lesions and the bacilloscopy [1]. In 2017, WHO introduced a new concept including nerve and skin involvement as follows: paucibacillary (PB) case with 1–5 skin lesions and without demonstrated presence of bacilli in a slit-skin smear (SSS); multibacillary (MB) case with more than five skin lesions or with nerve involvement (pure neuritis or any number of skin lesions and neuritis) or with demonstrated presence of bacilli in SSS regardless of the number of skin lesions [1, 2].

In 1985, a classification was developed by the HD control programme in Nepal based on the number of affected body areas. In this classification type, the body is divided into seven or nine areas and disease severity is graded according to the number of affected areas [4]. Studies conducted using the Nepalese classifications showed consistency with WHO Operational classifications: PB cases (up to five skin lesions) corresponded with the involvement of up to two body areas; MB cases (more than five skin lesions) with three or more body areas [5, 6].

There is overall correlation between the Ridley–Jopling, Madrid, and WHO Operational classifications. PB patients are comparable to the I, T, and TT forms of the other two classifications, some of the B from the Madrid classification, and BT (SSS negative) from the Ridley–Jopling classification—essentially, all forms in which bacilli have not been found in skin or nerve smears and/or histopathology. MB includes most of the Bs in the Madrid classification, the BTs (SSS positive) of Ridley–Jopling and all the BBs, BVs, Vs, and VVs—whenever the bacilli have been identified on skin or nerve smears and/or histopathology.

Detecting the clinical features of HD requires a methodical approach. The presentation is often subtle, especially in the indeterminate and tuberculoid forms. BT is the clinical form that can be most ambiguous because cases can present with single lesions but positive skin smears and histopathology consistent with MB forms.

2 Indeterminate Hansen's Disease (IHD)

All patients pass through this stage at the onset of HD, but it may or may not be noticeable. IHD is a clinical form that usually presents few lesions, represented by hypochromic, hyper/hypo- or anaesthetic macules, with imprecise borders, often with a more desquamative ('dry') appearance than the surrounding normal skin.

Lesions are most frequently found on the extensor surfaces of the limbs, buttocks, or face (Fig. 1). Lesions may heal spontaneously, remain unchanged for years, or progress to any other form of leprosy. There is no nerve trunk involvement; therefore, disability and deformity do not occur. The indeterminate form is most often seen in those parts of the world where HD is endemic or hyperendemic.

The main differential diagnoses are pityriasis versicolor, pityriasis alba, vitiligo, achromic nevus, and anaemic nevi (see chapter on differential diagnosis of skin lesions in Hansen's disease).

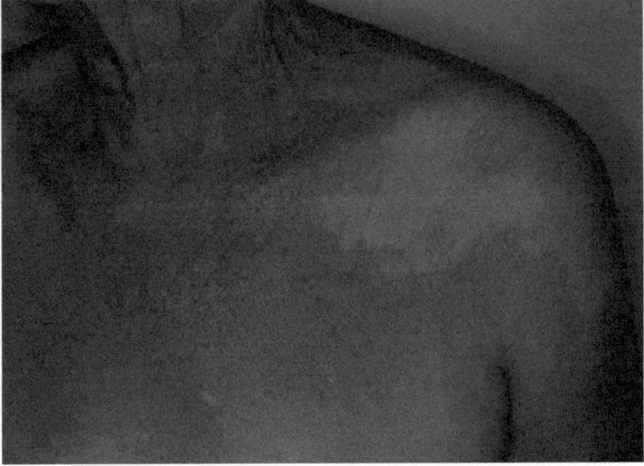

Fig. 1 Indeterminate HD hypochromic macula on left shoulder

It should be noted that, in the Ridley–Jopling classification, the indeterminate form (I) is that in which, after full investigation, a patient in whom HD has become manifest is nevertheless unclassifiable in any of the TT–VV spectrum groups because distinguishing features have not yet developed. Such patients would normally become classifiable if the infection is allowed to progress [3].

The exogenous histamine test may be useful for diagnostic suspicion. It consists of placing one or more drops of millesimal histamine solution on an affected area of skin, for example, a hypochromic patch, and on an area without lesions that acts as a control. Small punctures are made in the skin with a needle so that the histamine solution penetrates superficially into the skin.

The 'full histamine test' consists of the presence of erythema at the puncture site followed by larger erythema around the affected area (reflex erythema) followed by oedema at the puncture site. All these changes occur quickly, about 1–3 min after the start of the test. When reflex erythema is absent, the test is considered "incomplete." This occurs in cases of HD (Fig. 2) and is an additional finding that aids diagnosis. Beyond IHD, the histamine test can be useful when there are difficulties in obtaining responses to the skin-prick test, for example, in young children or people who have difficulties in understanding.

It is possible to carry out an endogenous histamine test if histamine solution is unavailable. This involves stimulating the release of histamine into the skin by linear compression with a blunt instrument, for example, the cap of a pen as used in dermographism, of normal and affected skin. As with the exogenous test, absence of reflex erythema in the area with skin lesions compared with the skin without lesion is consistent with HD.

SSS are negative in patients with IHD. The histopathological findings of IHD are a non-specific inflammatory infiltrate, consisting of undifferentiated lymphocytes and histiocytes, around the nerves and skin appendages, and few or no bacilli.

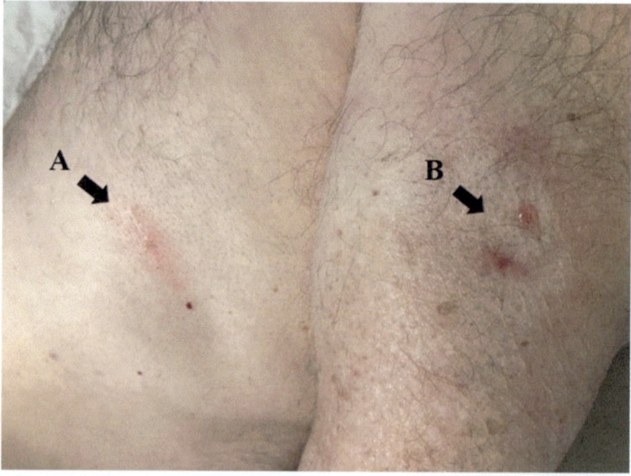

Fig. 2 Histamine test: (**a**) trunk control (presence of erythema reflex—histamine test complete); (**b**) HD hypochromic lesion on the arm (absence of the reflex erythema—histamine test incomplete—the lower erythematous area is a biopsy scar)

3 Tuberculoid Hansen's Disease (THD)

THD may result from the untreated form of IHD in patients with good immunological resistance to *M. leprae*. Lesions are usually erythematous plaques with well-defined borders, often atrophic and hypopigmented in the centre (Figs. 3 and 4).

In THD, the degree of resistance to the bacillus is high and the number of lesions is small, generally fewer than five. In most cases, THD manifests as a single lesion.

There is an alteration of thermal and painful sensitivity and, in older lesions, of tactile sensitivity, which in turn may be associated with altered motor function. There is hair loss and sweating is decreased or absent.

Skin nerves and peripheral nerve trunks are usually thickened in the region of the lesion (Fig. 5).

The predominance of the tuberculoid form in a region is an important epidemiological indicator of an increasing trend of the disease. Among the many differential diagnoses of the tuberculoid form are granuloma annulare and *tinea corporis* or dermatophytosis (see chapter on differential diagnosis of skin lesions in Hansen's disease).

In children under 7 years of age, nodular THD of childhood may occur. Here the skin lesion is an anaesthetic nodule on the face or trunk. In this form, there is no apparent peripheral nerve damage. It is important to distinguish nodular THD in children from American Tegumentary Leishmaniasis in an endemic area (see chapter on Hansen's disease in childhood).

SSS is negative in patients with THD. The main histopathological findings are granulomas with or without Langhans giant cells and damaged nerves infiltrated by the inflammatory process with epithelioid cells arranged side by side (Figs. 6 and 7a). The few bacilli will show complete phagocytosis and are seen almost exclusively in nerve trunks (Fig. 7b).

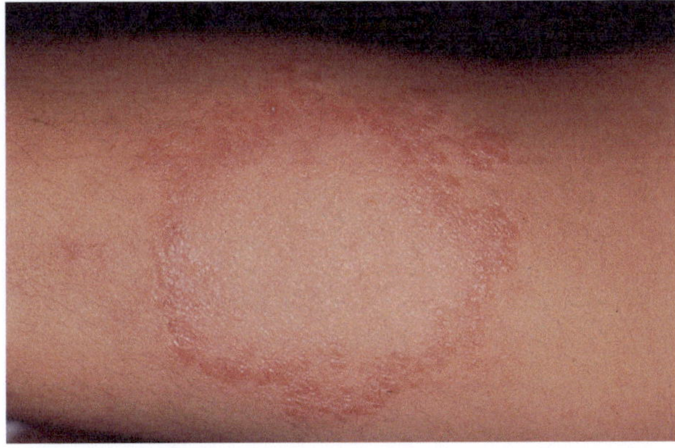

Fig. 3 Tuberculoid HD: erythematous plaque

Fig. 4 Tuberculoid HD: well-defined plaques on the face

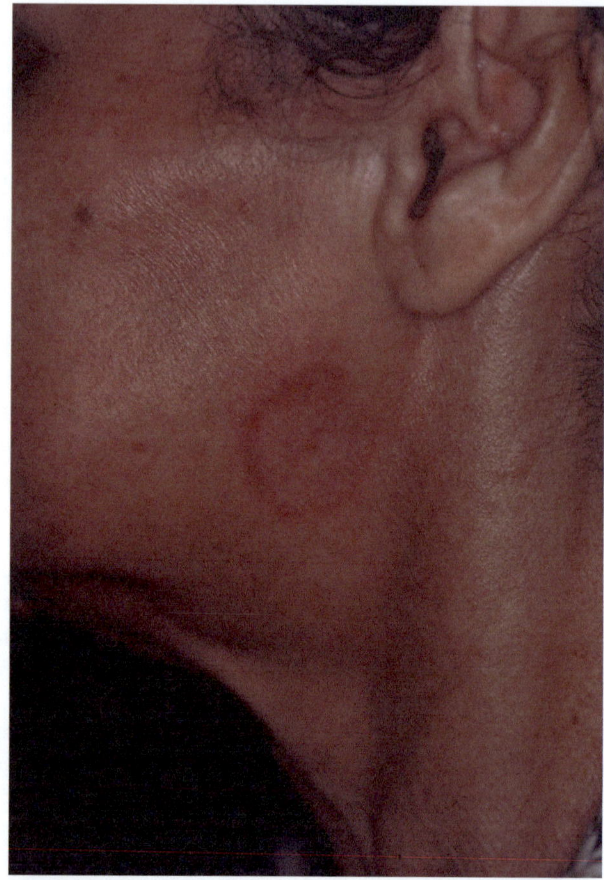

Fig. 5 Tuberculoid HD: ichthyosiform hyperchromic lesion and the thickened branch of the superficial fibular nerve

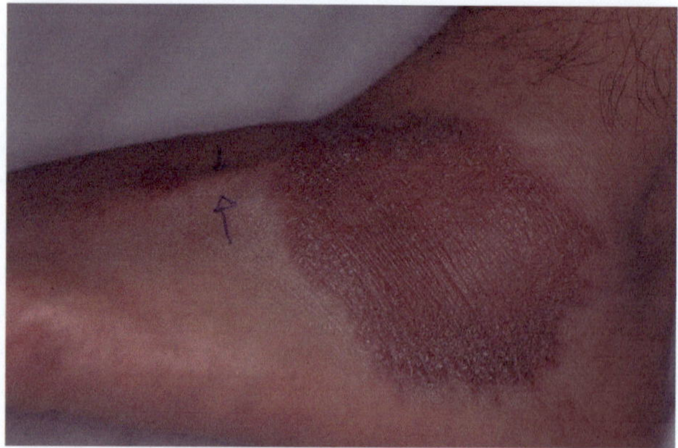

Fig. 6 Tuberculoid HD: superficial and deep tuberculoid granulomas, usually following the path of the neural branches (haematoxylin–eosin ×2)

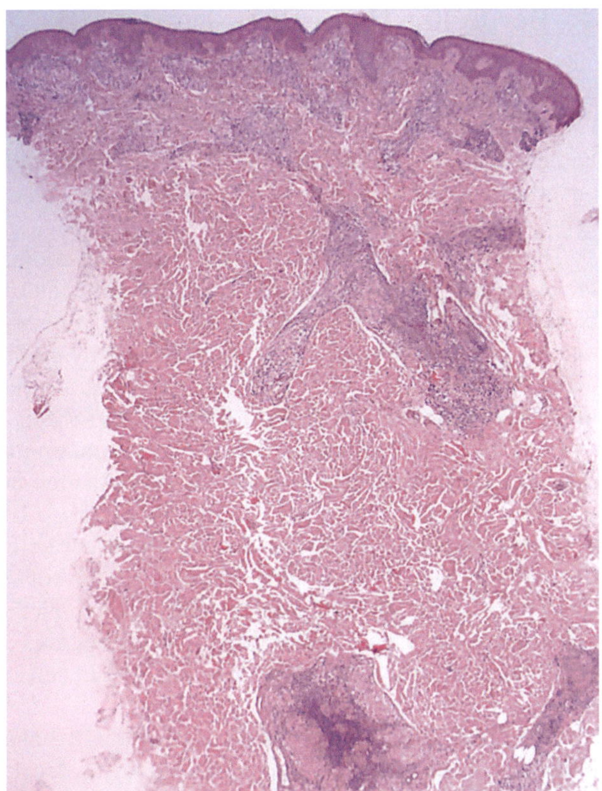

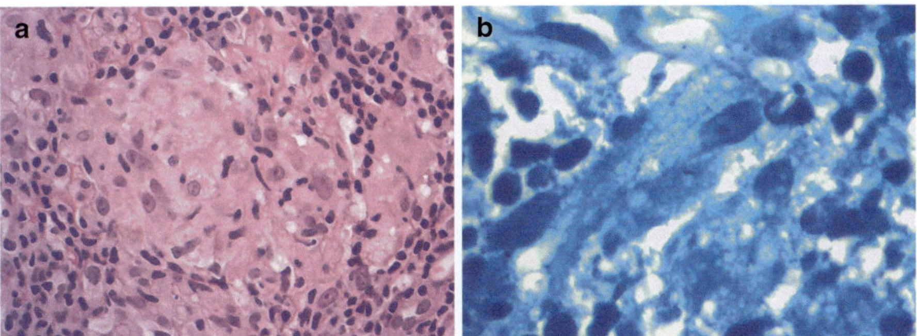

Fig. 7 Tuberculoid HD: (**a**) tuberculoid granuloma consisting of epithelioid macrophages in the centre and a lymphocytic mantle in the periphery (haematoxylin–eosin ×40); (**b**) bacilloscopy ranging from "0" to "1+". Presence of bacilli in the centre of the granuloma (Fite-Faraco ×100)

4 Borderline Hansen's Disease (BHD)

The borderline form is the most prevalent form of HD, with the immune response varying between the T and V poles. The form with the highest resistance among the borderline forms is BT, followed by BB and BV. Peripheral nerve damage is frequent in this form, causing most of the disabilities and deformities seen in HD. BHD is the form in which most HD reactions occur.

The clinical features observed in the different borderline forms resemble closely the respective polar forms as they approach either end of the spectrum. BTHD may be similar to THD or IHD both clinically and immunologically, but with a greater number of lesions (Fig. 8). It is characterized by erythematous plaques with well-defined borders and usually fewer than five lesions (Fig. 9a). Neural involvement may be present (Fig. 9b). In most BT cases, the SSS is negative.

Histopathological findings in BTHD are similar to those in tuberculoid leprosy, but with occasional bacilli usually in nerves. An area spared from the inflammatory process may occur in the subepidermal region (Figs. 10 and 11).

The cases in the middle of the spectrum, borderline-borderline (BB), present particular aspects with peculiar 'bumpy' or 'foveolar' or 'Swiss cheese' lesions (Figs. 12, 13, and 14), with borders clearly adjoining the central portion and imprecisely bordering the external portion. The lesions take on a characteristic rusty tone and there may be dryness of the skin (Fig. 15). In general, peripheral nerve involvement is frequent, causing severe disability.

Skin smear microscopy is usually positive in BB and BV HD. Histopathological findings in BHD are epithelioid cells, histiocytes, focal lymphocytes, increased cellularity in the nerves, presence of localized bacilli in the nerves, and spared subepidermal zone (Figs. 16 and 17).

BVHD differs very little from VVHD, with multiple plaques and infiltrated nodules (Figs. 18, 19, and 20).

Histopathological findings in Borderline-Virchowian HD are histiocytes, few epithelioid cells, foamy or Virchow cells (macrophages or histiocytes containing

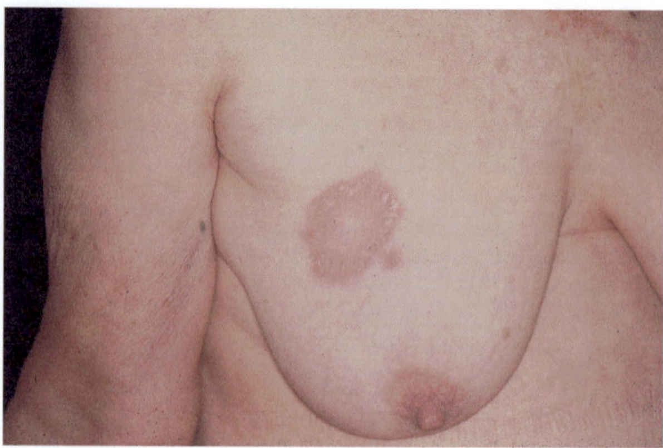

Fig. 8 Borderline-tuberculoid HD: "annular" erythematous plaque

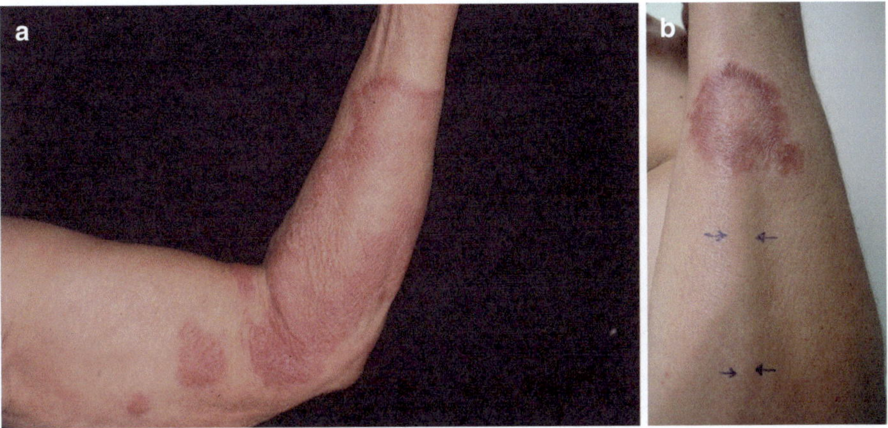

Fig. 9 Borderline-tuberculoid HD: (**a**) erythematous plaques; (**b**) neural involvement

Fig. 10 Borderline-tuberculoid Hansen's disease: superficial and deep tuberculoid granulomas, usually following the path of the neural branches, similar to tuberculoid HD (haematoxylin–eosin ×2)

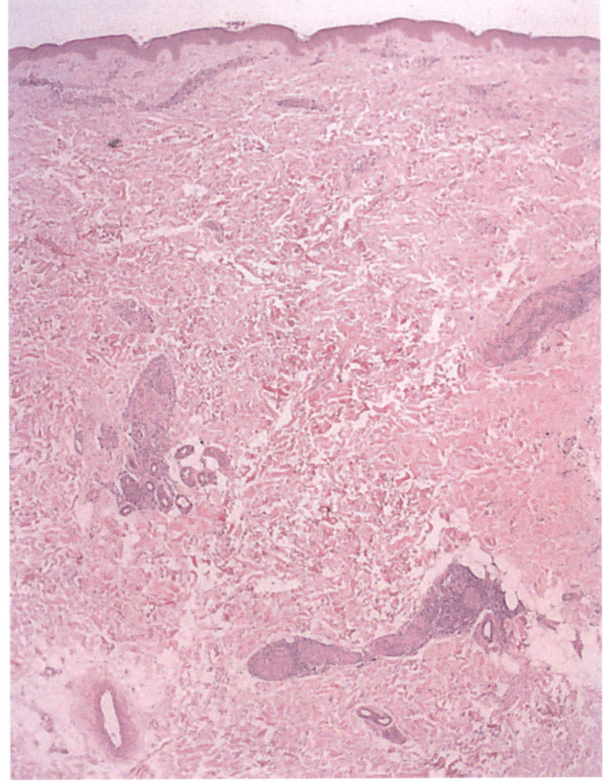

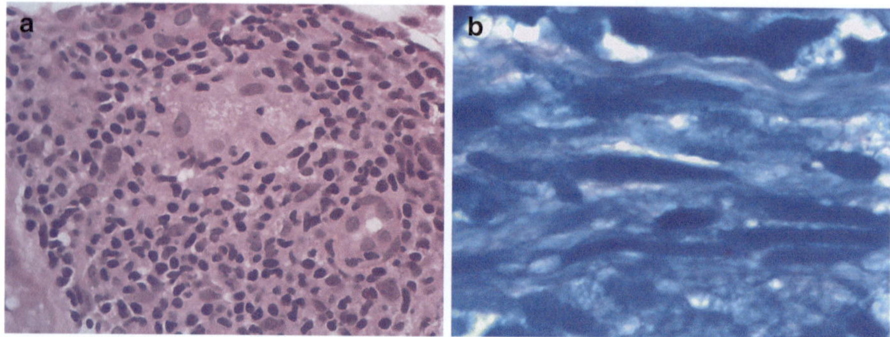

Fig. 11 Borderline-tuberculoid Hansen's disease: (**a**) tuberculoid granuloma consisting of epithelioid macrophages in the centre and a lymphocytic mantle in the periphery, similar to TT but with greater preservation of neural branches (haematoxylin–eosin ×40); (**b**) bacilloscopy ranging from "0" to "2+". Presence of bacilli in neural branches in the centre of the granuloma (Fite-Faraco ×100)

Fig. 12 Borderline-borderline HD: erythematous plaques with a 'foveolar' appearance

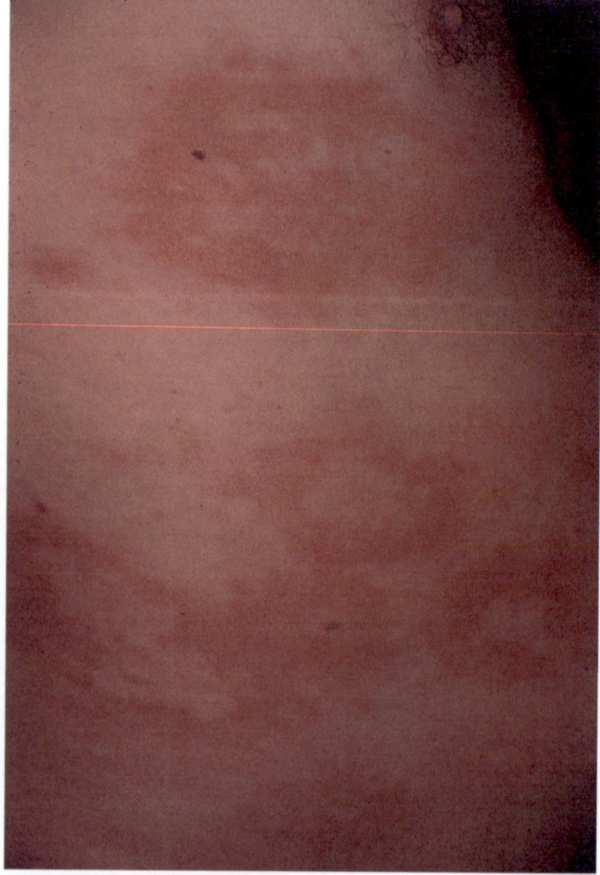

Fig. 13 Borderline-borderline HD: erythematous 'foveolar' plaques in the abdomen

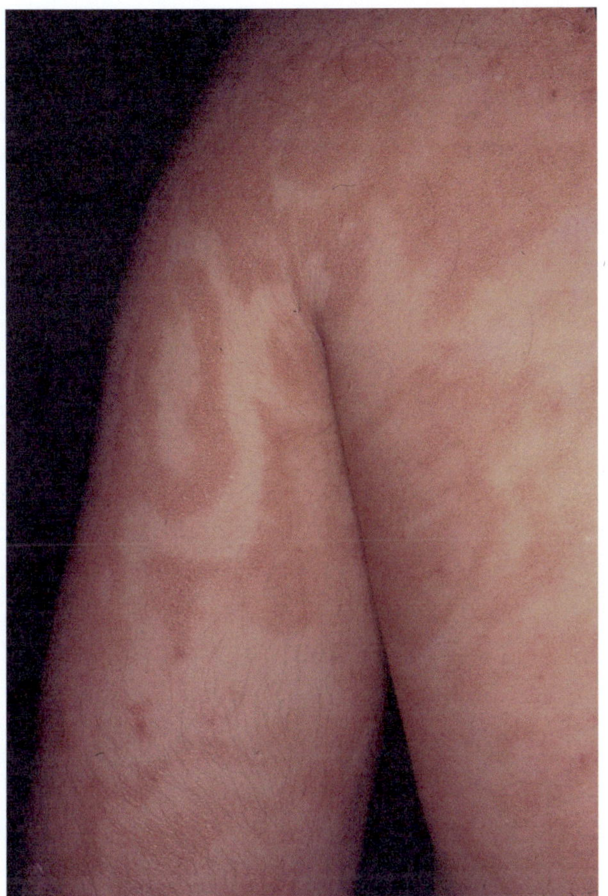

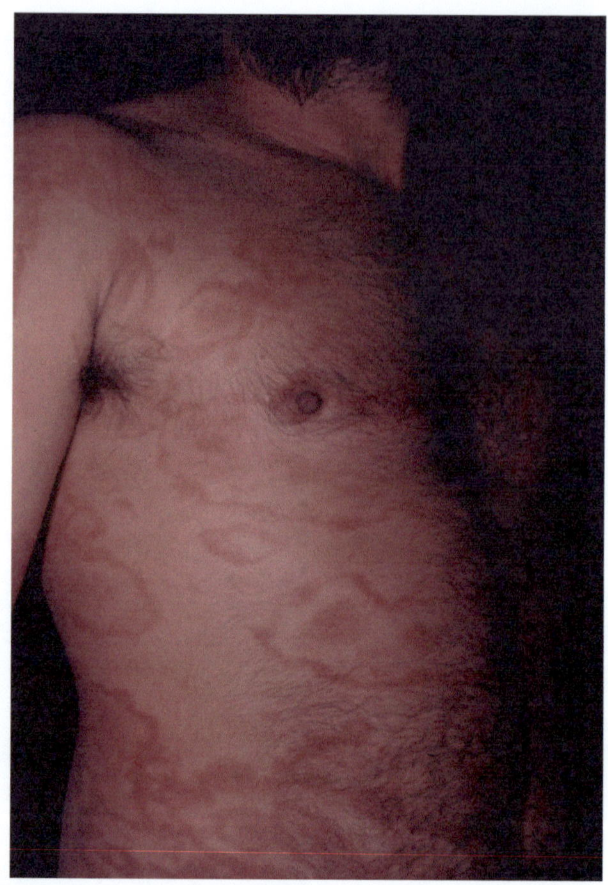

Fig. 14 Borderline-borderline HD: erythematous 'foveolar' plaques on trunk

Fig. 15 Borderline HD: dry skin with thickening of the ulnar nerve on palpation

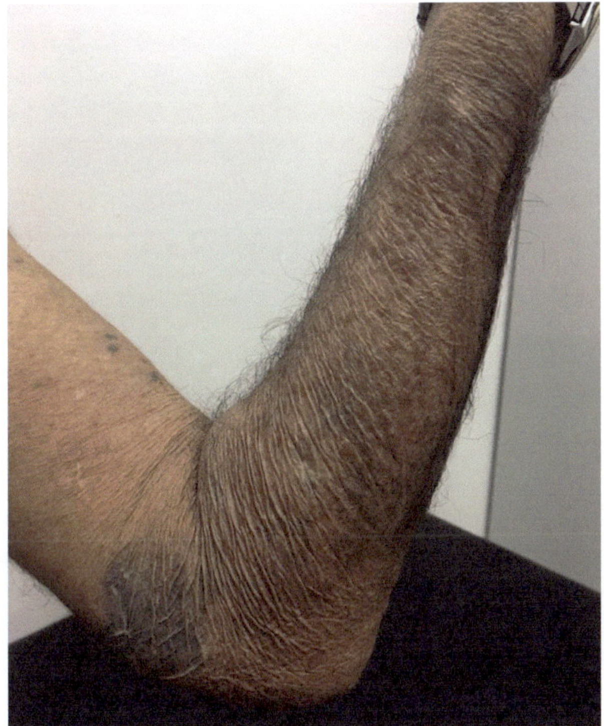

Fig. 16 Borderline HD: superficial and deep inflammatory infiltrate involving the neural branches, interstitium, and perivascular and perifollicular spaces (haematoxylin–eosin ×2)

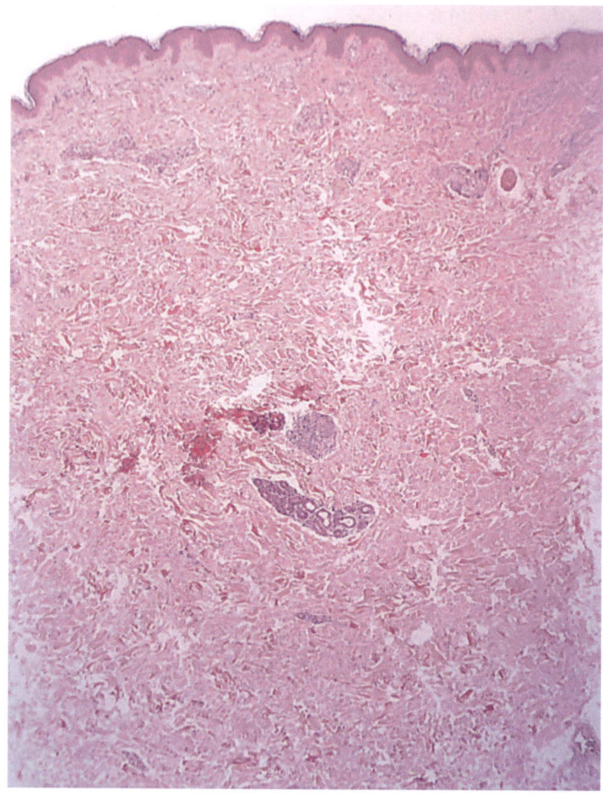

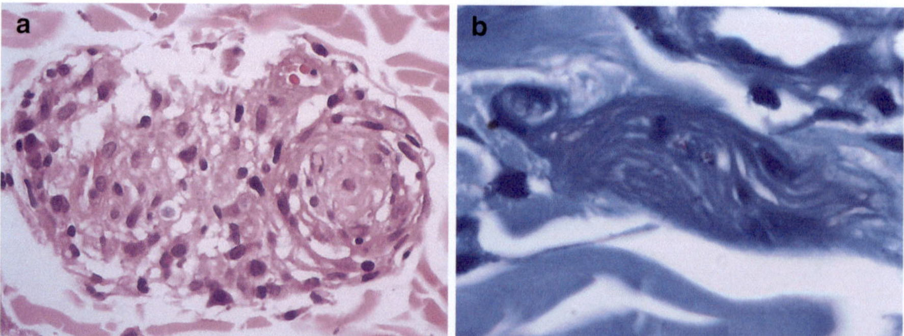

Fig. 17 Borderline HD: (**a**) inflammatory infiltrate consisting of macrophages and lymphocytes concentrically involving the neural branches, without destruction of the neural branch, and absence of tuberculoid granulomas as observed in tuberculoid and borderline-tuberculoid HD (haematoxylin–eosin ×40); (**b**) bacilloscopy ranging from "3+" to "5+". Presence of bacilli in neural branches (centre), macrophages, interstitial cells and in perivascular and perianexial inflammatory infiltrates (Fite-Faraco ×100)

Fig. 18 Borderline-Virchowian HD: erythematous 'foveolar' patches on trunk and upper limbs

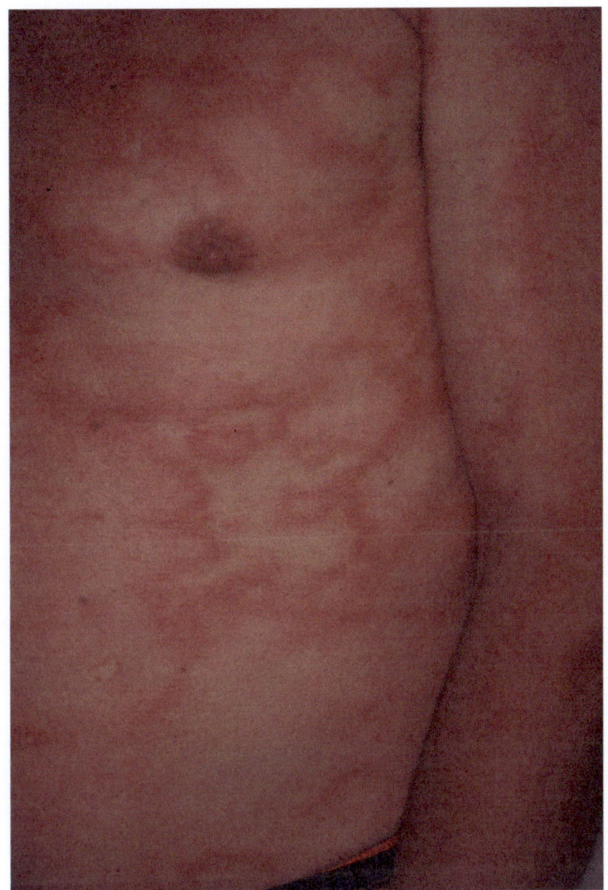

Fig. 19 Borderline-Virchowian HD: 'foveolar' patches on the upper limb

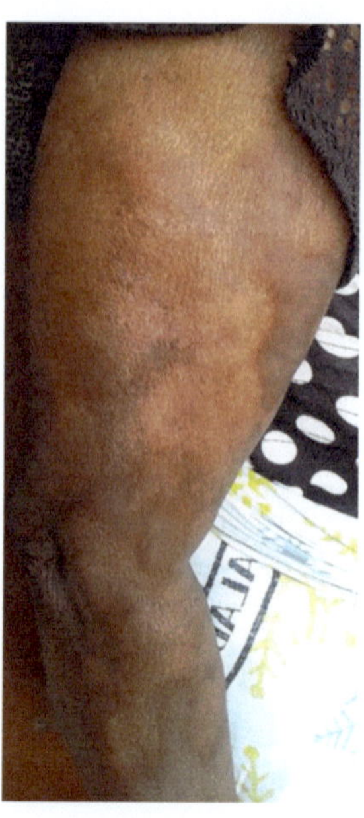

Fig. 20 Borderline-Virchowian HD: skin lesions on trunk and upper limbs

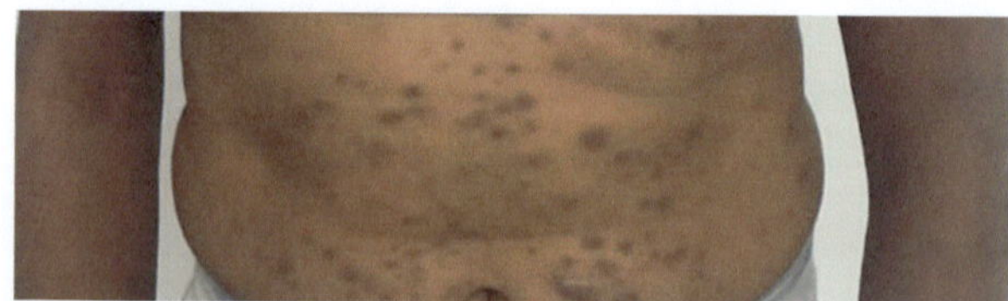

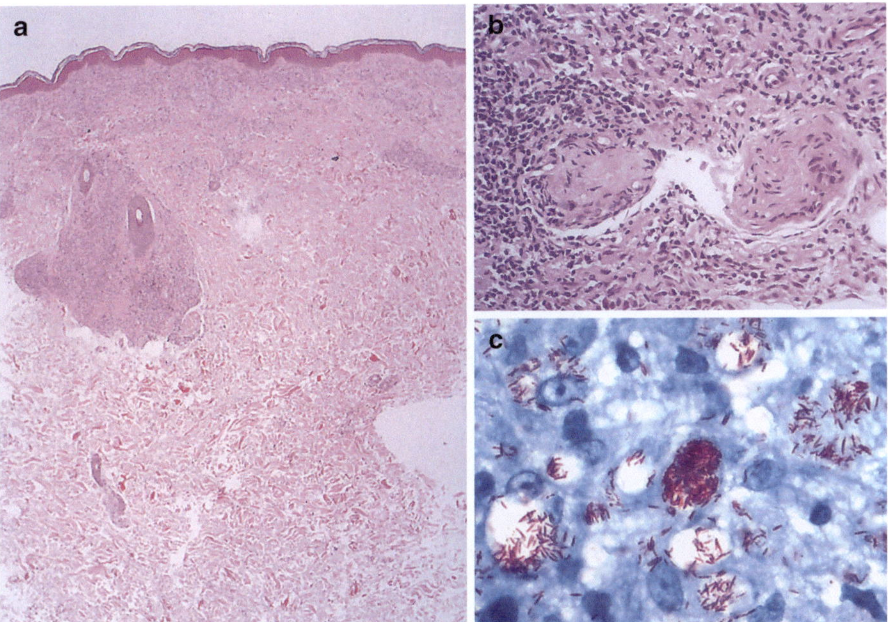

Fig. 21 Borderline-Virchowian HD: (**a**) superficial and deep inflammatory infiltrate, similar to those seen in borderline HD, but more extensive, involving the neural branches, interstitium, and the perivascular and perianexial spaces (haematoxylin–eosin ×2); (**b**) inflammatory infiltrate consisting of multivacuolated or fusiform macrophages permeated with lymphocytes and plasma cells concentrically involving the neural branches, without destruction of the neural branch. Tuberculoid granulomas such as those seen in tuberculoid and borderline-tuberculoid HD are absent (haematoxylin–eosin ×20); (**c**) bacilloscopy ranging from 4+ to 6+. Presence of bacilli in neural branches, macrophages, interstitial cells, in the perivascular and perianexial inflammatory infiltrates and occasionally in vessel walls and endothelium. In the centre, macrophages with intracytoplasmic vacuoles filled with numerous bacilli (globia) (Fite-Faraco ×100)

large numbers of bacilli), presence of bacilli in the nerves, and spared subepidermal zone (Fig. 21).

5   Virchowian Hansen's Disease (VHD)

In this form, infiltrated papules and/or nodules (HD nodules) are found over practically the whole skin, but more frequently in the 'cold' or cooler areas of the body, such as the ears, the central part of the face, and the extensor surfaces of the legs and arms. The so-called hot areas of the body like the scalp, armpits, and lumbar spine are generally spared.

The skin is erythematous or brownish, dry, and infiltrated with enlarged pores (orange peel appearance). The lesions are distributed symmetrically.

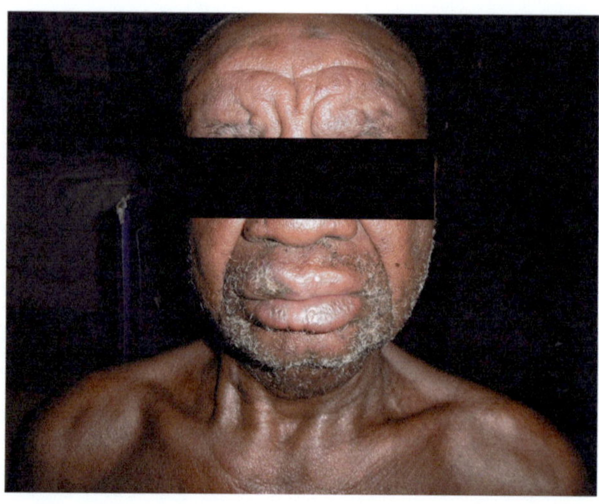

Fig. 22 Virchowian HD (VHD): infiltration of the forehead (glabella)

Nerve damage progresses slowly, and the person with VHD has numbness in the hands and feet. In more advanced stages, there is hair loss in some parts of the body, such as eyelashes and eyebrows, known as madarosis. Other areas that may be involved are the upper respiratory tract, mucous membranes, nerves, joints (joint effusion), bones (multibacillary bone marrow nodules), and other organs such as liver (hepatitis and periportal fibrosis), spleen, kidneys (glomerulonephritis with nephrotic syndrome and subsequent amyloidosis), lymph nodes, testicles, and eyes.

Polymorphic lesions with varying features (macules, papules, nodules, and infiltration) can also be found, being multiple, symmetrical, and erythematous in colour (Figs. 22, 23, 24, 25, 26, and 27). Oedema of the feet and hands are often seen. Loss of eyelashes, intense and diffuse infiltration leading to cutaneous induration and accentuation of the natural furrows, and preservation of hair alter the physiognomy, giving the aspect called 'leonine facies' (Fig. 24). The lesions can present themselves on the oral mucosa (Fig. 28a) and also on the lips (Fig. 28b).

Involvement of the nasal mucosa is frequent, causing symptoms such as nasal obstruction and epistaxis, with possible perforation of the nasal septum and deformation of the nose. Lesions in the mouth, tongue, pharynx, and larynx may also be found. Rhinomaxillary syndrome, first described in skulls of people affected by HD in the Middle Ages, can be identified in people with VHD by the presence of a saddle nose, nasal sinking, concavity of the middle third of the face, thinning of the maxilla, inversion of the upper lip, and loss of the central incisors (see chapter on ENT and mouth alterations in HD). In men, testicular damage may cause atrophy and consequent sterility, impotence, and gynaecomastia. It is important to be aware of young men with VHD who experience testicular pain due to orchitis.

There are alterations in sensation in the skin lesions, and nerve trunk involvement, but not as early and marked as in tuberculoid leprosy. Skin dryness and traumatic lesions are frequent, mainly on the hands (Fig. 29). SSS is usually strongly positive.

Fig. 23 Virchowian HD:
erythematous papules and
nodules on the face
and arm

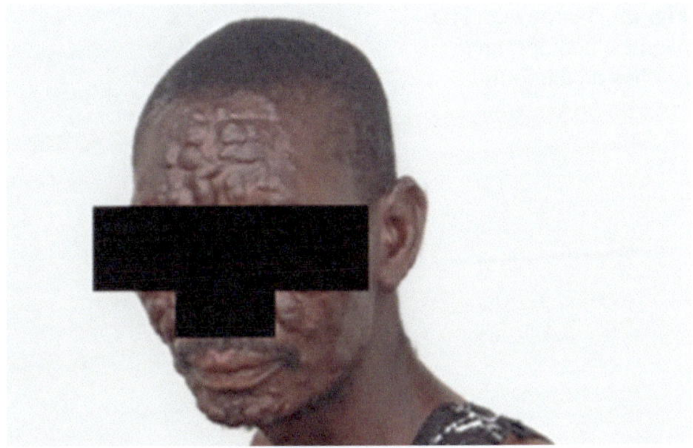

Fig. 24 Virchowian HD:
"leonine facies" -
infiltration of the face and
partial madarosis

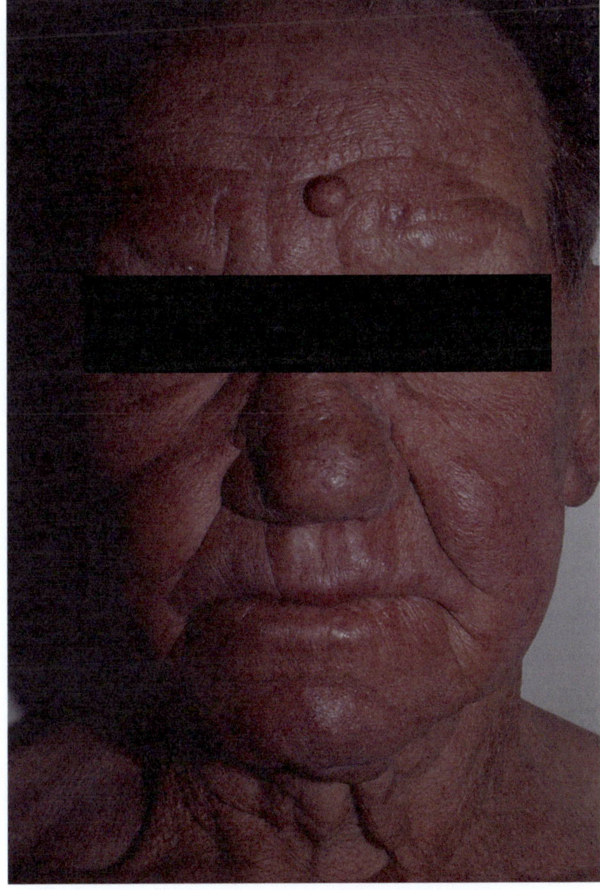

Fig. 25 Virchowian HD: papules, nodules, and patches on the foot

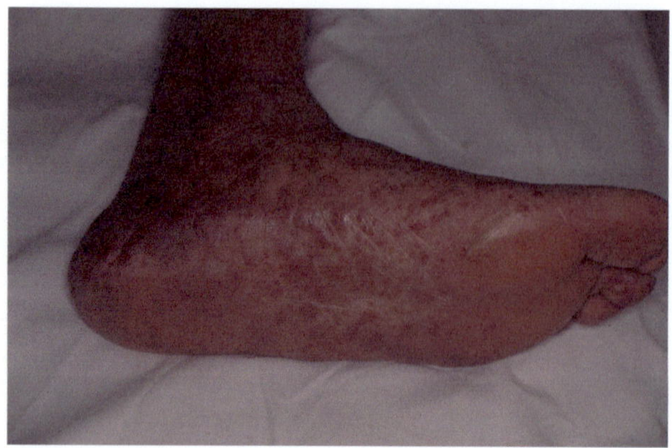

Fig. 26 Virchowian HD: diffuse papules and nodules on the skin

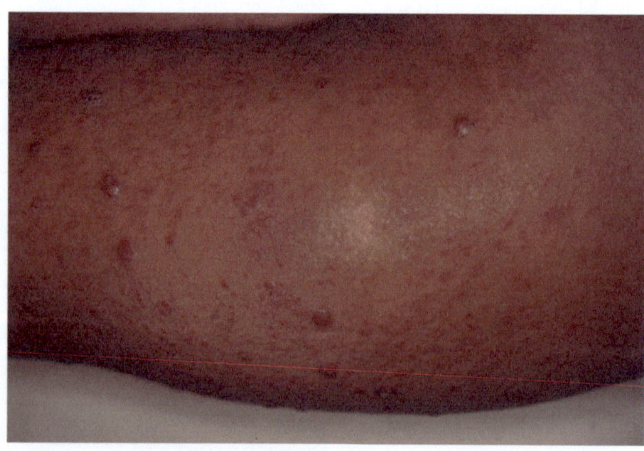

Fig. 27 Virchowian HD: nodules on the arm

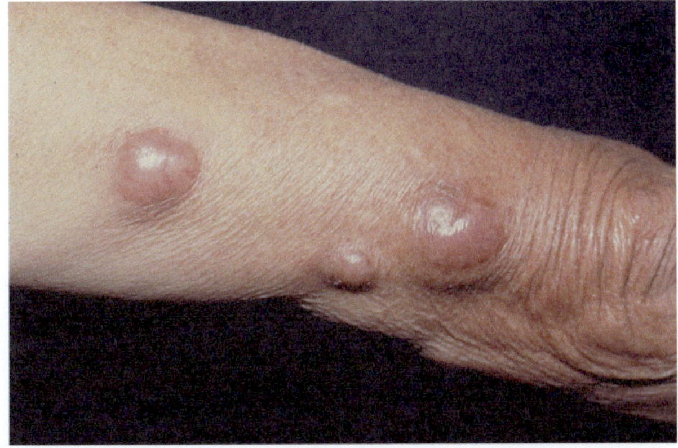

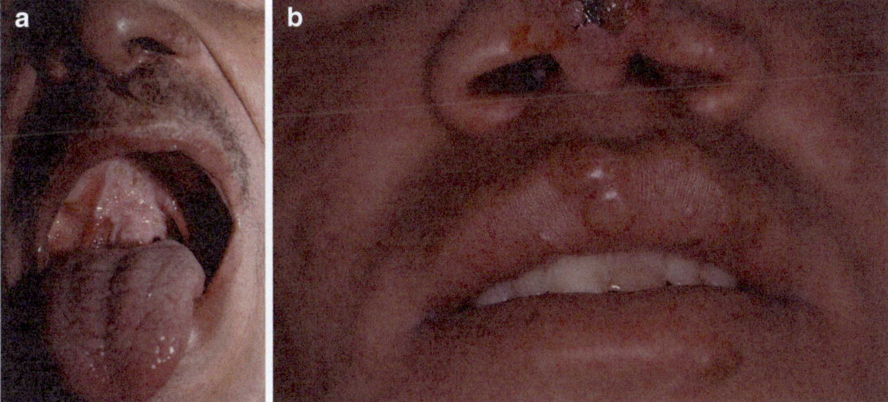

Fig. 28 Virchowian HD: (**a**) lesions of the oral mucosa (**b**) lip lesions

Fig. 29 Virchowian HD: Anaesthetized hands ('glove anaesthesia') showing intense dry scaling, oedema, fissures, ulcerations, and crusts

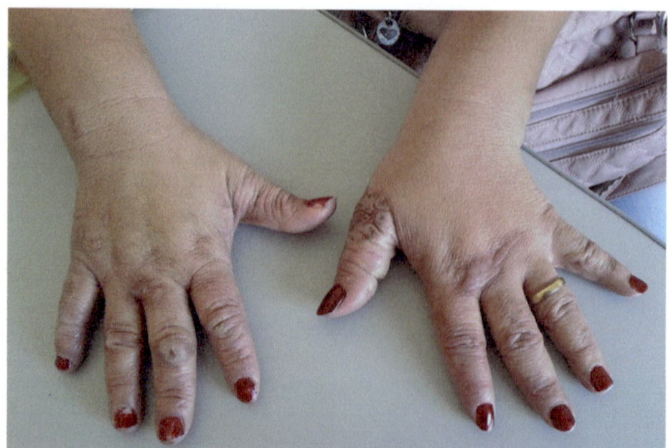

Fig. 30 Virchowian HD: superficial and deep inflammatory infiltrate involving all components of dermis and subcutaneous tissue. Atrophic epidermis with a subepidermal collagen band (Unna's band) (haematoxylin–eosin ×2)

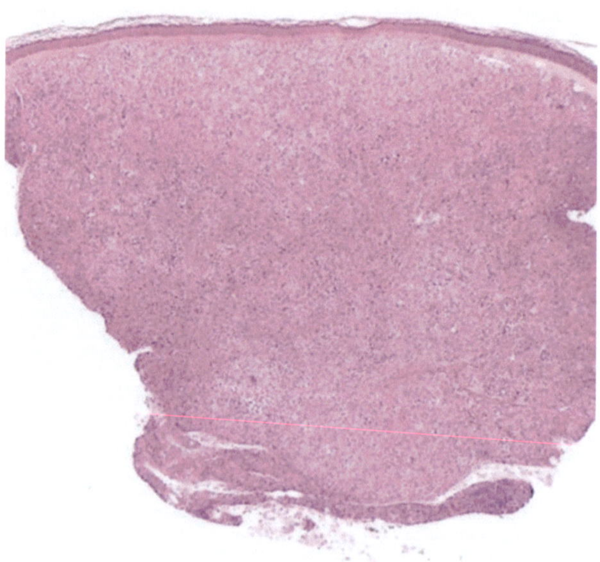

Histopathological findings in VHD are granuloma of the histiomonocytic type with presence of Virchow cells. The picture also comprises few lymphocytes, minimal intraneural cellular infiltration, and spared subepidermal zone (Figs. 30 and 31a). Tissue is strongly positive for AFB, including in the nerves (Fig. 31b).

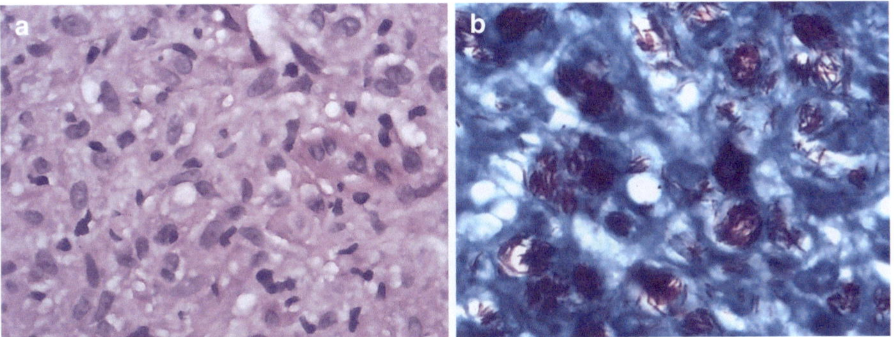

Fig. 31 Virchowian HD: (**a**) infiltrate consisting almost exclusively of multivacuolated or fusiform macrophages permeated with rare lymphocytes and involving all skin components, without destruction of the neural branch and absence of tuberculoid granulomas (haematoxylin–eosin ×40); (**b**) bacilloscopy ranging from '5+' to '6+'. Presence of bacilli in neural branches, macrophages, interstitial cells, in the perivascular and perianexial inflammatory infiltrates, vessel wall, endothelium, and occasionally in squamous epithelial and glandular cells of the skin annexes. In the centre (photo), several macrophages with intracytoplasmic vacuoles filled with numerous bacilli (globia) (Fite-Faraco ×100)

6 Histoid Variant of Virchowian Hansen's Disease

VHD may present as the histoid variant. This is seen infrequently and manifests with clinical keloid-like nodules (Figs. 32 and 33), whose histopathology shows fusiform histiocytes (similar to those that occur in dermatofibroma) and abundant bacilli with a predominance of typical bacilli (Fig. 34).

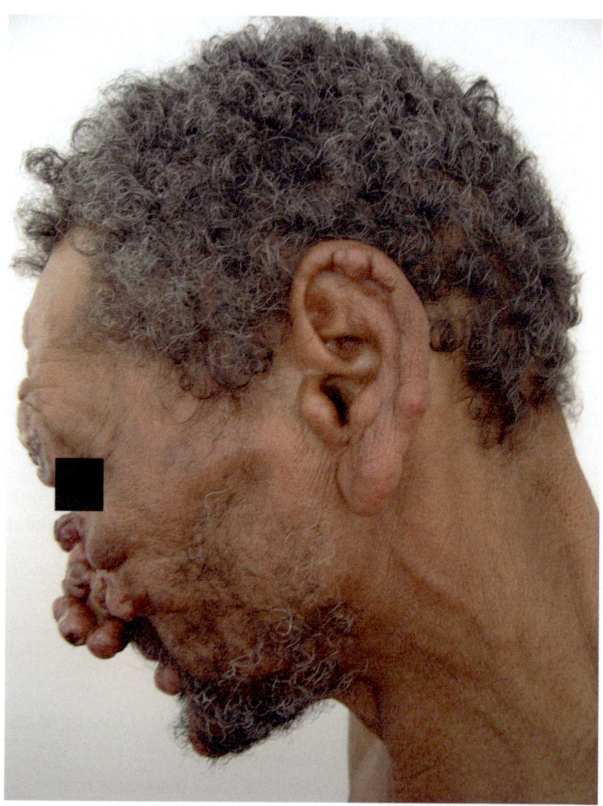

Fig. 32 Histoid variant of Virchowian HD: numerous papules and nodules on the face and ear

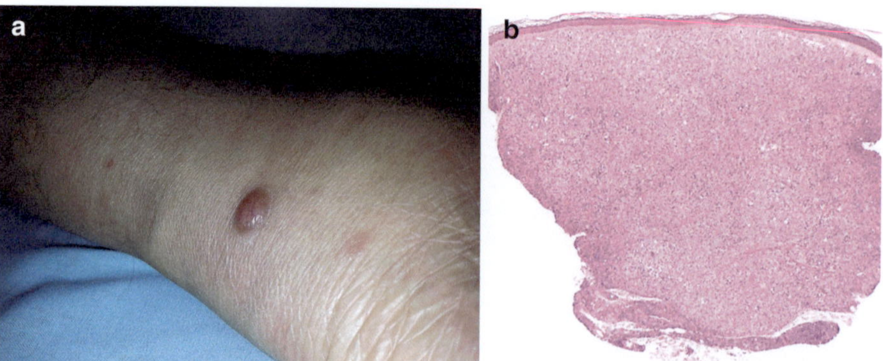

Fig. 33 Histoid variant of Virchowian HD: (**a**) individualized erythematous papules or small plaque-forming papules on the forearm; (**b**) histopathological aspect (haematoxylin-eosin x2)

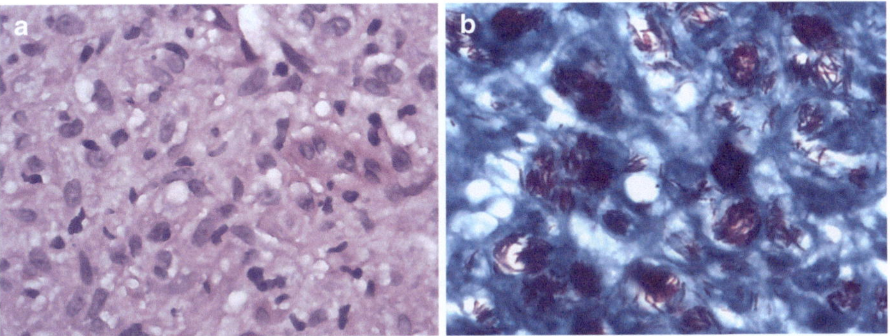

Fig. 34 Histoid variant of Virchowian HD: histopathological aspect showing spindle-shaped histiocytes (**a**). (haematoxylin–eosin x40) and abundant bacilli (**b**). (Fite-Faraco x100)

7 Diffuse Virchowian HD (DVHD)

This presentation of HD has been described in people from Mexico and is also known as diffuse HD of Lucio and Latapi. It is seen in untreated patients and is characterized by violaceous patches in which the lesions have a diffuse infiltrate that does not alter the patient's features, and by total superciliary and ciliary madarosis. This form is also known as *lepra bonita* ('pretty leprosy') because the myxedematous infiltration of the skin leads to an apparent reduction of expression wrinkles on the face of the patient. It may insidiously involve the nasal mucosa with oedema and telangiectasias, evolving to the formation of serosanguinous crusts, followed by ulceration and perforation of the nasal septum, collapse of the nasal pyramid and a saddle nose. In severe cases that remain untreated, the larynx may be involved, with dysphonia and even respiratory obstruction. There is significant visceral involvement and a large number of bacilli are detected.

An acute inflammatory event called Lucio's phenomenon, a type 2 HD reaction, can occur (see chapter on reactions in HD). In the Lucio's phenomenon occurs intense endothelial proliferation with narrowing of the vessel lumen, eventually with vasculitis. At an advanced stage, this is reflected clinically by skin infarcts, necrotic lesions, ulcers, thromboses, and haemorrhages.

Some studies point to *Mycobacterium lepromatosis* as the causative agent in several patients diagnosed with DVHD and Lucio's phenomenon, but these forms can also be caused by *M. leprae*.

8 Primary Neural HD

Primary neural HD (PNHD) or neuritic form (also called 'pure neural' by some authors), is characterized by peripheral neural involvement without skin lesions (Fig. 35). PNHD is not very prevalent, ranging from 2 to 13% of patients diagnosed with HD [7, 8]. It is a condition that may be present as single or multiple mononeuropathy, but also as polyneuropathy resulting from a confluence of mononeuropathies.

Diagnosis of PNHD requires the absence of other aetiological causes of neuropathy, absence of the skin lesions of HD, a negative SSS, and absence of significant histopathological changes in the skin area with loss of sensitivity or near the affected nerve. Neural involvement in PNHD may show any of the histological patterns or any of the forms of HD (Fig. 36). PNHD remains a nerve disease in most cases, but it may precede skin lesions by a few months and, if these appear, the diagnosis changes to one of the other forms of HD. Reactions may occur in the PNHD form, and it is not uncommon for a case of PNHD classified as BT or T to present with granuloma or a nerve abscess, which characterizes a type 1 HD reaction.

The nerves most commonly involved in PNHD are posterior tibial (sensory), ulnar (sensory and motor), median (sensory), and lateral popliteal (motor) [5, 9]. Claw hand is the most frequently observed disability.

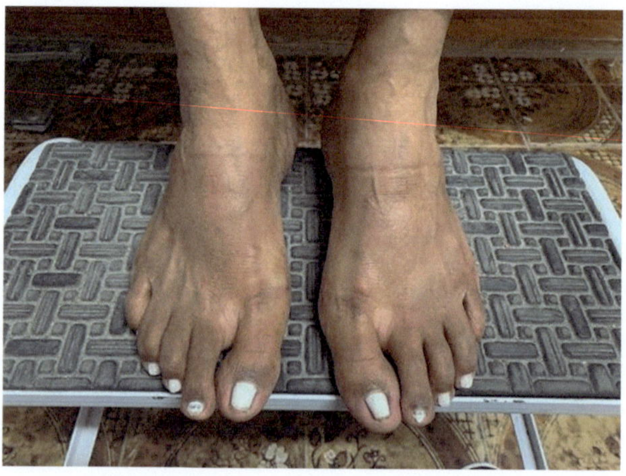

Fig. 35 Primary neural HD

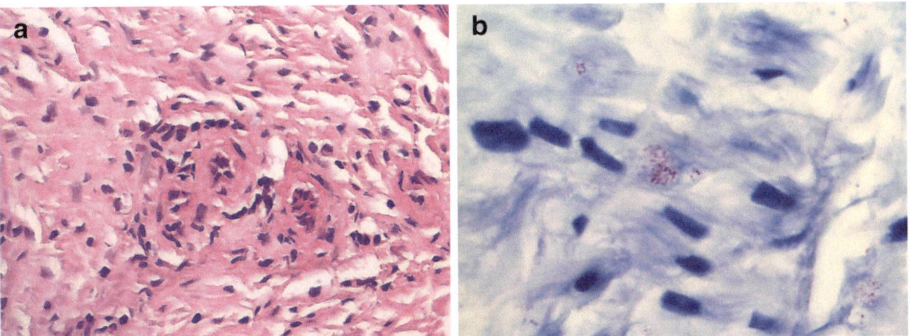

Fig. 36 Primary neural HD: (**a**) neural branch containing lymphocytes—neural involvement may show any of the patterns of the forms of HD (haematoxylin–eosin ×40); (**b**) bacilloscopy showing multiple bacilli within vacuoles in Schwann cells (Fite-Faraco ×100)

9 Subclinical Infection

Subclinical infection is a controversial subject. It describes the situation where infection does not progress to clinical manifestations (skin lesions and nerve damage). It is supposed that an infected person could remain in this stage and progress to a clinical form of HD or to self-cure. A 'healthy carrier' status has been suggested from the detection of *M. leprae* in nasal mucus using PCR [10, 11], and from the presence of anti-PGL-1 antibodies in healthy individuals. It is hypothesized that these persons are important in the chain of transmission of HD, especially in endemic areas [12].

References

1. World Health Organization. Global Leprosy Strategy 2016–2020. Accelerating towards a leprosy-free world. Monitoring and evaluation guide. Geneva: World Health Organization; 2017.
2. World Health Organization. Guidelines for the diagnosis, treatment and prevention of leprosy. Geneva: World Health Organization; 2018.
3. Ridley DS, Jopling WH. Classification of leprosy according to immunity. A five-group system. Int J Lepr Other Mycobact Dis. 1966;34:255–73.
4. International Nepal Fellowship (INF). Manual for the implementation of multi-drug therapy in the leprosy programme of Nepal. 1985.
5. Van Brakel WH, de Soldenhoff R, McDougall AC. The allocation of leprosy patients into paucibacillary and multibacillary groups for multidrug therapy, taking into account the number of body areas affected by skin, or skin and nerve lesions. Lepr Rev. 1992;63:231–46. https://doi.org/10.5935/0305-7518.19920028.

6. Rao PN, Sujai S, Srinivas D, Lakshmi T. Comparison of two systems of classification of leprosy based on number of skin lesions and number of body areas involved—a clinico-pathological concordance study. Indian J Dermatol Venereol Leprol. 2005;71:14. https://doi.org/10.4103/0378-6323.13779.

7. Garbino JA, Marques W, Barreto JA, et al. Primary neural leprosy: systematic review. Arq Neuropsiquiatr. 2013;71:397–404. https://doi.org/10.1590/0004-282X20130046.

8. Shukla B, Verma R, Kumar V, et al. Pathological, ultrasonographic, and electrophysiological characterization of clinically diagnosed cases of pure neuritic leprosy. J Peripher Nerv Syst. 2020;25:191–203. https://doi.org/10.1111/jns.12372.

9. Ramadan W, Mourad B, Fadel W, Ghoraba E. Clinical, electrophysiological, and immuno-pathological study of peripheral nerves in Hansen's disease. Lepr Rev. 2001;72:35–49. https://doi.org/10.5935/0305-7518.20010007.

10. Klatser PR, van Beers S, Madjid B, et al. Detection of *Mycobacterium leprae* nasal carriers in populations for which leprosy is endemic. J Clin Microbiol. 1993;31:2947–51.

11. Beyene D, Aseffa A, Harboe M, et al. Nasal carriage of *Mycobacterium leprae* DNA in healthy individuals in Lega Robi village, Ethiopia. Epidemiol Infect. 2003;131:841–8. https://doi.org/10.1017/s0950268803001079.

12. Guerrero MI, Arias MT, Garcés MT, León CI. Developing and using a PCR test to detect sub-clinical *Mycobacterium leprae* infection. Rev Panam Salud Publica. 2002;11:228–34. https://doi.org/10.1590/s1020-49892002000400004.

Reactions in Hansen's Disease

P. Narasimha Rao, Sujai Suneetha, and Santoshdev P. Rathod

1 Introduction

Immunologically mediated inflammatory episodes occurring in a leprosy patient during the course of the disease are collectively termed 'lepra reactions'. Any type of leprosy, except the indeterminate form, may undergo a sudden inflammatory phase of exacerbation as a part of the natural course of the disease. Lepra reactions are mainly of two types—type 1 reaction (T1R) and type 2 reaction (T2R), often referred to as ENL reaction [1]. A third type of reaction rarely seen in some parts of the world is the Lucio phenomenon. These may occur before, during, or even after the successful completion of MDT and up to 50% of leprosy patients experience at least one episode of reaction during the course of their disease [2].

Lepra reactions not only play a significant role in the morbidity associated with the disease, but they constitute a major risk factor for the development of disability and deformity in individuals affected by the disease. The importance of early and accurate identification of these episodes and the need for their optimal management cannot be over emphasized.

P. N. Rao (✉)
Bhaskar Medical College, Hyderabad, Telangana, India

S. Suneetha
Institute for Specialized Services in Leprosy (INSSIL), Nireekshana ACET, Hyderabad, India

S. P. Rathod
NHL Municipal Medical College, SCL Municipality General Hospital, Ahmedabad, India

P. D. Deps (ed.), *Hansen's Disease*, https://doi.org/10.1007/978-3-031-30893-2_10

2   Type 1 Reaction (T1R)

A type 1 reaction or 'reversal reaction' is expressed clinically by inflammatory exacerbation of the skin lesions and nerve trunks, consequently leading to sensory and motor alterations [3]. It occurs due to an acute upsurge in the cell-mediated immune response to *Mycobacterium leprae* antigens and is mainly observed in borderline tuberculoid (BT), mid-borderline (BB), and borderline lepromatous leprosy (BL) patients.

2.1   Incidence

Despite being an important event occurring in leprosy patients, accurate data on the incidence and frequency of occurrence of lepra reaction is not readily available. However, data available from institutional studies and studies carried by individual researchers indicates that, overall, the occurrence of T1R ranges in various studies from 20 to 40% in multibacillary (MB) patients [4]. The incidence of T1R in PB patients was found to be 20.4% in a study from north India [5]. Twenty-six percent of Brazilian patients who had positive slit-skin smears experienced a T1R during the 2 years period they were taking MDT [6]. Frequency of lepra reactions experienced by children with leprosy ranges from 3 to 34% [7, 8]. A recent study done in Brazil showed that the occurrence of T1R was as high as 52.9% [9]. In the nation-wide Dermlep study carried out in India, 26.1% of post-RFT patients experienced T1R [10].

2.2   Immunological Basis

T1R results from the activation of cell-mediated immunity (CMI) and represents a type IV Gell and Coombs *hypersensitivity reaction* wherein there is an exaggerated inflammatory response to *M. leprae* antigens, involving skin and nerves leading to sensory and motor Nerve Function Impairments (NFI). T1R often occurs after the start of treatment although it can be a presenting complaint in a significant proportion of new patients [11]. The cytokine expression pattern in T1R reflects this *upregulation* of the Th1 response along with an activation of CD4+ T cell-mediated cellular immune responses and the release of proinflammatory cytokines, such as TNF-α, IFN-γ, IL-1β, IL-6, lysosomal enzymes, and reactive oxygen species (Fig. 1), all of which cause leakiness in the endothelial barrier, tissue injury, and

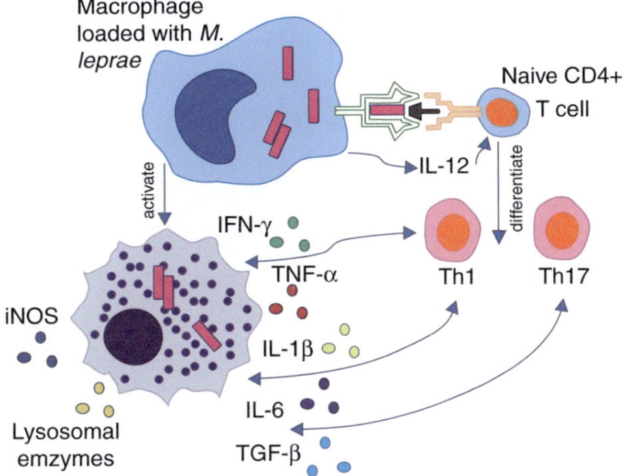

Fig. 1 Events in the pathogenesis of T1R (Adapted from Luo Y et al. 2021)—Open source

influx of activated lymphocytes and macrophages into the area [12–15]. The various risk factors for triggering T1R are summarized in Box 1.

Box 1 Risk factors for T1R

• Age of patient: ≥15 years • Sex: women carry higher risk than men and it is attributable to fluctuations in hormones, pregnancy, and delivery • Type of leprosy: borderline forms of leprosy with positive slit skin smear • Individuals who have WHO disability grades 1 or 2 at diagnosis • After starting treatment with multidrug therapy (MDT) • Skin lesions on the face and over nerve trunks	**Host-related immunological factors** TLR gene polymorphism – TLR2 and 4 gene polymorphisms, TLR4 SNP (1530G>T) predisposes to T1R [16]

2.3   Clinical Features

T1R is characterized by acute inflammation in pre-existing, or occasionally in newly appearing lesions, presenting as the sudden appearance of erythematous and raised skin lesions (Pictures 1, 2 and 3). Involvement of the peripheral nerves in T1R presents clinically as acute neuritis, with painful tender swelling of the affected nerve of sudden onset, often accompanied by sensory, motor, and/or autonomic NFI. A nerve abscess can rarely occur in severe T1R, observed as a localized tender nodular

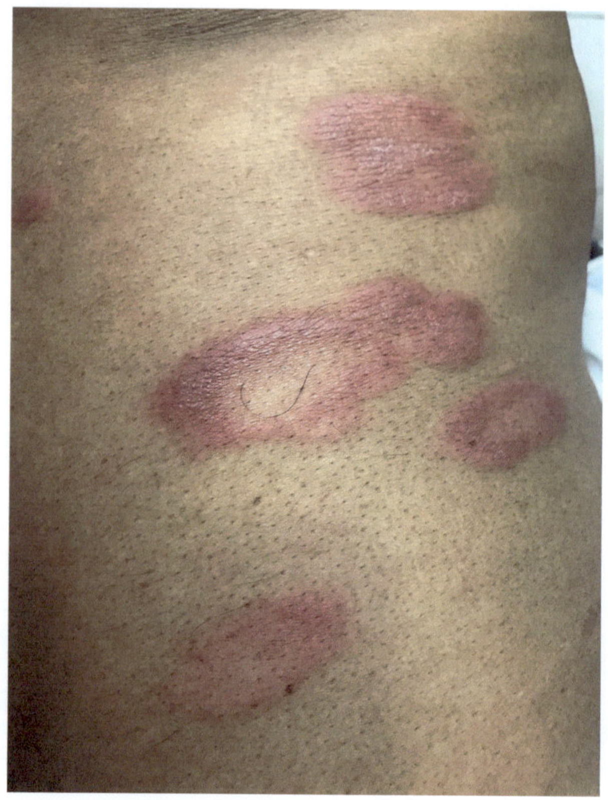

Picture 1 Type 1 reaction in skin lesions (borderline form. Note mild scaling in the centre of the lesion)

swelling of the nerve. Severe T1R of skin very seldom may progress to ulceration of skin.

T1R can occasionally be limited exclusively to either the skin or the nerves. Typically, when only skin is involved, T1R is considered a *mild reaction*. An episode of T1R manifesting with a new/sudden onset of motor weakness associated with thickened and tender nerve trunk and in some cases nerve abscesses is considered a *severe reaction*. Nevertheless, a reaction which is initially confined to the skin patches, often progresses to neuritis in one or more regional nerve trunks. Hence, a T1R limited to the skin may therefore be taken as a possible pointer of impending 'neuritis' [3, 11]. Special attention should be paid to T1R skin lesions of the face (Picture 4), especially in the malar region or around the eye as it is associated with a higher risk of facial motor paralysis, resulting in lagophthalmos and its sequelae [17].

Picture 2 Type 1 reaction in skin lesions

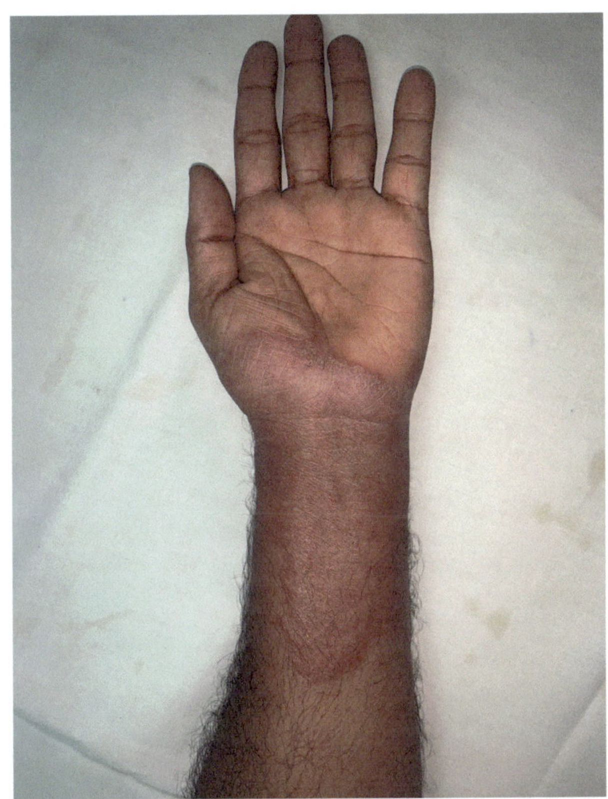

Picture 3 Type 1 reaction in skin lesions (Note swelling and erythema of the plaque along ulnar border of hand)

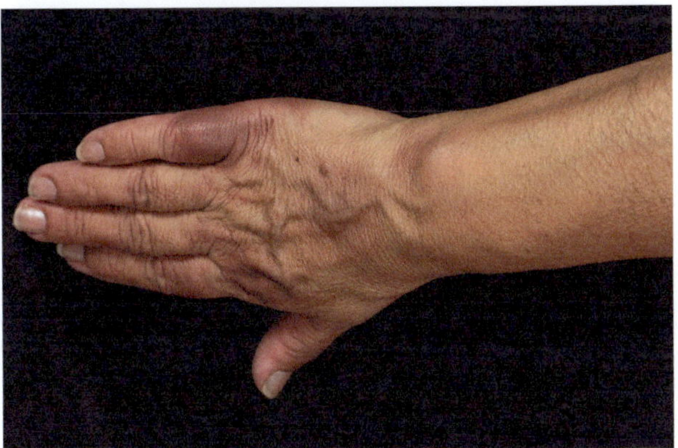

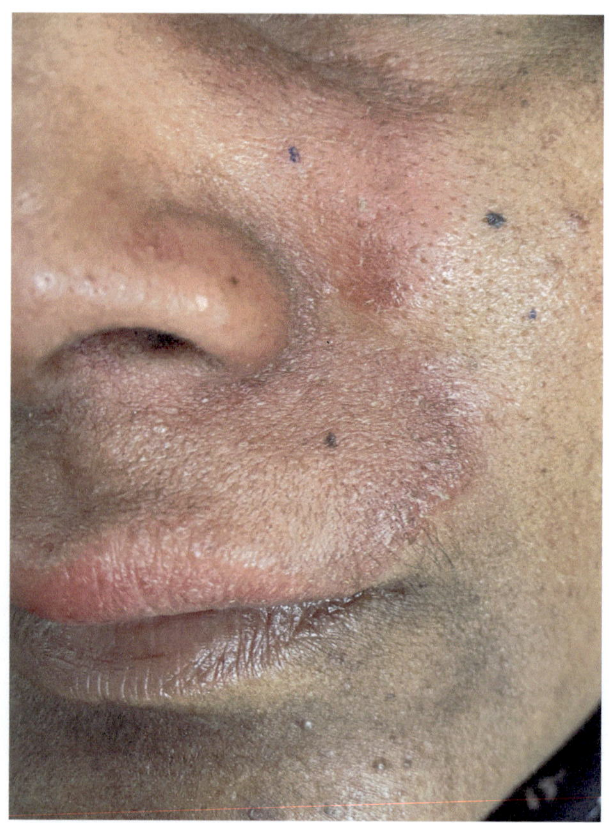

Picture 4 Type 1 reaction in BT. Patch of face involving lip

2.4 Histopathology

As previously mentioned T1R occurs mainly in the borderline spectrum of disease; BT and BB and sometimes in BL patients. On the background of this spectrum of disease, the histologic features that characterize T1R are the presence of oedema in the superficial dermis and in the granuloma, resulting in the disorganization of the granuloma, dilated vasculature, wide separation of dermal collagen, in addition to the presence of Langhans giant cells [18]. Rarely, epidermal erosion can occur when granuloma extends into the papillary dermis and invades the overlying epidermal layers. Severe reactions may be accompanied by fibrinoid necrosis and fibrosis [19].

Depending upon the changes observed in the histology T1R are further classified as 'upgrading' reaction and 'downgrading' reaction. When there are shift towards the tuberculoid spectrum with increased epithelioid cell differentiation, Langhans giant cell formation and a fall in AFB in the section it is indicative of an 'upgrading' T1R (or true reversal reaction), which is more often observed in patients on MDT and subsequent improvement in the immunity. *Downgrading reaction* usually occurs in patients who are not on treatment, wherein there is an increase in macrophage differentiation, fewer giant cells and increasing bacilli in histopathology is observed. However, clinically it is often very difficult to accurately identify upgrading or downgrading T1R and probably an unnecessary academic exercise, as the clinical course and complications do not differ between these two subtypes of T1R.

2.5 Differential Diagnosis

Morphological mimics of T1R include cellulitis, erysipelas, urticarial vasculitis, Sweet's syndrome, erythema multiforme and steroid modified dermatophytosis lesions which look inflamed with a red border. Differentiation of T1R from cellulitis/erysipelas can sometimes be difficult, nonetheless, the indolent course and cardinal features of leprosy will point to the correct diagnosis. Typical targetoid morphology of erythema multiforme and presence of itching in dermatophytosis distinguish them from T1R.

2.6 Diagnostic Procedures and Laboratory Tests

While clinical signs and symptoms of inflammation in a skin patch of leprosy are indicators of a clinical diagnosis of T1R, the confirmation of diagnosis can be done by histopathology. Histological diagnostic criteria are described in Sect. 2.5. Recently, dermoscopy is also being considered a supportive tool for the diagnosis of T1R. Orange-yellow globules with telangiectasia observed by dermoscopy are generally considered to be the representative of dermal granulomas. In T1R, a reddish background and white structureless areas with fine short linear blurry vessels, probably due to an increased number of lymphocytes and loss of normal granuloma organization are considered pointers of lepra reaction [20]. High-resolution ultrasonography of nerve trunks in T1R occasionally show massive increase in cross-sectional area (CSA) of the nerve accompanied by increased vascular signals within the affected nerves on use of colour Doppler that reflects intraneural vascular dilation due to inflammation associated with the lepra reaction in the nerve [21, 22].

2.6.1 Course and Duration of T1R

The natural course and duration of T1R varies depending on the clinical classification. It can be 3–9 months in BT patients, and far longer, up to 15 months in BL patients [23]. Patients who experience reappearance of reactional signs or symptoms after completion of a course of corticosteroid are diagnosed as having 'Recurrent Reaction'. The recurrence of T1R becomes a clinical and therapeutic problem, especially when they occur after the completion of treatment or after release from treatment (RFT) when there is no active surveillance of the patient [10]. T1R tend to recur less than T2R (ENL) reactions. However, studies have shown that about 1/3rd of all T1R patients can experience recurrence of reactional episodes [24]. BT patients with fewer skin lesions are most likely to have a single episode of T1R whereas BT and BL patients with multiple lesions and higher BI on smears are more likely to have a second and even a third episode of T1R [25].

2.7   Management

The objective of treatment for T1R is twofold; (a) to suppress and abate inflammation-mediated neuritis in order to prevent NFI; and (b) to restore normal nerve function if the damage has already occurred. In all patients of T1R with or without neuritis, standard MDT needs to be started and continued. The mainstay of the management of T1R is oral corticosteroid therapy. It is ideal that patients should receive an individualized treatment regime based on the severity of the reaction, but often in a field setting a semi-standardized approach may be more appropriate. The management of T1R in those with neuritis need closer monitoring and a more robust regimen for a longer duration [26]. It is important to explain to the affected individual the nature of the complication that can occur and the need for compliance to treatment.

2.7.1   Management of Mild T1R

For mild T1R limited to skin lesions, the objective is to reduce the inflammation and hence anti-inflammatory agents such as aspirin and other NSAIDs are drug of choice. Additionally, chloroquine, which acts by lysosomal membrane stabilization, inhibits prostaglandin synthesis, and complement activation, can also be tried.

2.7.2   Management of T1R with Neuritis

The aim of the treatment is to control the acute neural inflammation, ease pain, and reverse nerve damage. This objective of reducing intraneural inflammation and oedema is achieved by the judicious use of analgesics and corticosteroids. Rest, splinting, keeping the limb immobilized with a pad and bandage are basic general non-pharmacological measures. Oral corticosteroids while normalizing the intra-neural pressure also improve vascular and axoplasmic flow and allow recovery of nerve function. The starting dose for T1R in adults is 30–40 mg of prednisolone or its equivalents, preferably in a single or in two divided doses. While WHO publications suggest a duration of 12 weeks, in practice patients in T1R usually need oral corticosteroids for up to 6 months [27]. It is advisable to follow the checklist given in Box 2 before starting corticosteroids.

> **Box 2 Check list when starting corticosteroids**
> **Investigations**
> - Monitor BP and weight at each visit
> - Tests to exclude tuberculosis, as indicated (e.g. sputum examination, chest X-ray)
> - Tests to assess the possibility of diabetes (e.g. urine/blood sugar, test of glucose tolerance)
> - Stool examination
>
> **Drug Supplements**
> - Gastric protection with H2 blockers or proton pump inhibitor
> - Calcium supplementation (to prevent osteoporosis)
> - Prophylactic Albendazole or Ivermectin for *Strongyloides stercoralis* infection in endemic areas

The use of a semi-standardized tapering course of corticosteroids given on an out-patient basis opened up the wider use of steroids to treat T1R and neuritis on an out-patient basis in field conditions [28–30]. The once-a-day morning dosage is preferred as it causes less suppression of the hypothalamus–pituitary axis (HPA). It is vital to understand the importance of gradually tapering the steroid dose. This prevents many of the side effects of steroids as well as reduces the chances of HPA axis suppression and dependence. Future treatment options for patients with T1R are illustrated in Table 1.

Table 1 Future perspectives on management of T1R

Class of drugs	Proposed mechanism of action	Names
Type 1 interferons (IFNS)	Counteract antimicrobial effects of IFN-gamma and of inflammasome activation	– Betaferon/Betaseron and Rebif which are IFN-b and IFN-a, respectively
Drugs that target IL-1b	High level of this cytokine in sera of T1R patient	– IL1 receptor antagonist: Anakinra – IL1 blocking agents: Rilonacept, Canakinumab
PPAR agonist	PPAR-g gene expression is downregulated nTIR. Due to their diverse biological activities on keratinocytes, PAR agonists represent a potentially important source of investigation for the treatment of T1R	– Thiazolidinediones – Glitazones
IL 6 blockade	Uncontrolled production of IL-6 has been associated with the onset of TIR	– Tocilizumab

Various surgical techniques were developed to achieve surgical nerve decompression in severe recurrent neuritis of T1R, especially of the ulnar nerve. These include epineurotomy, medial humeral epicondylectomy, anterior ulnar nerve transfer, selective meshing of epineurium, partial or subtotal peri-neurectomy, and interfascicular decompression [31]. However, at present they are not being practiced widely, with the advent of effective corticosteroid therapy for T1R.

3 Type 2 Reaction or Erythema Nodosum Leprosum

3.1 Definition

Type 2 reaction (T2R) also known as Erythema nodosum leprosum (ENL) is an acute immune exacerbation encountered usually in smear positive MB patients and can occur before, during, or after multidrug treatment [5]. T2R occurs because of an antibody response to *M. leprae* antigens; the formation of antigen–antibody complexes which get deposited in the walls of capillary blood vessels and in other tissues triggering the complement cascade and inflammation. T2R is a neutrophil-mediated immune-complex reactional state, histologically defined by a prominent neutrophilic infiltrate throughout the granuloma with associated leukocytoclasis in the dermis and subcutis during the acute stage that is gradually replaced by lymphocytes with the evolution of the lesion.

3.2 Incidence

The incidence of T2R is increasing with the increasing number of multibacillary cases. T2R primarily affects individuals with LL and BL leprosy but may also occur in a small percentage of individuals with BB leprosy. Approximately 10% of patients with BL leprosy and up to 50–55% of those with LL leprosy are likely to develop ENL [6, 32].

Triggers Various factors have been implicated as triggers for the occurrence of T2R and include vaccinations, intercurrent infections such as malaria and typhoid, parasitic infestation, dental sepsis, pregnancy, parturition, severe psychological stress and hormonal changes. It is therefore prudent to look for and treat/manage these conditions in newly diagnosed smear positive MB patients to prevent the occurrence of ENL.

3.3   Etiopathogenesis

T2R is an immune complex-mediated systemic inflammatory response correspond-ing to Gell and Coombs Type III reaction that is triggered by the deposition of immune complexes; activation of complement system; and secretion of several pro-inflammatory cytokines in both skin lesions and peripheral blood. T2R is character-ized by high levels of TNF; intralesional neutrophil, eosinophil, and CD4+ T cell infiltrates; and prominent changes suggestive of vasculitis. Neutrophils are consid-ered as the 'signature cell' of T2R and contribute to the ENL-associated multi-sys-temic inflammation in multiple ways [33]. Bioinformatic pathway analysis of the gene expression profiles from ENL skin lesions have observed a role of an inte-grated axis comprising TLR2/FcR activation/neutrophil migration/inflammation as a mechanism of neutrophil recruitment in ENL [34]. Various steps in the immuno-pathogenesis of T2R are described in Fig. 2.

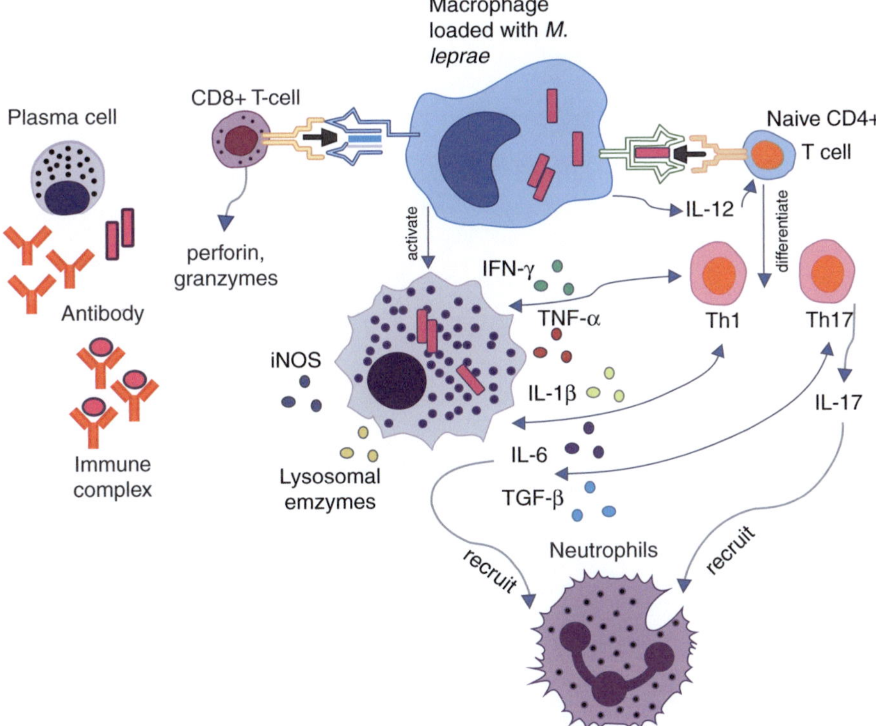

Fig. 2 Immunopathogenesis of ENL (Adapted from Luo Y et al. 2021)—Open source

3.4 Clinical Features

Various modes of onset are described for T2R [35]. It could be a *cutaneous onset* with multiple crops of evanescent, erythematous, tender nodules, and plaques commonly occurring over face, flexor aspect of forearms and medial aspects of the thighs (Picture 5). The lesions are often tender, warmer than the surrounding skin and blanch with light finger pressure. Some rare types include bullous, pustular, ulcerated, haemorrhagic, and erythema multiforme-like lesions (Picture 6). The *rheumatic onset type* typically presents with symmetrical involvement affecting the small joints of the hands and feet, in the so-called 'rheumatoid distribution'. Arthritis in T2R is usually acute in onset and lasts for a few weeks, and in most cases, resolves completely with treatment [36]. In the 'mixed onset' type both cutaneous and rheumatic symptoms are present simultaneously. T2R can also be associated with periostitis, usually involving the anterior aspect of the tibia. Neuritis is associated with T2R, which is usually insidious with episodes of acute flares.

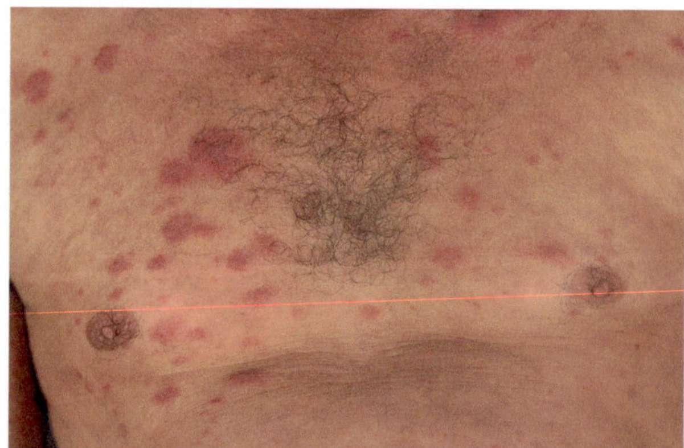

Picture 5 Type 2 reaction—erythematous nodules and plaques

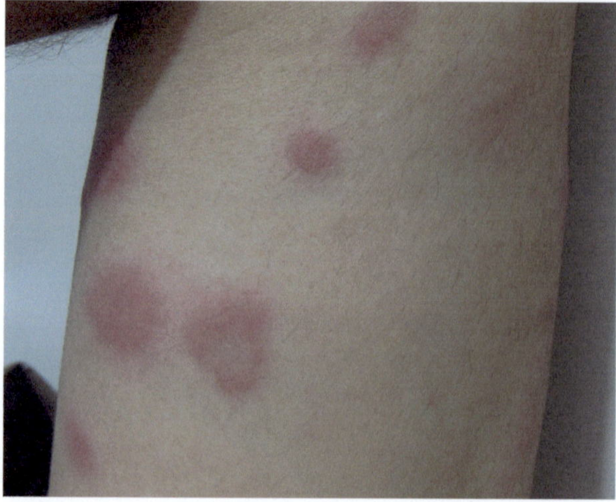

Picture 6 Type 2 reaction—erythema multiforme-like lesions (these lesions are difficult to perceive on the black skin)

While fever is regarded as one of the hallmarks of ENL, interestingly only 19.8% of patients had fever documented as a symptom. In severe T2R, there may be systemic involvement of other organs like testes with a reduction in testicular functions and eyes resulting in uveitis leading to blindness. Systemic involvement is less common now with the advent of MDT and early initiation of treatment. The natural course of untreated ENL is about 2–3 weeks, but the reaction can be recurrent with one episode overlapping another resulting in chronic ENL which may last many months and even after completion of FDT of 1 year [10, 37]. ENL is observed relatively common among younger females of childbearing age due to various biological reasons [38]. The clinical course of T2R is summarized in Box 3.

> **Box 3 Clinical course of T2R:**
> **Acute ENL**
> - It is one ENL episode lasting less than 6 months with a steady decrease in steroid tapering, no recurrence of ENL when receiving prednisolone, and no increase in severity requiring an increased steroid dose
>
> **Chronic ENL**
> - It is an episode lasting for more than 6 months
> - This could include single and multiple episodes
> - Patients with only one ENL episode with a borderline duration (5–6 months) can be considered as having chronic ENL if during the steroid tapering phase, they developed fresh ENL when receiving prednisolone and the steroid dose had to be increased
>
> **Steroid-Dependent ENL**
> - In these patients, tapering off the dose of systemic corticosteroids causes the patient to either get new ENL or had a worsening of their pre-existing ENL

3.4.1 Grading of ENL

An modified method to classify T2R has been developed by the ENLIST consortium based on the frequency of its occurrence. *Acute ENL*—A single episode lasting less than 2–4 weeks; *Recurrent ENL*—When a second or subsequent episode occurs after the treatment of the first acute episode. Recurrence rate of T2R is observed to be higher than T1R in leprosy patient [6]. *Chronic ENL*—When one episode overlaps another, and the patient requires continuous treatment for the T2R [39].

3.4.2 Complications

Neuritis occurs insidiously in T2R and not as an acute phenomenon as observed in T1R. However, patients who develop ENL reactions have a higher percentage of nerve complications when compared to non-reactional MB patients, as it leads to gradual deterioration in sensory, autonomic, and motor nerve function, occasionally to glove and stocking type of anaesthesia. Early recognition and treatment of T2R can stop the progress of NFI. Lepromatous patients who develop T1R are prone to develop more paralysed nerves than those who do not experience it.

ENL-associated uveitis occurs due to the direct effects of bacilli at the site as well as due to the *M. leprae* antibodies in the iris and anterior chamber. Left untreated it can produce adhesions to the lens, hypopyon and glaucoma leading to blindness. Effective treatment of the lepra reaction with corticosteroids, as well as use of mydriatics can be sight saving. The slow involvement of the testes in LL is heightened during T2R resulting in testicular pain and tenderness. Orchitis is usually associated with a drop in sperm count and can lead to sterility. In addition, as an immune complex disease, ENL can lead to synovitis, nephritis, hepatosplenomegaly, and lymphadenopathy. The intensity of these complications may vary from mild to severe and may last from a few weeks to months or even years.

3.4.3 Variants of ENL

Severe ENL includes necrotic ENL or erythema nodosum necroticans (ENN), which is a rare presentation seen in around 8% of patients. Other uncommon and severe variants of ENL, presenting with ulceronecrotic (Picture 7) and pustular lesions, have also been reported in the literature. This includes vesiculobullous, [40] Sweet's syndrome (SS)-like, (Picture 8) [41] erythema multiforme (EM)-like, Lucio phenomenon (LP), and reactive perforating type [42].

3.5 *Histopathology*

Histologically, the ENL lesion is characterized by an acute influx of polymorphs onto a background of macrophages which usually make up a lepromatous or borderline lepromatous histology. Dermal oedema and a mild rise in eosinophils and mast cells are present. Infiltration by neutrophils results in vasculitis, fibrinoid necrosis and panniculitis which are usual accompanying features [19]. As the reaction subsides, the acute stage cellular infiltrate is progressively replaced by lymphocytes and plasma cells. During ENL reactions, neutrophils may invade the nerves causing acute nerve abscesses which may cause extensive destruction of the nerve.

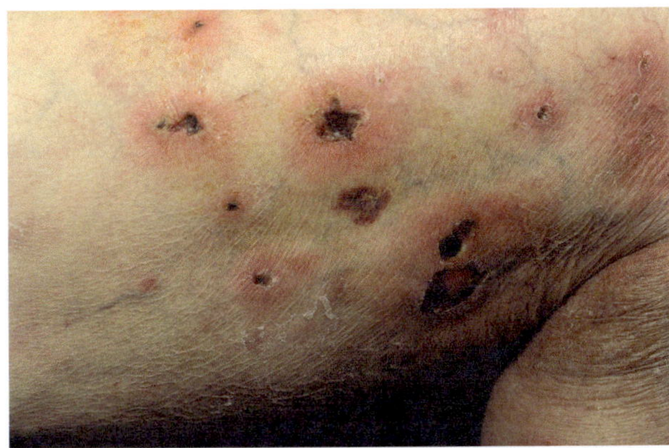

Picture 7 Type 2 reaction—ulceronecrotic lesions

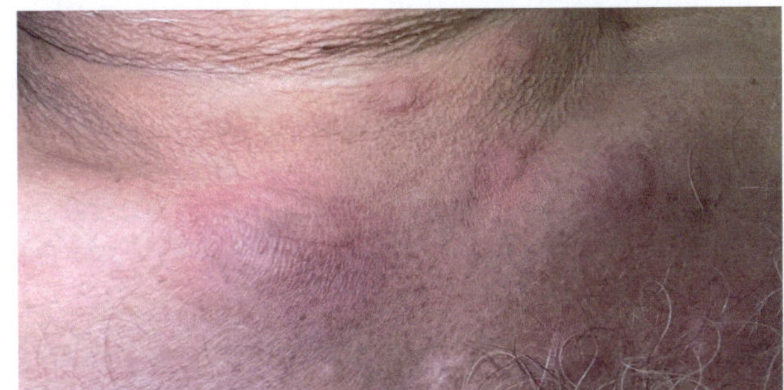

Picture 8 Type 2 reaction—Sweet's syndrome-like lesions

3.6 Differential Diagnosis

Nodular vasculitis, erythema nodosum, Sweet's syndrome, erythema induratum of Bazin and subcutaneous polyarteritis nodosa are important differentials in otherwise undiagnosed cases of leprosy. These can be differentiated based on characteristic clinical findings, and serological markers in case of autoimmune connective tissue diseases.

3.7 Laboratory Tests

Routine haematological investigations, kidney and liver function tests are needed in all suspected cases of T2R to know the extent of systemic involvement. They are also useful as screening investigations before corticosteroids/immunosuppressant drugs are given. Skin biopsy is often needed to confirm the diagnosis of ENL. Regular nerve function assessment is also indicated to monitor silent damage to nerves. A thorough ophthalmic examination is needed for all patients with ocular signs and symptoms, including a slit lamp examination, to identify early signs of uveitis and iridocyclitis.

3.8 Management of T2R

MDT should not be stopped in patients who develop T2R. The precipitating factors for reactions such as intercurrent infections and intestinal parasitic infestations should be appropriately treated. Corticosteroids forms the mainstay of therapy. The patient should be counselled about the symptoms and on the possible course of ENL. Ideally, they should be given a steroid card and steroid information leaflet that includes information on side effects, toxicity, and dangers of self-medication. It is important that patients are monitored by a clinician experienced in managing patients with ENL. The dose of corticosteroids required is dependent on the severity of the T2R and starting dose ranges from about 40–60 mg prednisolone per day (1 mg/kg body weight) for a duration for 3–6 weeks for each episode of ENL. However, as already mentioned, chronic ENL may need treatment up to 9 months or even beyond in patients with a high BI. A flow chart on how to start patients on corticosteroids for management of ENL along with dose optimization is given in the flowchart below. Weight gain, unmasking of diabetes, *Listeria monocytogenes* meningitis, cataracts in about 26% of patients and reactivation of tuberculosis in 3% are the major adverse effects associated with long-term use of corticosteroids. Steroid dependency due to adrenal insufficiency is a major challenge in management of chronic recurrent T2R and methods to overcome it is suggested in the flowchart of Box 4.

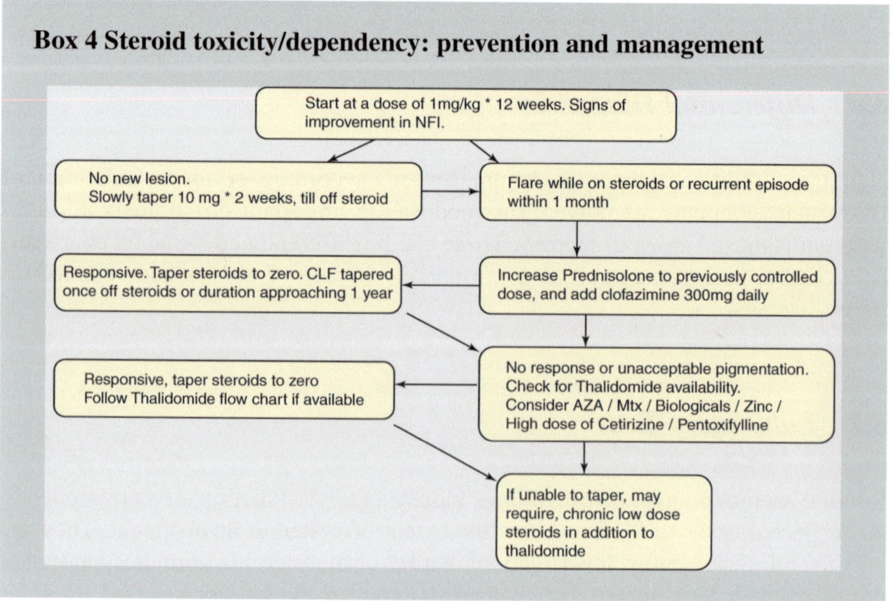

Clofazimine, which is an important component of MB MDT, also has anti-inflammatory properties and is useful in the treatment of T2R. The dosage recommended in T2R is a starting dose of 100 mg three times a day for 12 weeks, then reducing to 100 mg twice daily for the next 12 week and 100 mg once a day for 12 weeks. It is a slow-acting drug, and the effect is seen only after 4–6 weeks. Pigmentation of the skin and sclera as well as the crystallization with clofazimine is a major drawback with its use.

Thalidomide is an effective treatment for T2R and is a drug recommended by the World Health Organization (WHO) Expert Committee. Thalidomide is highly effective especially in the treatment of patients with chronic or recurrent ENL. It acts by inhibition of selective gene expression of tumour necrosis factor-α (TNF-α) which is involved in the pathogenesis of nerve damage in leprosy and by other mechanisms contributing to its anti-inflammatory effect [43]. Teratogenicity is a major risk with use of thalidomide and therefore is a good treatment option for males and post-menopausal females. If used in women of reproductive age group close monitoring is required involving counselling on avoiding pregnancy through use of double contraceptive methods. STEPS (System for Thalidomide Education and Prescribing Safety) monitoring protocol is one such online monitoring program.

The recommended starting dose of thalidomide is 300 mg per day, then reduced more slowly by 100 mg each month. During this period, the patient should be assessed to ensure that the ENL has not deteriorated. Any deterioration should be treated by increasing the thalidomide again for a few weeks. The patient should be stabilized on the lowest dose of thalidomide that controls the ENL and continue at this dose for a period of 2–3 months. Patients may require thalidomide for a duration of up to 1 year. Citing the risk of thrombosis with use of thalidomide, 75 mg of aspirin daily may be prescribed to prevent thrombosis. Major advantages of thalidomide are that it helps to attenuate steroid-induced morbidity and recurrence of ENL is lower (less than 6%) than with prednisolone (25%). Common adverse effects associated with the use of thalidomide are somnolence, constipation, nausea, headache, vertigo, pruritus, rash, and the inability to concentrate.

Other drugs found useful in different studies include Azathioprine, a purine antagonist which inhibits lymphocyte proliferation which has been used along with prednisolone for its steroid sparing effect. Few clinical studies have advocated a role for Methotrexate in the treatment of T2R; however, large trials are needed to confirm its benefit. Pentoxifylline acts by reducing the circulating levels of TNF-α, an action similar to thalidomide but not to the same effectiveness. Mycophenolate mofetil acts by inhibition of both B and T cell proliferation and blocking the production of guanosine nucleotides required for DNA synthesis, but it has doubtful benefit in type II but not in T1R (Table 2).

Table 2 Immunosuppressive agents for management of T2R

Immunosuppressive agent	Primary mechanism of action	Role
Corticosteroids	– Block transcription factors AP-1 and NF-kB – Inhibits synthesis of many pro-inflammatory cytokines	Treatment of choice
Thalidomide	Multiple dose-related mechanisms are described – Inhibits TNF – Stimulates IL-2. I – Inhibits IgM response – Promotes apoptosis in neutrophils	Treatment of choice
Methotrexate	– Anti-metabolite: inhibits lymphoid and myeloid proliferation	Beneficial
Cyclosporine	– Inhibits IL-2 and other cytokines	Good results, but not used in field conditions
Azathioprine	– Purine antagonist: inhibits lymphocyte proliferation: exact mechanism not known	Beneficial
Pentoxifylline	– Inhibits TNF and other cytokines	Conflicting results
Mycophenolate mofetil	– Blocks guanosine nucleotides. Inhibiting proliferation of T and B cells	Sparce data

Recently, the role of biological drugs, TNF-α inhibitors have been shown to play a role in the management of ENL. Etanercept 50 mg administered subcutaneously per week for 6 weeks and then tapered and given for 2 years has shown good response. Alternatively, Infliximab 5 mg/kg body weight can be used. Management options for the systemic involvement in ENL is summarized in Box 5.

Box 5 Management of multi-system involvement

Organ	Presentation	Appropriate referral + basic management
Eyes	Acute iridocyclitis Subacute uveitis	Referral to ophthalmologist is a must Rest to the eye with pad and bandage Mydriatics + local ocular corticosteroids, antibiotics
Joints	Arthralgia/arthritis	Thalidomide/corticosteroids Temporary immobilization Symptomatic treatment with analgesic
Bone	Periostitis: bone pain	Keeping the limb warm by pad and bandage/stockings Analgesics, sedatives, calcium
Testis	Orchitis	Bed rest. NSAIDS and oral corticosteroids Scrotal support using a wide triangular bandage

4 Lucio Phenomenon

4.1 Definition

Lucio Phenomenon (LP) sometimes referred to as type 3 lepra reaction is an uncommon reaction characterized by severe necrotizing cutaneous lesions that occurs in patients with Lucio's leprosy and lepromatous leprosy.

4.2 Epidemiology

Lucio phenomenon is one such rare reactional state seen peculiarly in the diffuse form of lepromatous leprosy (Lucio's leprosy) and less commonly in borderline forms. This phenomenon was first described by Lucio and Alvarado in Mexico in 1852 and further elaborated by Latapi and Zamora in 1948 [44] after the identification of histopathological changes involving multiple acute, necrotizing cutaneous vasculitis. It was considered a globally restricted phenomenon endemic to Mexico and Central America until sporadic cases were reported from non-endemic areas of the world, including the United States, Spain, Cuba, and countries in Southeast Asia, the Middle East, South America, and the South Pacific.

4.3 Etiopathogenesis

The most accepted hypothesis for the pathogenesis of LP is that bacterial liposaccharides stimulate active macrophages to release IL-1 and TNF-α which act on endothelial cells producing prostaglandins, IL-6 and coagulation factor-III, thus causing the formation of thrombi inside the vessels, promoting tissue necrosis, and a severe congestive vascular reaction which is usually haemorrhagic.

4.4 Clinical Features

Lucio phenomenon usually begins as painful purpuric lesions that evolve into well-defined, multi-angulated, jagged ulcerations with a geometric shape involving in the order of frequency—the feet, legs, hands, forearms, thighs, arms, and rarely, the trunk and face (Picture 9). Ulcers heal in about 2–8 weeks, leaving curvilinear jagged atrophic hypochromic scars with a surrounding halo of hyperpigmentation. There is an absence of associated fever, constitutional symptoms, and systemic involvement and neuritis.

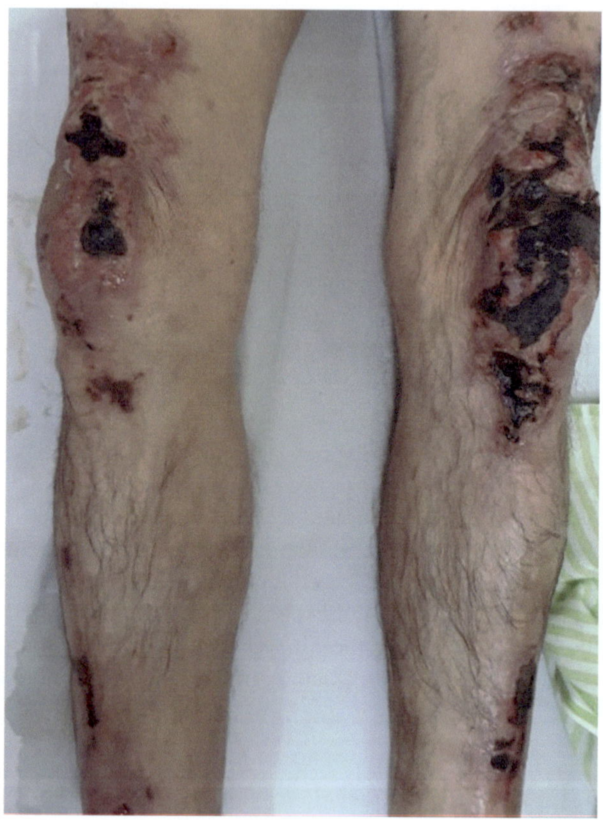

Picture 9 Lucio phenomenon

4.5 Histopathology

Lucio's phenomenon is characterized by a large number of AFB aggregates in the vascular endothelium, areas of fibrinoid necrosis, leukocytoclastic vasculitis, and ischemic epidermal necrosis. Lucio's phenomenon presents less neutrophil infiltration compared to erythema nodosum leprosum and confirmed colonization of endothelial cells by solid-staining AFB. Involvement of bone marrow and lymph nodes has been rarely described.

4.6 Differential Diagnosis

Lucio phenomenon should be differentiated from necrotizing erythema nodosum leprosum by following features; it occurs only in patients with non-nodular diffuse form of leprosy as erythematous spots of 0.5–1 cm in size, associated burning sensation and without localized infiltration which evolves into small superficial triangular or angular ulceration, that heals by leaving atrophic and hypochromic scars. It usually does not affect nerves, without any general symptoms or visceral damage.

4.7 Laboratory Diagnosis

Slit skin smear examination of Lucio phenomenon shows high positivity of bacteriological and morphological indices. Histopathology of the Lucio phenomenon is distinctive to distinguish it from ENL.

4.8 Management

Treatment of the Lucio phenomenon includes multibacillary multidrug therapy for leprosy, which includes rifampicin, dapsone, and clofazimine for 12 months. A short course of high-dose corticosteroids (1 mg/kg/day) can be effective in controlling the immune reaction in the initial phase, especially in severe cases. Unlike in classical ENL, thalidomide does not lead directly to clinical improvement in Lucio phenomenon, [45] compared to the use of corticosteroids.

References

1. Scollard DM, Smith T, Bhoopat L, Theetranont C, Rangdaeng S, Morens DM. Epidemiologic characteristics of leprosy reactions. Int J Lepr Other Mycobact Dis. 1994;62(4):559–67.
2. Walker SL, Lockwood DN. Leprosy type 1 (reversal) reactions and their management. Lepr Rev. 2008;79:372–86. https://doi.org/10.47276/lr.79.4.372.
3. Nery JA, Bernardes Filho F, Quintanilha J, Machado AM, de Oliveira SS, Sales AM. Understanding the type 1 reactional state for early diagnosis and treatment: a way to avoid disability in leprosy. An Bras Dermatol. 2013;88(5):787–92.
4. Walker SL. Chapter 2.2: Leprosy reactions. In: Scollard DM, Gillis TP, editors. International textbook of leprosy. Berlin: Springer; 2020. www.internationaltextbookofleprosy.org.
5. Kumar B, Dogra S, Kaur I. Epidemiological characteristics of leprosy reactions: 15 years experience from North India. Int J Lepr Other Mycobact Dis. 2004;72(2):125–33. https://doi.org/10.1489/1544-581X(2004)072<0125:ECOLRY>2.0.CO;2.
6. Nery JA, Vieira LM, de Matos HJ, Gallo ME, Sarno EM. Reactional states in multibacillary Hansen disease patients during multidrug therapy. Rev Inst Med Trop Sao Paulo. 1998;40(6):363–70. https://doi.org/10.1590/s0036-46651998000600005.
7. Jain S, Reddy RG, Osmani SN, Lockwood DN, Suneetha S. Childhood leprosy in an urban clinic, Hyderabad, India: clinical presentation and the role of household contacts. Lepr Rev. 2002;73(3):248–53.
8. Narang T, Kumar B. Leprosy in children. Indian J Paediatr Dermatol. 2019;20:12–24.
9. Bandeira SS, Pires CA, Quaresma JAS. Leprosy reactions in childhood: a prospective cohort study in the Brazilian Amazon. Infect Drug Resist. 2019;12:3249–57. https://doi.org/10.2147/IDR.S217181.

10. Rao PN, Suneetha S, Rathod SP, Narang T, Dogra S, Singal A, et al. Dermlep study part 3: post-RFT events in leprosy patients presenting to dermatologists. Indian Dermatol Online J. 2022;13:340–5.

11. van Brakel WH, Nicholls PG, Das L, Barkataki P, Suneetha SK, Jadhav RS, Maddali P, Lockwood DN, Wilder-Smith E, Desikan KV. The INFIR cohort study: investigating prediction, detection and pathogenesis of neuropathy and reactions in leprosy. Methods and baseline results of a cohort of multibacillary leprosy patients in North India [Erratum in: Lepr Rev 76(3):264]. Lepr Rev. 2005;76(1):14–34.

12. Lockwood DN, Suneetha L, Sagili KD, Chaduvula MV, Mohammed I, van Brakel W, Smith WC, Nicholls P, Suneetha S. Cytokine and protein markers of leprosy reactions in skin and nerves: baseline results for the North Indian INFIR cohort. PLoS Negl Trop Dis. 2011;5(12):e1327. https://doi.org/10.1371/journal.pntd.0001327.

13. Luo Y, Kiriya M, Tanigawa K, Kawashima A, Nakamura Y, Ishii N, Suzuki K. Host-related laboratory parameters for leprosy reactions. Front Med (Lausanne). 2021;22(8):694376. https://doi.org/10.3389/fmed.2021.694376.

14. Verhagen CE, Wierenga EA, Buffing AA, Chand MA, Faber WR, Das PK. Reversal reaction in borderline leprosy is associated with a polarized shift to type 1-like *Mycobacterium leprae* T cell reactivity in lesional skin: a follow-up study. J Immunol. 1997;159(9):4474–83.

15. Cooper CL, Mueller C, Sinchaisri TA, Pirmez C, Chan J, Kaplan G, Young SM, Weissman IL, Bloom BR, Rea TH, Modlin RL. Analysis of naturally occurring delayed-type hypersensitivity reactions in leprosy by in situ hybridization. J Exp Med. 1989;169(5):1565–81. https://doi.org/10.1084/jem.169.5.1565.

16. Misch EA, Macdonald M, Ranjit C, Sapkota BR, Wells RD, Siddiqui MR, et al. Human TLR1 deficiency is associated with impaired mycobacterial signaling and protection from leprosy reversal reaction. PLoS Negl Trop Dis. 2008;2:e231.

17. Hogeweg M, Kiran KU, Suneetha S. The significance of facial patches and type I reaction for the development of facial nerve damage in leprosy. A retrospective study among 1226 paucibacillary leprosy patients. Lepr Rev. 1991;62(2):143–9. https://doi.org/10.5935/0305-7518.19910016.

18. Lockwood DN, Lucas SB, Desikan KV, Ebenezer G, Suneetha S, Nicholls P. The histological diagnosis of leprosy type 1 reactions: identification of key variables and an analysis of the process of histological diagnosis. J Clin Pathol. 2008;61(5):595–600. https://doi.org/10.1136/jcp.2007.053389.

19. Suneetha S. Pathology of leprosy. In: Sacchidanand S, editor. IADVL Textbook of dermatology, vol 3. 5th ed. Mumbai: Balani Publishing House; 2022. p. 3747–57.

20. Ankad BS, Sakhare PS. Dermoscopy of borderline tuberculoid leprosy. Int J Dermatol. 2018;57(1):74–6. https://doi.org/10.1111/ijd.13731.

21. Chaduvula MV, Visser LH, Suneetha S, Suneetha L, Devaraju B, Ellanti R, Raju R, Jain S. High-resolution sonography as an additional diagnostic and prognostic tool to monitor disease activity in leprosy: a 2-year prospective study. Ultraschall Med. 2018;39(1):80–9. https://doi.org/10.1055/s-0042-108430.

22. Akita J, Miller LHG, Mello FMC, Barreto JA, Moreira AL, Salgado MH, Kirchner DR, Garbino JÁ. Comparison between nerve conduction study and high-resolution ultrasonography with color Doppler in type 1 and type 2 leprosy reactions. Clin Neurophysiol Pract. 2021;6:97–102. https://doi.org/10.1016/j.cnp.2021.02.003.

23. Rose P, Waters MF. Reversal reactions in leprosy and their management. Lepr Rev. 1991;62(2):113–21. https://doi.org/10.5935/0305-7518.19910013.

24. Lockwood DN, Vinayakumar S, Stanley JN, McAdam KP, Colston MJ. Clinical features and outcome of reversal (type 1) reactions in Hyderabad, India. Int J Lepr Other Mycobact Dis. 1993;61(1):8–15.

25. Roche PW, Theuvenet WJ, Britton WJ. Risk factors for type-1 reactions in borderline leprosy patients. Lancet. 1991;338(8768):654–7. https://doi.org/10.1016/0140-6736(91)91232-j.

26. Naafs B, Pearson JM, Wheate HW. Reversal reaction: the prevention of permanent nerve damage. Comparison of short and long-term steroid treatment. Int J Lepr Other Mycobact Dis. 1979;47(1):7–12.

27. WHO Technical Guidance Manual. Leprosy/Hansen disease: management of reactions and prevention of disabilities. Geneva: World Health Organization; 2020.
28. Kiran KU, Stanley JN, Pearson JM. The outpatient treatment of nerve damage in patients with borderline leprosy using a semi-standardized steroid regimen. Lepr Rev. 1985;56(2):127–34. https://doi.org/10.5935/0305-7518.19850016.
29. Kiran KU, Hogeweg M, Suneetha S. Treatment of recent facial nerve damage with lagophthalmos, using a semistandardized steroid regimen. Lepr Rev. 1991;62(2):150–4. https://doi.org/10.5935/0305-7518.19910017.
30. Naafs B. Treatment duration of reversal reaction: a reappraisal. Back to the past. Lepr Rev. 2003;74(4):328–36.
31. Virmond M, Joshua J, Solomon S, Duerksen F. Chapter 4.2: Surgical aspects in leprosy. In: Scollard DM, Gillis TP, editors. International textbook of leprosy. Berlin: Springer; 2017. www.internationaltextbookofleprosy.org.
32. Pocaterra L, Jain S, Reddy R, Muzaffarullah S, Torres O, Suneetha S, et al. Clinical course of erythema nodosum leprosum: an 11-year cohort study in Hyderabad, India. Am J Trop Med Hyg. 2006;74:868–79. https://doi.org/10.4269/ajtmh.2006.74.868.
33. Schmitz V, Tavares IF, Pignataro P, Machado ADM, Pacheco S, Schmitz V. Neutrophils in leprosy. Front Immunol. 2019;10:495. https://doi.org/10.3389/fimmu.2019.00495.
34. Lee DJ, Li H, Ochoa MT, Tanaka M, Carbone RJ, Damoiseaux R, et al. Integrated pathways for neutrophil recruitment and inflammation in leprosy. J Infect Dis. 2010;90095:558–69. https://doi.org/10.1086/650318.
35. Bhat RM, Vaidya TP. What is new in the pathogenesis and management of erythema nodosum leprosum. Indian Dermatol Online J. 2020;11(4):482–92. https://doi.org/10.4103/idoj.IDOJ_561_19.
36. Rai VM, Balachandran C. Necrotic erythema nodosum leprosum. Dermatol Online J. 2006;12:12.
37. Silva EA, Iyer A, Ura S, Lauris JR, Naafs B, Das PK, et al. Utility of measuring serum levels of anti-PGL-I antibody, neopterin and C-reactive protein in monitoring leprosy patients during multi-drug treatment and reactions. Trop Med Int Health. 2007;12:1450–8.
38. Negera E, Walker SL, Girma S, Doni SN, Tsegaye D, Lambert SM, et al. Clinicopathological features of erythema nodosum leprosum: a case-control study at ALERT hospital, Ethiopia. PLoS Negl Trop Dis. 2017;11(10):e0006011.
39. Walker SL, Sales AM, Butlin CR, Shah M, Maghanoy A, Lambert SM, et al. A leprosy clinical severity scale for erythema nodosum leprosum: an international, multicentre validation study of the ENLIST ENL severity scale. PLoS Negl Trop Dis. 2017;11:e0005716. https://doi.org/10.1371/journal.pntd.0005716.
40. Sethuraman G, Jeevan D, Srinivas CR, Ramu G. Bullous erythema nodosum leprosum (bullous type 2 reaction). Int J Dermatol. 2002;41:362–4.
41. Kou TT, Chan HL. Severe reactional state in lepromatous leprosy simulating Sweet's syndrome. Int J Dermatol. 1987;26(8):518–20. https://doi.org/10.1111/j.1365-4362.1987.tb02293.x.
42. Gunawan H, Yogya Y, Hafinah R, Marsella R, Ermawaty D, Suwarsa O. Reactive perforating leprosy, erythema multiforme-like reactions, sweet's syndrome-like reactions as atypical clinical manifestations of type 2 leprosy reaction. Int J Mycobacteriol. 2018;7(1):97–100. https://doi.org/10.4103/ijmy.ijmy_186_17.
43. Tadesse A, Abebe M, Bizuneh E, Mulugeta W, Aseffa A, Shannon EJ. Effect of thalidomide on the expression of TNF-alpha m-RNA and synthesis of TNF-alpha in cells from leprosy patients with reversal reaction. Immunopharmacol Immunotoxicol. 2006;28:431–41.
44. Vargas-Ocampo F. Diffuse leprosy of Lucio and Latapí: a histologic study. Lepr Rev. 2007;78(3):248–60.
45. Souza CS, Roselino AM, Figueiredo F, Foss NT. Lucio's phenomenon: clinical and therapeutic aspects. Int J Lepr Other Mycobact Dis. 2000;68(4):417–25.

Hansen's Disease in Children

Jerome S. Leonard and Jessica K. Fairley

1 Introduction

Pediatric Hansen's disease (HD-Leprosy), defined as cases that occur in individuals less than 15 years of age, is an important consideration for clinicians working in or with patients from endemic regions, as it represents active community transmission. The WHO designates HD as a neglected tropical disease (NTD) and reported 15,000 new pediatric cases, representing 7.4% of the total cases in 2019 [1]. The majority of pediatric cases are detected in India, Indonesia, and Brazil, with the remainder of cases primarily throughout southeast Asia and Africa [2]. However, Micronesia, Kiribati, the Comoros, and the Marshall Islands carry the highest per capita rate of pediatric disease [2].

In addition, there were 370 children reported with grade 2 disability (G2D) annually, signifying delayed diagnosis [1, 3]. The nerve damage and deformity caused by HD is irreversible and continues to carry significant social stigma, placing undue burdens on families and significantly affecting children's mental health and quality of life. With a variety of presentations, a prolonged incubation period and poor diagnostic measures, pediatric cases can be difficult to detect early and often require active contact tracing and community surveillance.

J. S. Leonard (✉) · J. K. Fairley
Emory University, Atlanta, GA, USA
e-mail: Jerome.stephen.leonard@emory.edu; Jessica.fairley@emory.edu

133

P. D. Deps (ed.), *Hansen's Disease*, https://doi.org/10.1007/978-3-031-30893-2_11

2 Epidemiology/Demographics

Children at the greatest risk of contracting Hansen's disease are those with prolonged, direct contacts of known cases, including immediate family members and those within living within the same household [4]. Some research has shown potential genetic susceptibility to HD [3] although the contribution of this genetic component remains unclear. Regardless, it is important to screen for HD among family and household contacts of detected cases and to have heightened clinical suspicion in the event of a family history of Hansen's disease.

Most studies demonstrate a slight prevalence of pediatric cases among males vs females [4–6]. Age does not appear to influence susceptibility, infants and adolescents are at the same risk of contracting HD. However, greater than 70% of pediatric cases are detected in the 10–15-year-old age group [4], which is likely due to the prolonged incubation period of the disease, and delay in seeking treatment until more advanced symptoms have developed [2, 5, 6].

3 Diagnostic Considerations

Due to its wide variety of potential presentations and differential diagnoses, HD can be misdiagnosed even at advanced stages. Children can present at any stage on the Ridley-Jopling scale (tuberculoid, borderline tuberculoid, borderline, borderline lepromatous, lepromatous), or the WHO scale, of paucibacillary (<5 lesions, no neuronal involvement) or multibacillary (≥5 lesions or neuronal involvement); however, they are more likely than adults to have paucibacillary disease [5].

The most common presentation in children is hypopigmented hypoesthetic macules [3, 4, 6] (Fig. 1). While hypoesthesia is the pathognomonic symptom, the hypoesthesia may be incomplete or difficult to elicit in younger children, resulting in lesions that are difficult to distinguish from other common rashes such as tinea,

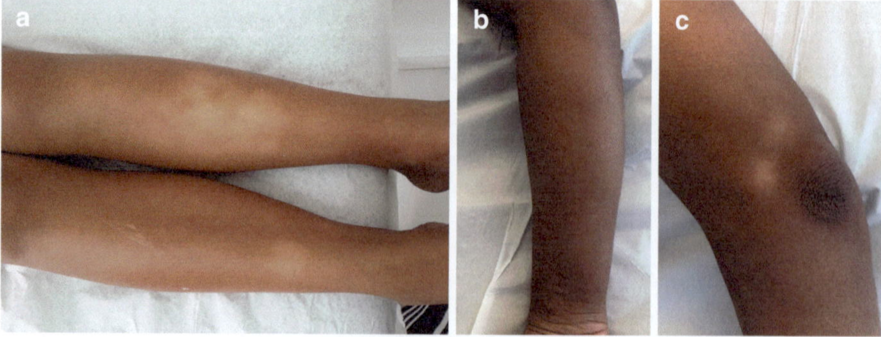

Fig. 1 HD hypochromic lesions on the legs and arm. (**a**) Indeterminate HD. (**b** and **c**) Borderline Tuberculoid HD

pityriasis, or vitiligo. Lesions can also appear as raised erythematous patches with or without central clearing, papules, or nodules but the hypoesthesia remains the primary diagnostic criteria. TT leprosy can present with papules or tubercles that may group in a few well-demarcated plaques or annular lesions and may or may not be associated with erythema. It has been noted that nodular HD (also known as infantile nodular leprosy), a subset of tuberculoid disease is a presentation almost exclusively seen in children, and often consists of a single nodular lesion commonly on the face [7].

Another common symptom useful to differentiate HD from other common rashes is anhydrosis [4, 6] which can be helpful in establishing diagnosis especially when hypoesthesia is difficult to elicit or absent. While lesions can appear anywhere *M. leprae* has a predilection for peripheral nerves in cooler areas of the body, commonly upper and lower limbs and the face. Figure 1 shows some typical skin lesions in children.

Laboratory diagnostics, such as slit-skin smears and biopsies, can be helpful but have low sensitivity in children. Slit-skin smears are relatively easy to obtain but lesions are rarely positive for bacilli in paucibacillary cases. While biopsies are more sensitive, only about 50% of cases have histopathology consistent with diagnosis [5], and biopsies can be difficult to obtain in endemic areas.

It is important to keep in mind that families may not seek treatment until later stages of disease when there is notable neuronal involvement, development of disability or during a Type 1 (lepra, or reversal reaction) or Type 2 (erythema nodosum leprosum) reaction. Detecting grade 1 disability (G1D), (anesthesia without visible deformity) and grade 2 disability (G2D) (physical impairments or deformity) are key to preventing worsening pediatric morbidity. G2D commonly presents as hand, foot, or ocular deformity. Hand disability includes "claw hand" due to ulnar nerve involvement, contractures, or atrophy of thenar or hypothenar muscles. Foot involvement typically presents as foot drop or ulceration on the soles of the feet. Ocular involvement is rare but generally presents as lagophthalmos, and in advanced cases, loss of vision [4, 8].

Type 1 reactions present additional complications for morbidity in that they can initiate or rapidly exacerbate neurologic or physical disability and can present at any time during illness or treatment. Type 1 reactions (T1R) and Type 2 erythema nodosum leprosum reactions (T2R or ENL) appear to be slightly less common overall in pediatric disease when compared with adults [9]; however, reactions may also be more common in children with paucibacillary or single lesion disease when compared to adults with similar disease burden [9].

Type 1 reactions are due to a robust cell-mediated response with acute neuritis, swelling of cutaneous or neuronal lesions, or development of new lesions. Signs of reaction are usually localized to the original lesions with fever and systemic involvement uncommon [3]. While rare, children with lesions on the face are at increased risk of developing lagophthalmos and ocular involvement in the event they develop a type I reaction [10].

Erythema nodosum leprosum reactions are due to a systemic immune complex deposition and presents similarly to erythema nodosum with the development of tender papules and nodules across the body, not limited to sites of lesions, fever and systemic involvement are common including migrating polyarthralgia's, lymphadenitis, bone pain, and in rare cases, nephritis [6, 10, 11].

Close follow-up and neurologic monitoring during treatment is important to detect these reactions. Follow-up visits should always include full neurologic evaluation and monitoring of muscle strength and light sensation with monofilaments to detect any worsening of symptoms, in order to promptly initiate treatment.

4 Prevention

Prevention of HD is a difficult task but the Bacillus Calmette–Guérin (BCG) vaccine at birth and single dose rifampicin (SDR) therapy in exposed contacts have shown some efficacy at prevention; however, while endorsed by the WHO, this has not been adopted in many countries including Brazil and the USA. The BCG vaccine at birth has shown about 55% reduction in risk for contracting Hansen's disease [3] and is recommended at birth for all high-burden countries by the WHO.

For children >2 years exposed to Hansen's disease, the WHO recommends using a single dose of rifampicin (SDR) as chemoprophylaxis, which has shown a 57% reduction in Hansen's disease over 2 years and 30% reduction over 5 years [3]. When used in a patient who has also received the BCG vaccine, the risk reduction improves to 80% over 2 years with single dose rifampicin. This intervention is recommended by the WHO only once TB and Hansen's disease are excluded, and only for programs that can both obtain the consent of the index case to disclose their disease status and ensure adequate management of contacts.

5 Pediatric Treatment Considerations

The standard treatment regimen for Hansen's disease of rifampin or rifampicin, dapsone, and clofazimine are all recommended as first-line in pediatric patients. Weight-based dosage is recommended instead of standard adult doses. The WHO does provide pediatric dosed "blister packs" of rifampicin, dapsone, and clofazimine for children 10–14 years old and >40 kg for both paucibacillary and multibacillary treatment regimens.

For resistant strains requiring alternate treatment regimens, tetracyclines such as minocycline are not recommended in children under 9 years of age due to the risk of enamel hypoplasia and permanent tooth discoloration, and fluoroquinolones (levofloxacin, moxifloxacin) are not recommended for use in pediatric patients due to risk of tendon rupture and arthralgias.

References

1. World Health Organization. Towards zero leprosy. Global leprosy (Hansen's Disease) strategy 2021–2030. 2021
2. World Health Organization. World Health Organization's Global Health Observatory Leprosy Database. 2022. Accessed Aug 2022. https://www.who.int/data/gho/data/themes/topics/leprosy-hansens-disease
3. World Health Organization. Guidelines for the diagnosis, treatment and prevention of leprosy. 2018.
4. Rodrigues TS, Gomes LC, Cortela DC, Silva EA, Silva CA, Ferreira SM. Factors associated with leprosy in children contacts of notified adults in an endemic region of Midwest Brazil. J Pediatric (Rio J). 2020;96(5):593–9. https://doi.org/10.1016/j.jped.2019.04.004.
5. Ghunawat S, Relhan V, Mittal S, Sandhu J, Garg VK. Childhood leprosy: a retrospective descriptive study from Delhi. Indian J Dermatol. 2018;63(6):455–8. https://doi.org/10.4103/ijd.IJD_99_17.
6. American Academy of Pediatrics. Committee on Infectious Diseases. Red book: report of the committee on infectious diseases. Elk Grove Village, IL: American Academy of Pediatrics; 2018.
7. Fakhouri R, Sotto MN, Manini MI, Margarido LC. Nodular leprosy of childhood and tuberculoid leprosy: a comparative, morphologic, immunopathologic and quantitative study of skin tissue reaction. Int J Lepr Other Mycobact Dis. 2003;71:218–26.
8. Rusyati LM. Characteristics of Grade 2 disability in Indonesian children with leprosy: a five-year multicenter retrospective study. Clin Cosmet Investig Dermatol. 2021;14:1149–53. https://doi.org/10.2147/CCID.S325858. PMID: 34511959; PMCID: PMC8420076
9. Sehgal VN, Chaudhry AK. Leprosy in children: a prospective study. Int J Dermatol. 1993;32(3):194–7.
10. World Health Organization. Leprosy/Hansen Disease: Management of reactions and prevention of disabilities. 2020.
11. Scollard DM, Martelli CM, Stefani MM, Maroja Mde F, Villahermosa L, Pardillo F, Tamang KB. Risk factors for leprosy reactions in three endemic countries. Am J Trop Med Hyg. 2015;92(1):108–14. https://doi.org/10.4269/ajtmh.13-0221. Epub 2014 Dec 1. PMID: 25448239; PMCID: PMC4347363

Neuropathophysiology in Morbus Hansen or Hansen's Disease: Mechanisms of Nerve Injury

Bernard Naafs and Marlous L. Grijsen

1 Nose and Skin

Morbus Hansen (MH) is caused by *Mycobacterium (M). leprae* and *M. lepromatosis*. The infection is believed to be acquired through the nasal mucosa and/or small skin injuries. When the infection with live, dead, or fragmented bacilli has entered, these bacilli come in blood and lymph where they are phagocytosed by macrophages. *M. leprae* bacilli can multiply in these macrophages and other phagocytic cells (Schwann cells), at least in those individuals whose host cells can be turned on to support *M. leprae* bacilli [1].

When the antigens circulate in blood and lymph, they are exposed to the immune system. Together with the innate, both the humeral and the cellular adaptive immune system will respond, whether the host will develop "MH" or not.

B. Naafs (✉)
Stichting Global Dermatology Munnekeburen, Friesland, The Netherlands

Regional Dermatology Training Centre (RDTC), Moshi, Tanzania

Instituto Lauro de Souza Lima (ILSL), Bauru, São Paulo, Brazil
e-mail: benaafs@dds.nl

M. L. Grijsen
Centre for Tropical Medicine and Global Health, Nuffield Department of Medicine, University of Oxford, Oxford, UK

Eijkman-Oxford Clinical Research Unit, Jakarta, Indonesia

P. D. Deps (ed.), *Hansen's Disease*, https://doi.org/10.1007/978-3-031-30893-2_12

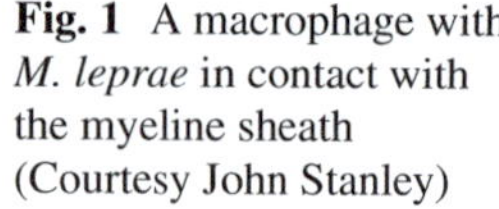

Fig. 1 A macrophage with *M. leprae* in contact with the myeline sheath (Courtesy John Stanley)

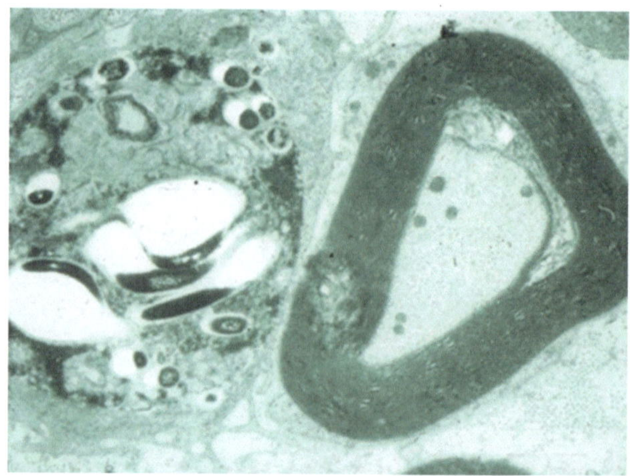

2 The Nerve

M. leprae has a predilection for Schwann cells and macrophages in the skin and peripheral nerves. The bacilli survive and multiply in places with a relatively low temperature (32–35 °C). It is difficult for the bacilli to enter the nerve fibres because there are no lymph vessels in the endoneurium. They must enter through the bloodstream and pass the so-called blood–nerve barrier. Graham Weddell observed that MH-related damage occurred at locations where there is movement, for example, the wrist, elbow, knee, and ankle (personal communication). Nerves move there against bone or tunnel wall, such movements cause friction and lead to microtraumata triggering an reparation response.

The endothelial cells of the blood vessels in the endoneurium then express adhesion molecules [2]. Macrophages, some loaded with *M. leprae* antigens will adhere to the endothelial cells and enter via diapedesis into the endoneurium, where they encounter the Schwann cells (Fig. 1). *M. leprae* then invades the Schwann cells as suggested by Anura Rambukkana, using PGL-1 and other surface molecules, leading to proliferation and/or demyelination [3].

3 Damage due to *M. Leprae* Antigens

It is shown that PGL-1 alone, expressed by macrophages, can cause demyelination [4]. Nawal Bahia El Idrissi, et al. showed that another important *M. leprae* surface antigen, lipoarabinomannan, can cause demyelination by complement activation (membrane attack complex (MAC)) [5]. These findings suggest that the presence of antigens alone, without live bacilli, might be a sufficient cause for segmental demyelination, which is the hallmark of MH.

It is important to note that PGL-1 is broken down relatively quickly, whereas lipoarabinomannan may be present for years and may continue to cause damage [6].

Similarly, Toll-like receptors on the Schwann cells such as TLR9, which binds to circulating DNA, and TLR1, 2 and 4, which bind to mycobacterial antigens, maybe a persistent cause of MH-related pathology [7]. This could explain why MH contacts can develop damage without having MH as actual disease [8].

4   Nerve Damage due to Reactions

Most of the MH-related damage occurs during reactions, episodes of exacerbated inflammation in the chronic phase of the infection when there is an increase in immune reactivity. Cell-Mediated Immunity (CMI) at the tuberculoid pole (Th1 response) Type−1-MH Reaction (T-1-MHR) as opposed to the humeral (Th2 response) Type-2-MH Reaction (T-2-MHR) at the lepromatous pole [9, 10].

Nerve damage may occur at three levels:

1. at the skin where the nerve endings are affected
2. at the subcutaneous nerves
3. at the nerve trunks

4.1   In the Skin

The histopathology of reactional tuberculoid MH [11] shows granuloma formation high in the dermis and dermal papillae. This infiltrate may erode the epidermis and destroys the nerve endings in the papillae. It is not unlikely that the driving force behind these damaging reactions is antigenic determinants in the epidermis and in the nerve endings, which are identical to those of *M. leprae* (antigenic mimicry). This reaction could be an autoimmune phenomenon (Fig. 2) [12].

In borderline MH, the nerves of the lower dermis and especially those located around the adnexa are most often involved. Granuloma formation can be seen in and

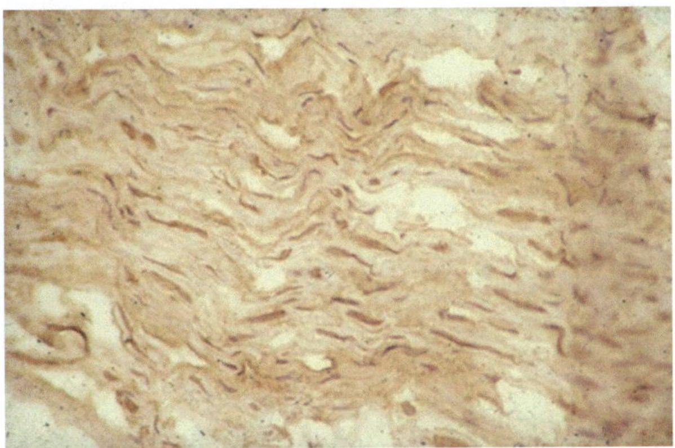

Fig. 2 A normal nerve stained with monoclonal antibodies against *M. lepra* (Courtesy Ben Naafs)

around these nerves together with a proliferation of Schwann cells in and around the perineurium. Damage can be attributed to compression and destruction of the nerve fibres by the epithelioid granuloma. During the reactional episode, there is an influx of immunocompetent cells with oedema formation and expanding granuloma. This contributes to further nerve damage, especially when extracellular oedema accumulates inside the thickened neural sheaths, converting it into a rigid tube compromising the axons inside [13].

4.2 In Large Subcutaneous Nerves and Nerve Trunks

The mechanisms that occur here are more complicated. At the tuberculoid end of the spectrum, these processes are like those in the skin, with massive granuloma formation with occasional colliquation and abscess formation. Further into the borderline range, these features are usually less distinct and often even absent. Frequently only oedema is observed [13].

Damage to cutaneous and subcutaneous nerves causes loss of sensation in the affected areas and loss of autonomic nerve function like sweating and regulation of vascular tone. However, it is the damage to the peripheral nerve trunks which is the major consequence of reactions. This damage is partly caused by the immune system, but mechanical factors are also involved [13] (Fig. 3). During a T-1-MHR (increased CMI), inflammation and consequently oedema occurs in the nerve. The reaction leads to oedema located within the interstitial tissues of the epi-, peri-, and

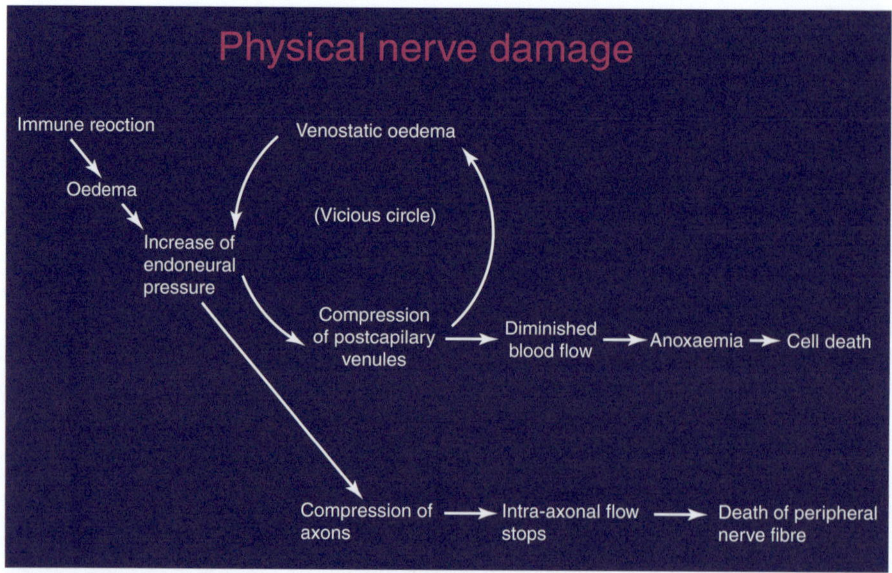

Fig. 3 Immune damage leading to physical damage (Courtesy Ben Naafs)

endoneurium. Unlike the skin, the nerve cannot expand much, limited by its sheaths. The perineurium, which is largely impermeable to fluids, forms a rigid compressing tube around the expanding endoneurium. This results in an increase in pressure within the nerve. As a result, the axons in the endoneurium are compressed by the increased pressure and stop conducting leading to loss of muscular strength, sensation, and autonomic functions (Fig. 3). The intra-axonal flow which brings nutrients from the cell body to the peripheral nerve ending is interrupted, and sooner or later the nerve fibre dies and is destroyed [14].

When the pressure on and the tension along the perineurium increase due to the increase of the pressure in the endoneurium, there is an increase in the pressure on the blood vessels, which transverse obliquely through the perineurium. These blood vessels then become compressed, the venules with relatively low pressure more than the arterioles with higher pressure. The compression of the venules will lead to higher pressure in the capillaries of the endoneurium, which may start "leaking" and thus increase the pressure in the endoneurium. This "venostatic oedema" can maintain itself even when the immunological events subside [14] (Figs. 3 and 4).

In T-2-MHR, the mechanisms leading to tissue destruction, i.e. activation of granulocytes, contribute to damage of nerves fibres and endings. It also has been shown that the cytokines involved are able to demyelinise the nerve fibres. Demyelination seems to be the major nerve damage in multibacillary MH as shown by nerve conduction studies. The damage in multibacillary leprosy may also be caused by lipoarabinomannan that on its own can lead to demyelination by complement activation and MAC formation when in contact with the Schwann cells [5]. Moreover, in the large nerve trunks, the immunological processes may give rise to venostatic oedema with compression of axons similar as described for T-1-MHR.

A recent report may support parts of the above-presented theories: "We observed that viable and dead bacteria distinctly modulate Schwann cell genes, with emphasis to viable bacilli upregulating transcripts related to glial cell plasticity, dedifferentiation and anti-inflammatory profile, while dead bacteria affected genes involved

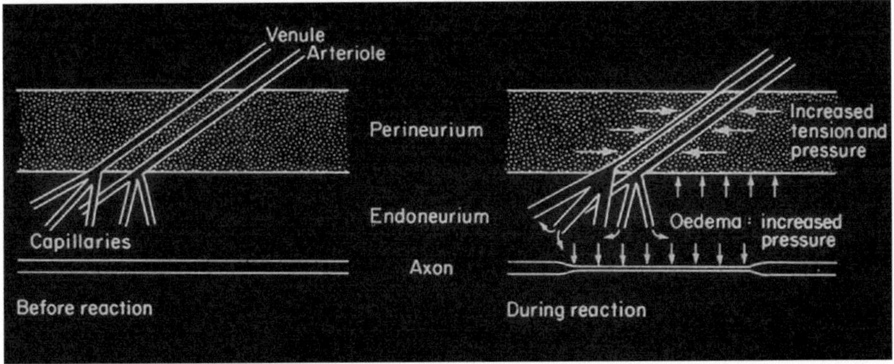

Fig. 4 The pressure on the perineurium compresses the venules more than arterioles which both pass obliquely through the perineurium because the pressure in the venules is lower (Courtesy Ben Naafs)

in neuropathy and pro-inflammatory response. In addition, dead bacteria also upregulated genes associated with nerve support, which expression profile was similar to those obtained from leprosy nerve biopsies. These findings suggest that early exposure to viable and dead bacteria may provoke Schwann cells to behave differentially, with far-reaching implications for the ongoing neuropathy seen in leprosy patients, where a mixture of active and non-active bacteria are found in the nerve microenvironment" [15].

After all these occurrences, the nerve may end as a fibrotic string and the patient is severely disabled. With the knowledge available this can be prevented, provided there are clinicians to diagnose the disease and complications in time and provide proper treatment.

References

1. Naafs B. Why can't we control Morbus Hansen? Info Hansen. 2020. https://en.infohansen.org/resources/blog/morbus-hansen.
2. Scollard DM. Endothelial cells and the pathogenesis of lepromatous neuritis: insights from the armadillo model. Microbes Infect. 2000;2(15):1835–43.
3. Rambukkana A, Zanazzi G, Tapinos N, Salzer JL. Contact-dependent demyelination by mycobacterium leprae in the absence of immune cells. Science. 2002;296(5569):927–31.
4. Madigan CA, Cambier CJ, Kelly-Scumpia KM, Scumpia PO, Cheng T-Y, Zailaa J, et al. A macrophage response to mycobacterium leprae phenolic glycolipid initiates nerve damage in leprosy. Cell. 2017;170(5):973–985.e10.
5. Bahia El Idrissi N, Das PK, Fluiter K, Rosa PS, Vreijling J, Troost D, et al. M. Leprae components induce nerve damage by complement activation: identification of lipoarabinomannan as the dominant complement activator. Acta Neuropathol (Berl). 2015;129(5):653–67.
6. Verhagen C, Faber W, Klatser P, et al. Immunohistological analysis of in situ expression of mycobacterial antigens in skin lesions of leprosy patients across the histopathological spectrum. Association of Mycobacterial lipoarabinomannan (LAM) and mycobacterium leprae phenolic glycolipid-I (PGL-I) with leprosy reactions. Am J Pathol. 1999;154(6):1793–804.
7. Polycarpou A, Holland MJ, Karageorgiou I, et al. Mycobacterium leprae Activates Toll-Like Receptor-4. Signaling and Expression on Macrophages Depending on previous Bacillus Calmette-Guerin Vaccination. Front Cell Infect Microbiol. 2016;6:72. Published 2016 Jul 8. https://doi.org/10.3389/fcimb.2016.00072.
8. Shetty VP, Mehta LN, Antia NH, et al. Teased fibre study of early nerve lesions in leprosy and in contacts, with electrophysiological correlates. J Neurol Neurosurg Psychiatry. 1977;40(7):708–11.
9. Verhagen CE, Wieringa EEA, Buffing AAM, et al. Reversal reaction in borderline leprosy is associated with a polarized shift to Type-1-like mycobacterium leprae T cell reactivity in lesional skin: a follow-up study. J Immunol. 1997;159:4474–83.
10. Naafs B. Leprosy reactions: new knowledge. Trop Geogr Med. 1994;46:80–4.
11. Noto S, Clapasson A, Nunzi E. Classification of leprosy: the mystery of reactional tuberculoid. G Ital Dermatol Venerol. 2007;142:294–5.
12. Naafs B, Kolk AHJ, Lien Ram CA, et al. Anti-mycobacterium leprae monoclonal antibodies cross-reactive with human skin. An alternative explanation for the immune responses in leprosy. J Invest Dermatol. 1990;94:685–8.

13. Naafs B. Nerve damage and repair. Hyderabad, India (AIFO): International leprosy congress; 2008. http://www.aifo.it/english/resources/online/books/leprosy/ila-india08/nerve-damageBen_Naafs.pdf
14. Naafs B, Van Droogenbroeck JBA. Décompression des névrites réactionnelles dans la lèpre: justification physopathologique et méthodes objectives pour en apprécier les résultats. Méd Trop. 1977;37:763–70.
15. Junqueira de Souza B, Abud Mendes M, Sperandio da Silva GM, et al. Gene Expression Profile of Mycobacterium leprae contribution in the pathology of leprosy neuropathy. Front Med. 2022;2022:929. https://doi.org/10.3389/fmed.2022.861586.

Neurological Alterations In Hansen's Disease

Francisco Almeida

1 Introduction

Once *Mycobacterium leprae* infection is established, there is lymphatic and hematogenous spread by the pathogen. Admittedly, there is an early affinity for parasitism to the Schwann's cell. Despite the emphasis on skin lesions caused by Hansen's disease, it is fundamentally important to emphasize that the disease is primarily a neural pathology [1].

Thus, the extensive network of innervation that is distributed throughout the skin promotes the occurrence of visible or merely autonomous skin changes. However, peripheral nerve trunks are affected together with the skin or separately, for reasons not yet satisfactorily elucidated, characterizing cases of primary neural Hansen's disease [2].

The inflammatory process resulting from infection in the peripheral nerves is responsible for the various clinical manifestations of Hansen's disease neuropathy, which are worsened during reactional episodes [3].

All peripheral nerves in addition to target organs such as the eyeball and testicles can be compromised by Hansen's disease, but the affected extremities (hands and feet) exhibit the severe neural compromise of Hansen's disease that leads to permanent and irreversible disabilities. The involvement of the extremities can be verified with several patterns described, from multiple mononeuropathies or polyneuropathies [4–6].

All clinical forms of the disease will present neural involvement. Although classically not described in indeterminate Hansen's disease, there are articles that demonstrate cases where clinically and histopathologically, skin lesions compatible with the indeterminate clinical form showed significant involvement of peripheral nerve trunks [7].

F. Almeida (✉)
Mauricio de Nassau University Center, Recife, Pernambuco, Brazil

P. D. Deps (ed.), *Hansen's Disease*, https://doi.org/10.1007/978-3-031-30893-2_13

Thus, considering leprosy as a systemic infection, it can be assumed that there is no involvement of a single isolated nerve although there may be a greater or lesser clinical expression in a particular nerve, without ruling out the involvement of other nerves.

This chapter is dedicated to describing the clinical neurological alterations of Hansen's disease, which, when not evidenced in a timely manner, may represent a lack of early diagnosis, resulting in an advanced disease involvement.

2 Upper Limb Innervation and Alterations Caused by Hansen's Disease

2.1 The Ulnar Nerve

The ventral branch of the C8 and T1 nerve roots join to form the inferior nerve trunk of the brachial plexus. This lower nerve trunk, in turn, is divided into anterior and posterior, giving rise to the ulnar nerve fibers from the anterior division. These fibers run from the *axillae* to the medial aspect of the anterior compartment of the upper arm. The ulnar nerve is a mixed nerve, which contains both motor and sensory axons. It is fundamentally clinically important the recognition of the anatomical site to access possible changes in relation to its consistency and/or diameter, as well as the terminal areas that will in turn lead to the sensory-motor changes in Hansen's disease (Fig. 1a) [8, 9].

Initial sensory changes will lead to loss of sensitivity in the dermatome highlighted in Fig. 1c, d, which can be measured using Siemens-Weinstein monofilaments, according to the World Health Organization disability (WHO) scale [10].

The ulnar nerve supplies all the muscles in the hypothenar region. When crossing the deep part of the hand, it also supplies all the interosseous muscles and the third and fourth lumbrical muscles. Finally, it also innervates the adductor *pollicis* and the medial head of the flexor *pollicis brevis*. This musculature will suffer amyotrophy, which will induce the evident semiflexion of the fifth and fourth fingers as well as a loss of strength in the regions responsible for its innervation, limiting and disabling the execution of many movements (Fig. 1b). Pain is a striking symptom in most patients who are going through episodes of acute or chronic neuritis [11, 12].

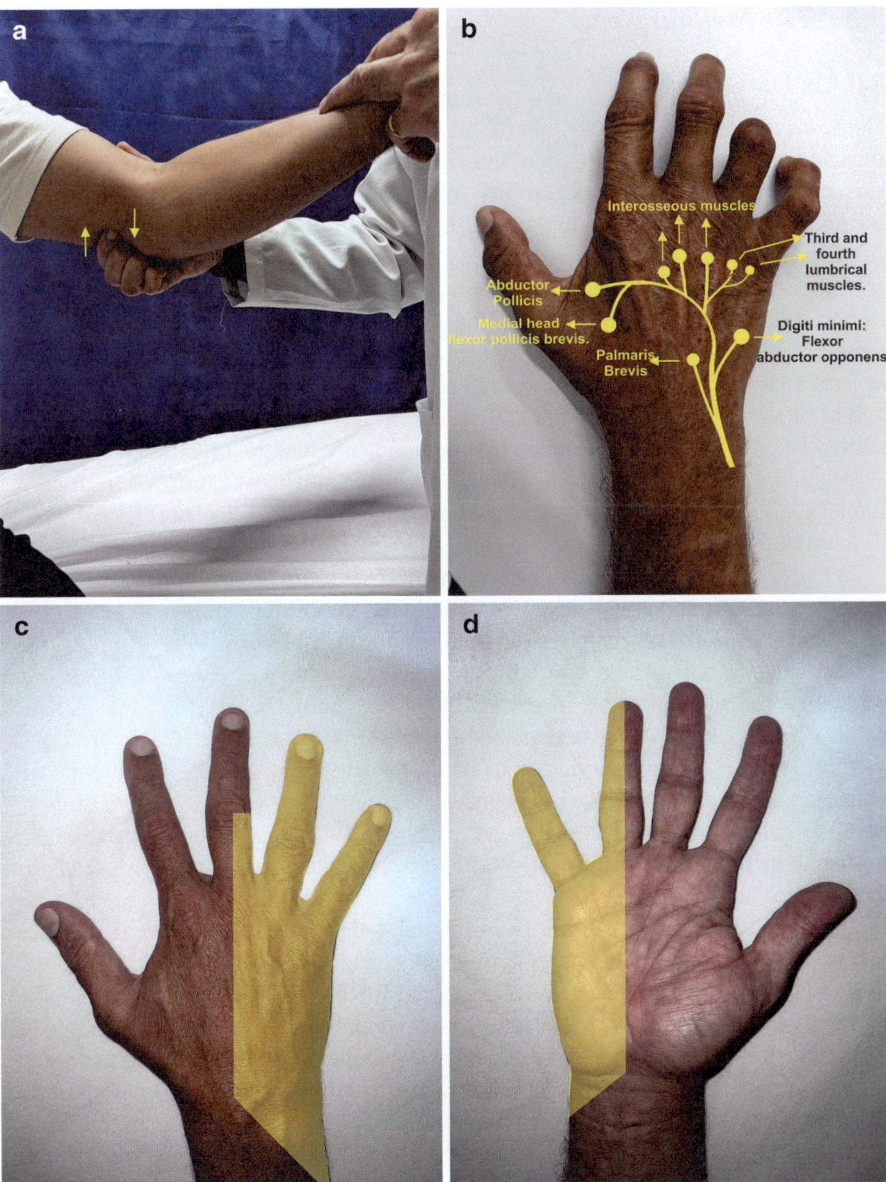

Fig. 1 Ulnar nerve. (**a**) Semiotic technique of palpation of the ulnar nerve. Slightly above and medially to the epitroclean gutter, search the ulnar nerve with gentle up and down movements, gradually increasing the pressure until you feel the nerve under the distal phalanges of the second and third fingers. (**b**) Motor innervation of the hand supplied by the ulnar nerve. Note the amiotrophies and involuntary flexion of the fingers. (**c**) Sensory territory of the dorsum of the hand supplied by the ulnar nerve. (**d**) The sensory territory of the palmar region supplied by the ulnar nerve

2.2　*The Median Nerve*

The median nerve is also a sensory-motor nerve that is usually also affected by Hansen's disease. It is responsible for a large area of tenderness on the palm side of the hand, from the central region of the wrist to the hypothenar region. On the dorsal surface of the hand, the responsibility for the sensitivity of the distal phalanges of the second and third fingers and medially 50% of the distal phalanx of the second finger is verified [13].

It is responsible for pronation, flexion of the first three fingers and wrist, in addition to antepulsion and opposition of the pollux (Fig. 2b). From the beginning of its course in the brachial plexus to its terminal branches, this nerve passes through several anatomical regions where it can be compressed, mainly in the carpal tunnel and in the pronator teres. Anatomical variations have been described, with the possibility of communication between the median nerve and the ulnar nerve [14].

Median nerve involvement in Hansen's disease is usually confused with carpal tunnel syndrome (CTS), even with the knowledge that most cases of CTS are related to traumatic, vascular, or metabolic causes [15].

When affected by Hansen's disease, median nerve involvement can be followed by ulnar nerve involvement, even in subclinical conditions, often evidenced only with well-conducted electrophysiological studies [16, 17].

Ultrasonography can be a good tool to help distinguish between CTS of other etiologies and median nerve involvement by Hansen's disease (Fig. 3a). Nagappa et al. (2021) analyzed 26 patients with Hansen's disease and CTS, finding an increase in the cross-sectional area at all measurement points in patients with Hansen's disease, with a maximum increase of 2 cm proximal to the wrist crease and gradual proximal reduction. In patients with CTS, this observed increase was maximal in distal wrist crease. Neural decompression surgery can demonstrate these observations [18].

Sensitive alterations resulting from median nerve involvement can also be seen in the corresponding innervation dermatomes (Fig. 5). It is important to mention that in Hansen's disease, due to the precarpal involvement, the sensory loss is not restricted to the areas of the distal extremities of the fingers, but also to the region of the palms of the hands. This fact can contribute to the differential diagnosis between the two conditions, especially with the use of Semmes-Weinstein monofilaments (MFSW) (Fig. 2c, d) [19].

Motor impairment in Hansen's disease leads to functional loss, mainly affecting pinch and grip functions. In severe cases, there is also retraction of the third finger, almost always followed by involvement of the ulnar nerve, with retraction of the fourth and fifth fingers accompanying the changes. Palmar amyotrophies will also be present [20].

Therefore, within an epidemiological scenario where Hansen's disease is present, one of the main etiological suspicions of CTS when other possibilities are ruled out, should be Hansen's disease making the investigation of all peripheral innervation mandatory.

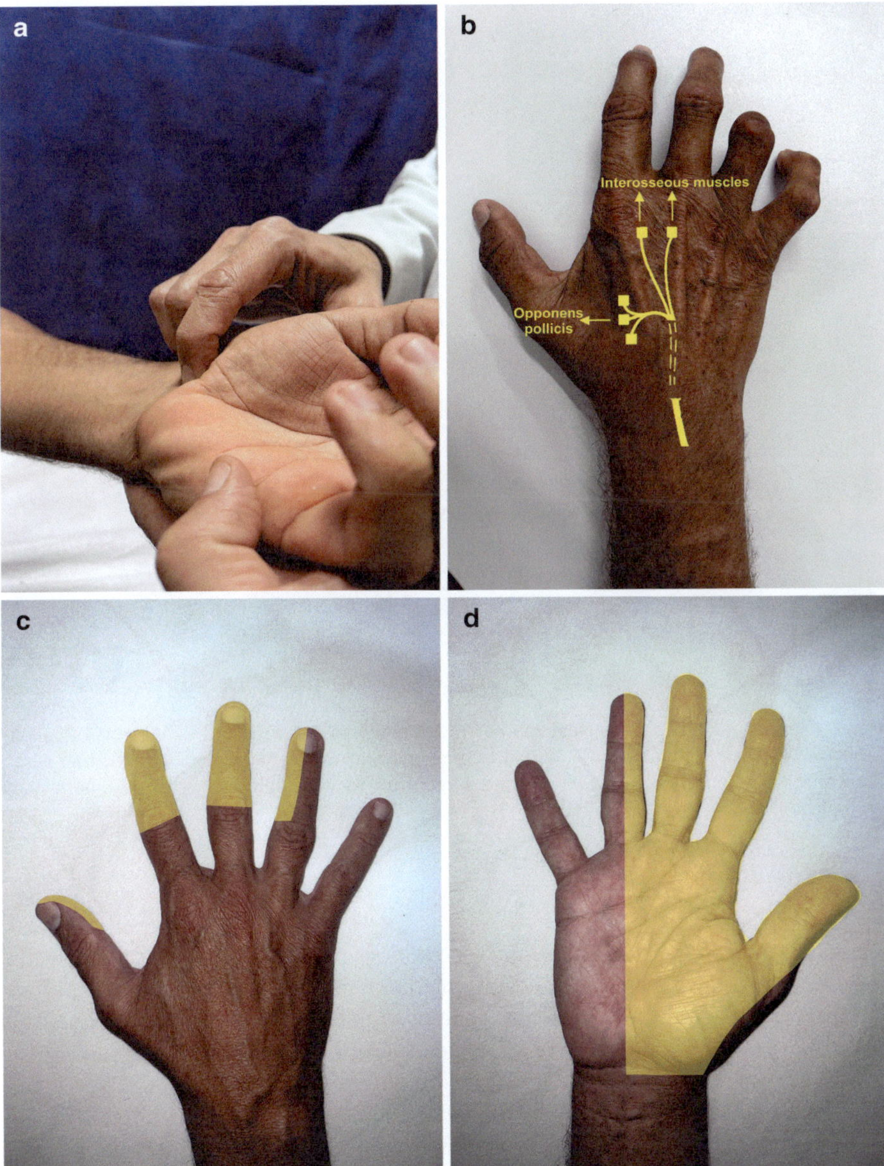

Fig. 2 Median nerve. (**a**) Semiotic technique to check the median nerve. This nerve is hardly palpated. Just below the scaphoid bone and between the tendons of the palmaris longus and the *flexor carpi radialis* muscles, this nerve can be perceived. As a rule, percussion is used to check it. When affected, Tinel's sign may be verified. (**b**) Motor innervation of the hand supplied by the median nerve. The same patient in Fig. 1 has ulnar and median nerve involvement. (**c**) Sensory territory of the dorsum of the hand supplied by the median nerve. (**d**) The sensory territory of the palmar region supplied by the median nerve

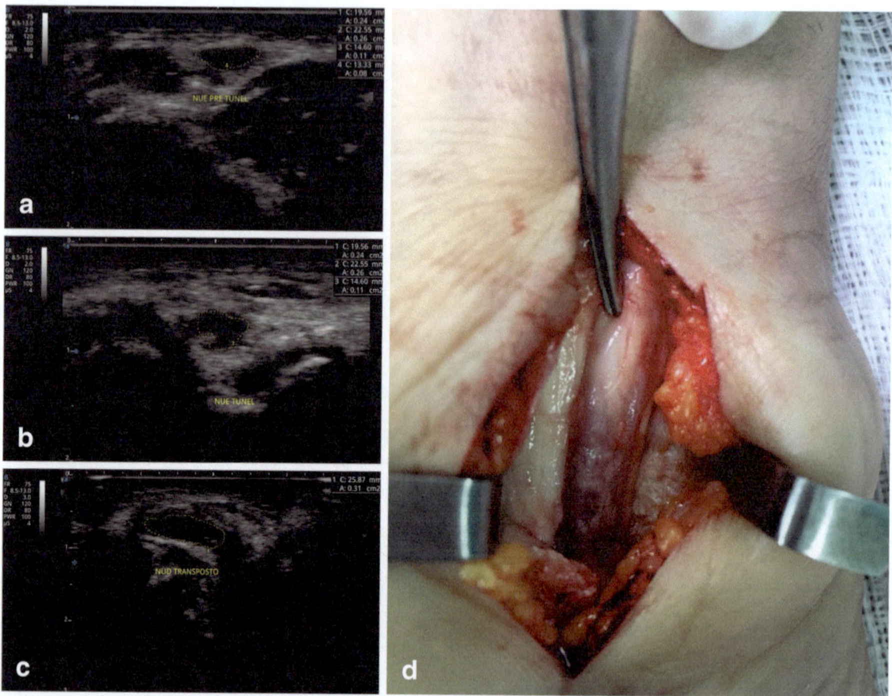

Fig. 3 Ultrasonography and surgical approach to the median nerve. (**a–c**) Median nerve thickening before the carpal tunnel, in the carpal tunnel, and after the carpal tunnel. (**d**) Median nerve thickening found on ultrasonography during surgery for its decompression. (Images courtesy of Dr. Sideval Pontes—Recife, PE—Brazil)

2.3   *The Radial Nerve*

The radial nerve has its origin from the posterior cord of the brachial plexus. After crossing the axilla, it passes posterior to the humeral diaphysis in the spiral groove and pierces the lateral intermuscular septum to enter the anterior compartment of the arm. Close to the elbow, it is subdivided into the posterior interosseous nerve and the sensory radial nerve [21].

Consensually, radial nerve involvement in Hansen's disease is less frequent and usually occurs after involvement of the ulnar and median nerves. The radial sensory nerve is most often cited as affected by Hansen's disease. Its impairment leads to sensory changes in the corresponding dermatome (Fig. 7) while motor impairment

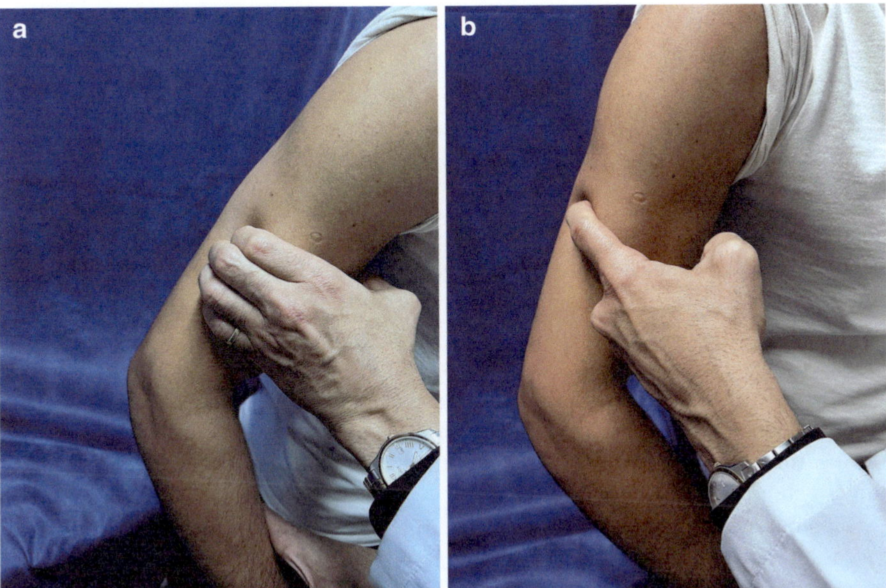

Fig. 4 Radial nerve. (**a, b**) Semiotic technique to check the radial nerve before its subdivision. You must search the radial nerve halfway between the greater humeral tuberosity and the lateral epicondyle, initially by exerting greater pressure with your fingers, between the long head and the lateral head of the triceps muscle until you locate it. Later, this nerve can be perceived only with the second examiner's second finger

even later leads to a progressive weakness of the dorsiflexor capacity of the carpus [22].

Palpation of the radial nerve is not always easy to perform. Even before its subdivision, it can closely be found thickened approximately halfway between the greater humeral tuberosity and the lateral epicondyle. Individuals with robust muscle mass or obese individuals with a large adipose tissue make it difficult to palpate (Fig. 4) [23, 24].

Distally close to the wrist, palpation of the radial nerve can be performed, commonly between the radial styloid process and the dorsal tubercle of the radius, except for individual anatomical variations. When thickened, this nerve can be visible even by mere inspection [25].

In the clinical experience of this author in the field, when correctly approached before its subdivision, the involvement of the radial nerve may be more frequent than what is described in the literature, and may even contribute to the early diagnosis of Hansen's disease.

3   The Innervation of the Lower Limbs and the Alterations Caused by Hansen's Disease

3.1   *The Common Peroneal Nerve and its Ramifications: Superficial Peroneal Nerve and Sural Nerve*

The common peroneal nerve represents the terminal lateral branch of the sciatic nerve, which runs lateral to the lateral head of the gastrocnemius muscle. It surfaces posteriorly near the head of the fibula, where it is easily accessible to palpation, except in individuals with robust adipose tissue (Fig. 5) [26, 27].

Just below the fibular head, this nerve subdivides into two branches which are the deep peroneal nerve and the superficial peroneal nerve. The deep peroneal nerve is responsible for innervating the muscles of the anterior and lateral compartments of the leg: the tibialis anterior muscle, the extensor *hallucis longus* muscle and the long finger extensor muscle [28].

This nerve is frequently compromised in Hansen's disease and leads to relevant motor alterations, although it also responds together with the superficial common peroneal nerve, through the cutaneous innervation of the leg. The progressive impairment caused by Hansen's disease initially leads to sensory losses in the leg, in the aforementioned territories, and later the motor impairment will lead to the inability to perform foot dorsiflexion, leading to "foot drop" [29].

These changes, in turn, lead to gait disturbances, with hip abduction occurring in a compensatory manner to allow greater distance between the foot and the ground. Another no less important motor alteration is the loss of ankle eversion capacity. In cases of significant thickening, due to vascular compression, a decrease in distal arterial pulses can still be perceived [30].

Just above and slightly anterior to the lateral malleolus, the superficial deep peroneal nerve arises. This nerve bifurcates into its two terminal branches, represented by the medial dorsal cutaneous nerve and the intermediate dorsal cutaneous nerve. The latter, as a rule, is considered to be only the superficial fibular nerve properly known and is easily verified by simple semiotic techniques [31].

The superficial peroneal nerve is responsible for skin sensitivity in an extensive range along the lower limb, extending over the entire dorsum of the foot, with the exception of a small area between the hallux and the second toe, which is the responsibility of the deep fibular nerve. This nerve location may represent a good region to measure the initial involvement of this nerve, considering that the sensory fibers intermingle with the superficial fibular nerve in the lateral region of the leg (Fig. 6a) [32].

These changes, in turn, lead to gait disturbances, with hip abduction occurring in a compensatory manner to allow greater distance between the foot and the ground. Another no less important motor alteration is the loss of ankle eversion capacity. In cases of significant thickening, due to vascular compression, a decrease in distal arterial pulses can still be perceived and may represent a good region to measure the

Fig. 5 The common peroneal nerve. Semiotic technique to check the common peroneal nerve before its subdivision. This nerve is easily located just behind the head of the *peroneum.* Using the distal phalanx of the second finger, the examiner wraps the head of the fibula until it meets the common peroneal nerve, performing up and down movements, with the leg's patient positioned at right angles to the thigh

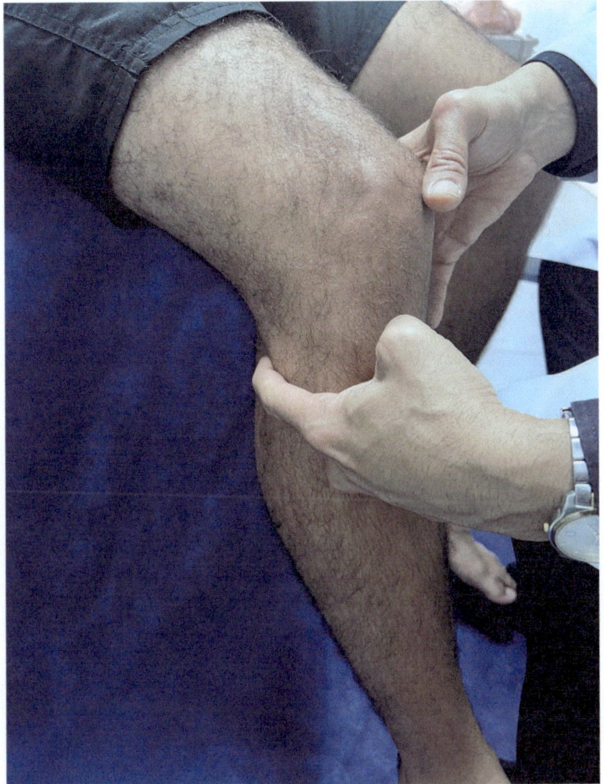

initial involvement of this nerve, considering that the sensory fibers intermingle with the superficial fibular nerve in the lateral region of the leg [33].

This nerve also has a motor component. The motor component is responsible for the innervation of the peroneus longus and peroneus brevis muscles, which in turn perform light plantar flexion and foot eversion, helping to maintain the physiological plantar arch [34].

The semiotic examination can be performed through inspection and palpation. Upon inspection, the patient should preferably be seated with the leg at a 90° angle to the thigh and with the feet flat on the floor. When frankly thickened, its visualization will be possible (Fig. 8). If the thickening is not evident in this way, inspection and subsequent palpation can be obtained by performing maximum plantar flexion and eversion with the individual sitting on the stretcher with the feet suspended or supported on the examiner's lap without the plantar region touching any surface of the foot support (Fig. 6b, c) [35].

Examination of the superficial peroneal nerve is very useful and may represent the possibility of early diagnosis of Hansen's disease [36].

The distal sural nerve arises most frequently from the union of the medial sural cutaneous nerve and the peroneal communicating nerve although there are

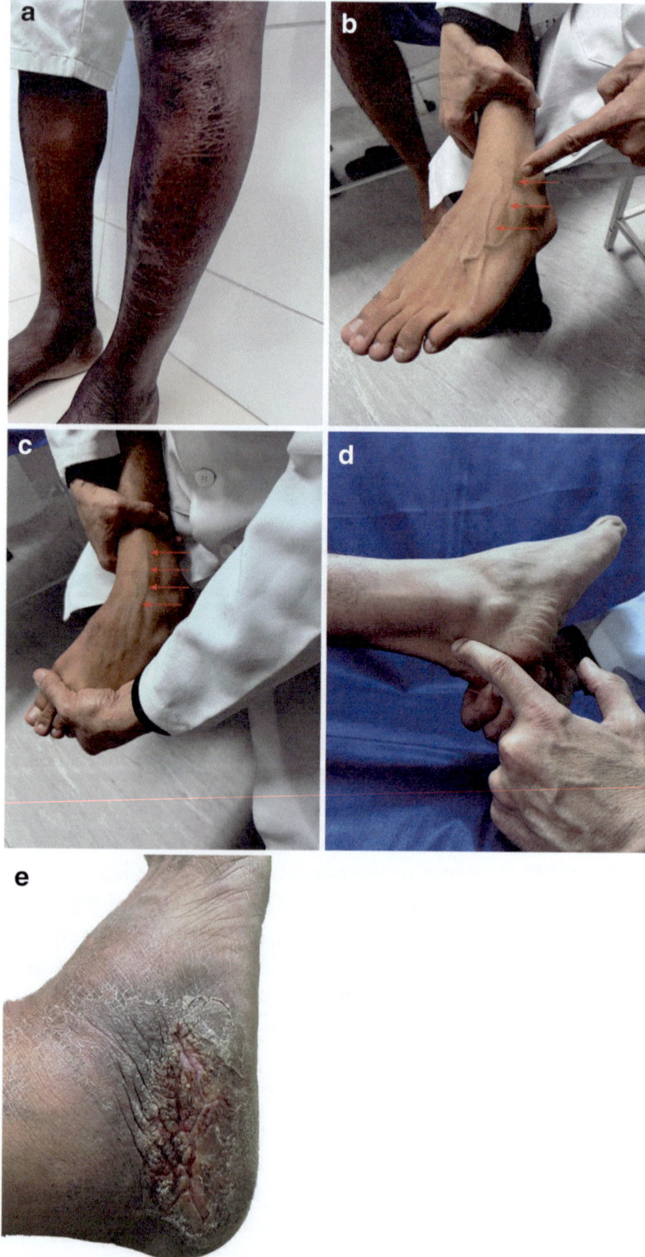

Fig. 6 The superficial peroneal nerve and the sural nerve. (**a**) Cutaneous dermatome corresponding to the compromised superficial peroneal nerve. Note the exuberant cutaneous xerosis. (**b**) Slightly above and anterior to the medial malleolus, the nerve can be visualized on mere inspection. (**c**) Maximum eversion of the foot makes the nerve even more evident along the dorsum of the foot. (**d**) Between the lateral malleolus and the Achilles tendon, the sural nerve can be seen by inspection and palpation. (**e**) Cutaneous ulceration due to loss of sensation in the sural nerve territory

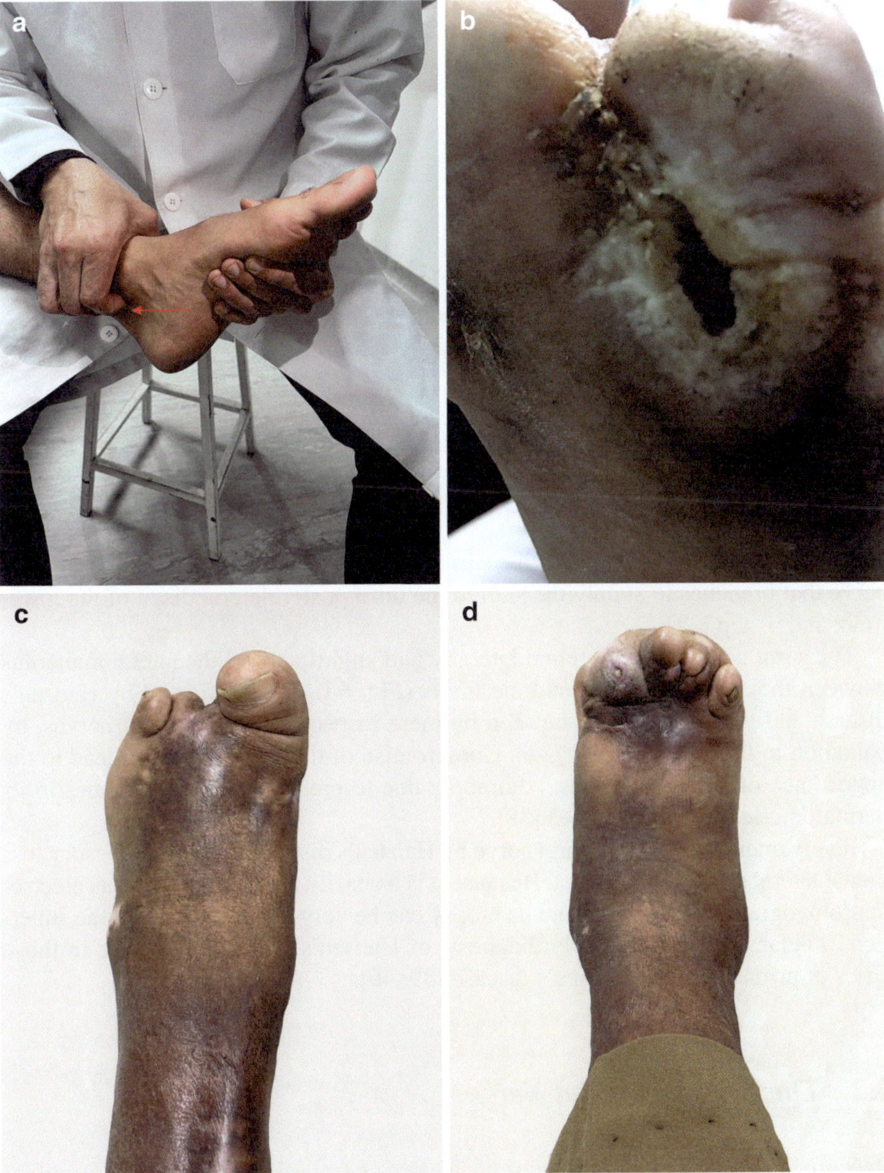

Fig. 7 The posterior tibial nerve. (**a**) Semiotic technique of palpation of the posterior tibial nerve. This nerve is easily found between the medial malleolus and the Achilles tendon. (**b**) Large and profound plantar ulceration present on the right foot of the same patient of images C and D. (**c, d**) Dorsal view of patient's both feet, exhibiting osteolysis, bone resorption, and deformity due to loss of sensation. In this severe case, Hansen's disease compromises all feet's nerves

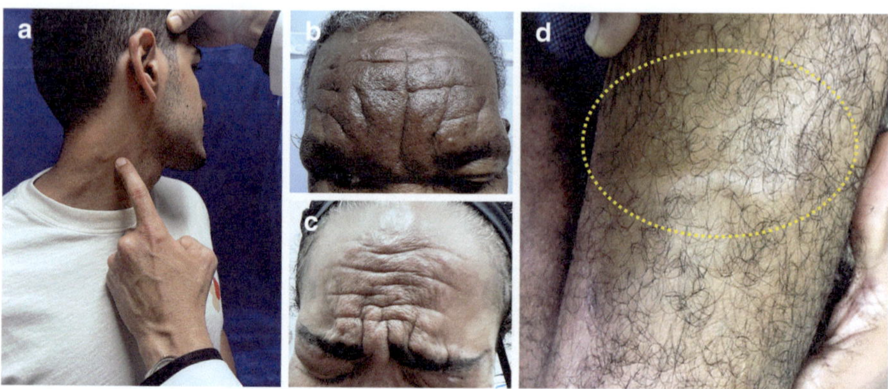

Fig. 8 Other nerves affected by Hansen's disease. (**a**) Magnus auricular nerve, perceived on inspection, lateralizing the patient's head, parallel to the external jugular vein. (**b, c**) Exuberant supraorbital nerves infiltration. (**d**) Thickened cutaneous femoral nerve visible on inspection in the middle of the left thigh, highlighted in the yellow circle

anatomical variations well described in the literature. It is essentially a sensory nerve that branches to supply the skin in the third posterolateral distal of the lower limb, and instep [37].

The sural nerve is easily found laterally and slightly above the lateral malleolus between the Achilles tendon and the fibula (Fig. 6d). When affected by Hansen's disease and thickened, it can be seen by mere inspection or, like other nerves, by palpation in this anatomical region. Compromise of the sural nerve can lead to the appearance of skin ulcerations, commonly due to pressure exerted by shoes in its dermatomeric territory (Fig. 6e) [38].

Involvement of the distal sural nerve by Hansen's disease can lead to sensory loss on the lateral surface of the foot. Because it is an easily accessible nerve, its electro-neuromyography, ultrasound and its biopsy can be very useful, as well as the superficial fibular nerve, in the early diagnosis of Hansen's disease as well as in those cases of primary neural Hansen's disease [39, 40].

3.2 The Posterior Tibial Nerve

Recently, it was found that the most appropriate terminology of the posterior tibial nerve is just "tibial nerve." However, both propositions can be used and to avoid confusion, this chapter will use the most common terminology in Hansen's disease [41].

The posterior tibial nerve arises from the sciatic nerve and is its largest terminal branch. Classically, when mentioning the posterior tibial nerve in Hansen's disease, one remembers the entrance of the tarsal tunnel behind the medial malleolus [42].

The preference of *Mycobacterium leprae* for the coldest areas of the body justifies that, in fact, this anatomical region of the tibial nerve is the most affected by Hansen's disease, with the deleterious thickenings and subsequent impairment of plantar sensitivity. However, it is already known that the proximal parts of the nerve, from its bifurcation in the popliteal fossa, may also be affected in a spurt, although clinically difficult to detect [43].

Access to this nerve in the tarsal tunnel is performed between the medial malleolus and the Achilles tendon (Fig. 7a) and the main way to verify its involvement, if no morphological changes are detected, is through the measurement of plantar sensitivity. For this purpose, routinely the MFSW assess the tactile sensitivity and may contribute to the early diagnosis of Hansen's disease [44].

The impairment of plantar sensitivity is dramatic for patients affected by Hansen's disease, leading to deep chronic plantar ulcerations that are difficult to heal, in addition to repeated trauma and its consequences, requiring the use of adapted shoes or surgeries for neural decompression and symptom improvement (Fig. 7b–d) [45].

4   Other Nerves Affected by Hansen's Disease

As mentioned, all peripheral innervation may be compromised. Therefore, changes in other nerves can still be perceived. Worth mentioning:

- The supraorbital nerves: Supraorbital nerves Neurological alterations, in Hansen's diseases upraorbital nerves can be clearly seen thickened upon mere inspection. When frankly compromised, they can lead to external supraciliary madarosis (Fig. 8a, b) [46];
- The great auricular nerve, Great auricular nerve Neurological alterations, in Hansen's disease great auricular nerve whose thickening can be verified by placing the head laterally parallel to the external jugular vein (Fig. 8c) [47];
- The anterior cutaneous femoral nerve Anterior cutaneous femoral nerve Neurological alterations, in Hansen's disease anterior cutaneous femoral nerve visualized and/or palpated along the antero-distal aspect of the thigh (Fig. 8d) [48].
- And trigeminal and facial nerves, whose impairment is classically identified by checking the corneopalpebral reflex, as part of eyeball changes in Hansen's disease. The affected trigeminal nerve leads to corneal anesthesia and the affected facial nerve, due to the impairment of the *orbicularis oculi muscles*, leads in turn to *lagophthalmos* [49].

5   Complementary Tests in Hansen's Disease Neuropathies

Despite Hansen's disease being an essentially neural pathology, early cases of Hansen's disease with subtle manifestations and/or cases of neural involvement without thickening may go unnoticed when using the described semiotic techniques. In this way, complementary exams can become a good ally to aid in the diagnosis, even collaborating with the possible differential diagnoses.

Electroneuromyography is a recognized technique in the diagnosis of Hansen's disease. It has proven to be a tool for early diagnosis of Hansen's disease, including among asymptomatic household contacts [50].

Ultrasonography, especially high resolution, can help in the diagnosis of neural impairment in Hansen's disease, showing morphometric alterations of the nerves even in the impossibility of detection on palpation, with neural elastography being able to collaborate to increase the sensitivity of the technique. Confirmation of asymmetry between right and left (bilateral) peripheral nerve (CSA), in addition to the parameters of the absolute values of the CSA measurements, other authors [51, 52] suggest the asymmetry index [Δ CSA = (> CSA right or left) - (< CSA right or left)] in the evaluation of Hansen's disease neuropathy. The asymmetry index between the right and left peripheral nerves has high sensitivity and specificity in the differentiation between nerves of healthy individuals and nerves of patients with leprosy [51–53].

Neural biopsy is consecrated for the diagnosis of Hansen's disease, even in the absence of apparent clinical manifestations, whether dermatological and/or neurological. However, it requires specialized training and sophisticated techniques that are not widely available in the field. The same comment is appropriate for diagnostic techniques involving molecular biology and anti-PGL-I serology, which together can contribute to the early diagnosis of the neurological manifestations of Hansen's disease, not only in patients diagnosed with the disease, but also in apparently healthy household contacts [54, 55].

6   Final Considerations

Within the spectrum of neurological manifestations of Hansen's disease, in addition to the peripheral nervous system, it is noteworthy that there are reports of central nervous system (CNS) involvement by the disease (Table 1), and this possibility cannot be disregarded, and may be more frequent than is believed to date.

Table 1 CNS involvement by Hansen's disease

Authors	Year	Main findings
Aung T, Kitajima S, Nomoto M, et al.	2007	In 67 post-mortem lepromatous cases, 44 (67%) had vacuolar changes of motor neurons either in medulla oblongata (nucleus ambiguous or hypoglossal nucleus) or spinal cord. PGL-I was positive in vacuolated areas. PCR revealed *Mycobacterium leprae*-specific genomic DNA in 18 of 19 cases (95%) with vacuolated changes and 5 of 8 (63%) without vacuolated changes [56]
Lee KH, Moon KS, Yun SJ, et al.	2014	A cystic lesion was removed from the right patient's frontal lobe and the material reveals fragmented-acid-fast bacilli with *Mycobacterium leprae*-specific genomic DNA [57]
Sharma D, Gupta A, Chhabra SS, Jain S. A	2017	Involvement of cranial nerve nuclei along with seventh cranial nerve in the case of facial paralysis in a patient diagnosed with borderline-tuberculoid leprosy [58]
Baveja, Sukriti; Sandhu, Sunmeet; Vashisht, Deepak	2019	A lesion identified by MRI on the dorsal aspect of left pontomedullary junction, with no postcontrast enhancement, suggestive of vacuolar degeneration of leprosy [59]
Polavarapu K, Preethish-Kumar V, Vengalil S, et al.	2019	MRI showed eight patients with Hansen's disease with involvement of the facial nucleus, nucleus ambiguous, and spinal cords [60]
Bhoi SK, Naik S, Purkait S	2021	Pure neuritic Hansen's disease in the CNS in three patients with bilateral foot drop with the involvement of posterior column and cranial nerves. MRI T2W sequence of cervico-dorsal cord showed dorsal column hyperintensity in two patients. Diffusion-weighted MR revealed decrease fractional anisotropy and an increase in the apparent diffusion coefficient. Similar findings were also noted in the optic nerves [38]

7 Conclusion

Knowledge of peripheral cutaneous innervation about semiotic techniques for adequate physical examination and its alterations are essential for physicians to correctly perform the neurological examination of Hansen's disease. The finding of a single compromised nerve, according to the WHO, modifies the operational classification of the patient who must be treated for at least 12 months with multidrug theraphy, regardless of the number or presence of skin lesions and the acid-fast bacilli in slit skin smear [61].

Acknowledgements To Dr. Fred Nietto (Ph.D.) for the collaboration in the English translation; to the patients who kindly provided their images; to the medical doctor's students Rafael Bezerra and Matheus Melo for the effort in the production of the photographs for the demonstration of the semiotic techniques. Finally, to the author M.D. Ph.D. Patrícia Deps for the invitation to write this chapter.

References

1. Spierings E, De Boer T, Zulianello L, Ottenhoff TH. The role of Schwann cells, T cells and *Mycobacterium leprae* in the immunopathogenesis of nerve damage in leprosy. Lepr Rev. 2000;71(Suppl):S121–9.
2. Pannikar VK, Arunthathi S, Chacko CJ, Fritschi EP. A clinico-pathological study of primary neuritic leprosy. Lepr India. 1983;55(2):212–21.
3. de Freitas MR, Said G. Leprous neuropathy. Handb Clin Neurol. 2013;115:499–514. https://doi.org/10.1016/B978-0-444-52902-2.00028-X.
4. Pitta IJR, Hacker MAV, Andrade LR, et al. Follow-up assessment of patients with Pure Neural Leprosy in a reference center in Rio de Janeiro-Brazil. PLoS Negl Trop Dis. 2022;16(1):e0010070. https://doi.org/10.1371/journal.pntd.0010070.
5. Gunawan H, Achdiat PA, Rahardjo RM, Hindritiani R, Suwarsa O. Frequent testicular involvement in multibacillary leprosy. Int J Infect Dis. 2020;90:60–4. https://doi.org/10.1016/j.ijid.2019.10.013.
6. Dos Santos AR, Silva PRS, Steinmann P, Ignotti E. Disability progression among leprosy patients released from treatment: a survival analysis. Infect Dis Poverty. 2020;9(1):53. https://doi.org/10.1186/s40249-020-00669-4.
7. Mishra B, Mukherjee A, Girdhar A, Husain S, Malaviya GN, Girdhar BK. Neuritic leprosy: further progression and significance. Acta Leprol. 1995;9(4):187–94.
8. Spinner M. Injuries to the major branches of peripheral nerves of the forearm. Philadelphia: WB Saunders; 1978.
9. Polatsch DB, Melone CP Jr, Beldner S, Incorvaia A. Ulnar nerve anatomy. Hand Clin. 2007;23(3):283–v.
10. Brandsma JW, Van Brakel WH. WHO disability grading: operational definitions. Lepr Rev. 2003;74(4):366–73.
11. Rajan P, Premkumar R, Rajkumar P, Richard J. The impact of hand dominance and ulnar and median nerve impairment on strength and basic daily activities. J Hand Ther. 2005;18(1):40–5. https://doi.org/10.1197/j.jht.2004.10.011.
12. Giesel LM, Pitta IJR, da Silveira RC, et al. Clinical and neurophysiological features of leprosy patients with neuropathic pain. Am J Trop Med Hyg. 2018;98(6):1609–13. https://doi.org/10.4269/ajtmh.17-0817.
13. Soubeyrand M, Melhem R, Protais M, Artuso M, Crézé M. Anatomy of the median nerve and its clinical applications. Hand Surg Rehabil. 2020;39(1):2–18. https://doi.org/10.1016/j.hansur.2019.10.197.
14. Kozin SH. The anatomy of the recurrent branch of the median nerve. J Hand Surg [Am]. 1998;23(5):852–8. https://doi.org/10.1016/S0363-5023(98)80162-7.
15. Tosti R, Ilyas AM. Acute carpal tunnel syndrome. Orthop Clin North Am. 2012;43(4):459–65. https://doi.org/10.1016/j.ocl.2012.07.015.
16. Vital RT, Illarramendi X, Antunes SL, et al. Isolated median neuropathy as the first symptom of leprosy. Muscle Nerve. 2013;48(2):179–84. https://doi.org/10.1002/mus.23731.
17. Nagappa M, Pujar GS, Keshavan AH, et al. Sonographic pattern of median nerve enlargement in Hansen's neuropathy. Acta Neurol Scand. 2021;144(2):155–60. https://doi.org/10.1111/ane.13432.

18. Sedal L, McLeod JG, Walsh JC. Ulnar nerve lesions associated with the carpal tunnel syndrome. J Neurol Neurosurg Psychiatry. 1973;36(1):118–23. https://doi.org/10.1136/jnnp.36.1.118.

19. Yildirim P, Gunduz OH. What is the role of Semmes-Weinstein monofilament testing in the diagnosis of electrophysiologically graded carpal tunnel syndrome? J Phys Ther Sci. 2015;27(12):3749–53. https://doi.org/10.1589/jpts.27.3749.

20. Sapage R, Pereira PA, Vital L, Madeira MD, Pinho A. Surgical anatomy of the radial nerve in the arm: a cadaver study. Eur J Orthop Surg Traumatol. 2021;31(7):1457–62. https://doi.org/10.1007/s00590-021-02916-2.

21. Vishwanath G, et al. Isolated radial nerve involvement in leprosy. Med J Armed Forces India. 2001;57(3):237–8. https://doi.org/10.1016/S0377-1237(01)80052-6.

22. Tornetta P III, Hochwald N, Bono C, Grossman M. Anatomy of the posterior interosseous nerve in relation to fixation of the radial head. Clin Orthop Relat Res. 1997;345:215–8.

23. Cox CL, Riherd D, Tubbs RS, Bradley E, Lee DH. Predicting radial nerve location using palpable landmarks. Clin Anat. 2010;23(4):420–6. https://doi.org/10.1002/ca.20951.

24. Robson AJ, See MS, Ellis H. Applied anatomy of the superficial branch of the radial nerve. Clin Anat. 2008;21(1):38–45. https://doi.org/10.1002/ca.20576.

25. Kumar N, Garg RK, Malhotra HS. Ulnar and superficial radial nerve swellings in two patients with leprosy. Am J Trop Med Hyg. 2018;98(4):939–40. https://doi.org/10.4269/ajtmh.17-0940.

26. Hardin JM, Devendra S. Anatomy, bony pelvis and lower limb, calf common peroneal (fibular) nerve. In: StatPearls. Treasure Island (FL): StatPearls Publishing; 2021.

27. Nori SL, Stretanski MF. Foot Drop. In: StatPearls. Treasure Island (FL): StatPearls Publishing; December 15, 2021.

28. Anderson JC. Common fibular nerve compression: anatomy, symptoms, clinical evaluation, and surgical decompression. Clin Podiatr Med Surg. 2016;33(2):283–91. https://doi.org/10.1016/j.cpm.2015.12.005.

29. JGA. Foot drop in leprosy. Lepr Rev. 1964;35:41–6. https://doi.org/10.5935/0305-7518.19640006.

30. Garrett A, Geiger Z. Anatomy, bony pelvis and lower limb, superficial peroneal (fibular) nerve. In: StatPearls. Treasure Island (FL): StatPearls Publishing; 2021.

31. Ribak S, Fonseca JR, Tietzmann A, Gama SA, Hirata HH. The Anatomy and morphology of the superficial peroneal nerve. J Reconstr Microsurg. 2016;32(4):271–5. https://doi.org/10.1055/s-0035-1568881.

32. Thevenon A, Serafi R, Fontaine C, Grauwin MY, Buisset N, Tiffreau V. An unusual cause of foot clonus: spasticity of fibularis longus muscle. Ann Phys Rehabil Med. 2013;56(6):482–8.

33. De Maeseneer M, Madani H, Lenchik L, Kalume Brigido M, Shahabpour M, Marcelis S, de Mey J, Scafoglieri A. Normal anatomy and compression areas of nerves of the foot and ankle: US and MR imaging with anatomic correlation. Radiographics. 2015;35(5):1469–82.

34. de Leeuw PA, Golanó P, Blankevoort L, Sierevelt IN, van Dijk CN. Identification of the superficial peroneal nerve: anatomical study with surgical implications. Knee Surg Sports Traumatol Arthrosc. 2016;24(4):1381–5. https://doi.org/10.1007/s00167-016-4063-8.

35. Vaidyanathan EP, Vaidyanathan SI. Superficial peroneal nerve thickening as an early diagnostic sign in leprosy. Lepr Rev. 1978;49(2):149–51. https://doi.org/10.5935/0305-7518.19780018.

36. Ramakrishnan PK, Henry BM, Vikse J, et al. Anatomical variations of the formation and course of the sural nerve: A systematic review and meta-analysis. Ann Anat. 2015;202:36–44. https://doi.org/10.1016/j.aanat.2015.08.002.

37. Manchanda R, Dhar N, Kumar M, Kumar N, Tiwari A. Thickened sural nerve in Hansen's disease. QJM. 2021;114(3):202–3. https://doi.org/10.1093/qjmed/hcaa216.

38. Bhoi SK, Naik S, Purkait S. Pure neuritic leprosy with bilateral foot drop and central nervous involvement: a clinical, electrophysiological, and MR correlation. Neurol India. 2021;69(5):1349–53. https://doi.org/10.4103/0028-3886.329620.

39. Haimanot RT, Mshana RN, McDougall AC, Andersen JG. Sural nerve biopsy in leprosy patients after varying periods of treatment: histopathological and bacteriological findings on light microscopy. Int J Lepr Other Mycobact Dis. 1984;52(2):163–70.

40. Wagenaar I, Post E, Brandsma W, et al. Early detection of neuropathy in leprosy: a comparison of five tests for field settings. Infect Dis Poverty. 2017;6(1):115. https://doi.org/10.1186/s40249-017-0330-2.

41. Palande DD, Azhaguraj M. Surgical decompression of posterior tibial neurovascular complex in treatment of certain chronic plantar ulcers and posterior tibial neuritis in leprosy. Int J Lepr Other Mycobact Dis. 1975;43(1):36–40.

42. Krishna G. Popliteal fossa. In: Chaurasia BD, editor. Human Anatomy (Regional and Applied Dissection and Clinical) Volume 2—Lower limb, abdomen, and pelvis. 5th ed. India: CBS Publishers and Distributors Pvt Ltd; 2010. p. 86,87,120, 131. ISBN 978-81-239-1864-8.

43. Richard B, Khatri B, Knolle E, Lucas S, Turkof E. Leprosy affects the tibial nerves diffusely from the middle of the thigh to the sole of the foot, including skip lesions. Plast Reconstr Surg. 2001;107(7):1717–24. https://doi.org/10.1097/00006534-200106000-00012.

44. Khambati FA, Shetty VP, Ghate SD, Capadia GD. Sensitivity and specificity of nerve palpation, monofilament testing and voluntary muscle testing in detecting peripheral nerve abnormality, using nerve conduction studies as gold standard; a study in 357 patients. Lepr Rev. 2009;80(1):34–50.

45. Cordeiro TL, Frade MA, Barros AR, Foss NT. Baropodometric Evaluations and Sensitivity Alterations in Plantar Ulcer Formation in Leprosy. Int J Low Extrem Wounds. 2014;13(2):110–115. https://doi.org/10.1177/1534734614536034.

46. Massone C, Clapasson A, Gennaro S, Nunzi E. Enlarging plaque on the face with enlarged supraorbital nerve. Dermatol Pract Concept. 2013;3(1):17–20. Published 2013 Jan 31. https://doi.org/10.5826/dpc.0301a05.

47. Gupta N, Vinod KS, Singh G, Nischal N. Bilateral greater auricular nerve thickening in leprosy. QJM. 2020;113(8):579. https://doi.org/10.1093/qjmed/hcz287.

48. Neto FBA, Neto RA, Cardoso LMC. The first report of pure neuritic leprosy with involvement of the anterior femoral cutaneous nerve. Neurol Int. 2019;11(2):8001. Published 2019 Jun 18. https://doi.org/10.4081/ni.2019.8001.

49. Grzybowski A, Nita M, Virmond M. Ocular leprosy. Clin Dermatol. 2015;33(1):79–89. https://doi.org/10.1016/j.clindermatol.2014.07.003.

50. Santos DFD, et al. Revisiting primary neural leprosy: clinical, serological, molecular, and neurophysiological aspects. PLoS Negl Trop Dis. 2017;11(11):e0006086. https://doi.org/10.1371/journal.pntd.0006086.

51. Frade MA, Nogueira-Barbosa MH, Lugão HB, Furini RB, Marques Júnior W, Foss NT. New sonographic measures of peripheral nerves: a tool for the diagnosis of peripheral nerve involvement in leprosy. Mem Inst Oswaldo Cruz. 2013;108(3):257–62. https://doi.org/10.1590/S0074-02762013000300001.

52. Lugão HB, Nogueira-Barbosa MH, Marques W Jr, Foss NT, Frade MA. Asymmetric nerve enlargement: a characteristic of leprosy neuropathy demonstrated by ultrasonography. PLoS Negl Trop Dis. 2015;9(12):e0004276. Published 2015 Dec 8. https://doi.org/10.1371/journal.pntd.0004276.

53. Nogueira-Barbosa MH, Lugão HB, Gregio-Júnior E, et al. Ultrasound elastography assessment of the median nerve in leprosy patients. Muscle Nerve. 2017;56(3):393–8. https://doi.org/10.1002/mus.25510.

54. Dos Santos DF, Antunes DE, Dornelas BC, et al. Peripheral nerve biopsy: a tool still needed in the early diagnosis of neural leprosy? Trans R Soc Trop Med Hyg. 2020;114(11):792–7. https://doi.org/10.1093/trstmh/traa053.

55. Santos DFD, Mendonça MR, Antunes DE, et al. Molecular, immunological and neurophysiological evaluations for early diagnosis of neural impairment in seropositive leprosy household contacts. PLoS Negl Trop Dis. 2018;12(5):e0006494. Published 2018 May 21. https://doi.org/10.1371/journal.pntd.0006494.

56. Aung T, Kitajima S, Nomoto M, et al. Mycobacterium leprae in neurons of the medulla oblongata and spinal cord in leprosy. J Neuropathol Exp Neurol. 2007;66(4):284–94. https://doi.org/10.1097/nen.0b013e31803d597e.

57. Lee KH, Moon KS, Yun SJ, et al. Brain involvement by leprosy presenting as a frontal cystic lesion. J Neurosurg. 2014;121(1):184–8. https://doi.org/10.3171/2014.1.JNS131429.
58. Sharma D, Gupta A, Chhabra SS, Jain S. A unique case of concomitant intra and extra-cranial Hansen's disease. Acta Neurochir. 2017;159(2):205–8. https://doi.org/10.1007/s00701-016-3008-9.
59. Baveja S, Sandhu S, Vashisht D. A rare case of possible vacuolar degeneration of leprosy in brain with segmental necrotizing granulomatous neuritis and horner's syndrome. Indian Dermatol Online J. 2019;10(4):444–6. https://doi.org/10.4103/idoj.IDOJ_388_18.
60. Polavarapu K, Preethish-Kumar V, Vengalil S, et al. Brain and spinal cord lesions in leprosy: a magnetic resonance imaging-based study. Am J Trop Med Hyg. 2019;100(4):921–31. https://doi.org/10.4269/ajtmh.17-0945.
61. WHO. Guidelines for the diagnosis, treatment and prevention of leprosy. New Delhi: World Health Organization, Regional Office for South-East Asia; 2017. Licence: CC BY-NC-SA 3.0 IGO.

Evaluation, Monitoring and Prevention of Disabilities in Hansen's Disease

Marcos Tulio Raposo and Susilene Maria Tonelli Nardi

1 Who Disability Grade and Eye-Hand-Foot Score

It is estimated that between 3 and 4 million people worldwide live with visible deformities caused by Hansen's disease (HD) [1]. Nerve damage resulting from the direct action of *Mycobacterium leprae*, inflammatory and immune-mediated responses, traumatic mechanical factors, and edema [2] can lead to permanent disabilities, and severe social consequences [1].

The assessment of nerve function in HD is focused on the "eyes, hands and feet" examination. From this, the "World Health Organization Disability Grade" (DG) is defined and the disabilities are graded on an increasing scale: Grade 0 (G0D), Grade 1(G1D), and Grade 2(G2D). The DG assigned to the person is defined as the maximum value given to any of the sites assessed [3, 4]. The sum of the grades assigned to each of the six structures evaluated is equivalent to the eye-hand-foot score (EHF score), which details the disabilities at the individual level, and can range from 0 (no disability) to 12 points (maximum severity) [5–7]. Figure 1 shows the DG classification according to the structures, the description of the signs and/or symptoms and expresses the EHF score.

M. T. Raposo (✉)
Universidade Estadual do Sudoeste da Bahia, Jequié, Brazil
e-mail: tulio.raposo@uesb.edu.br

S. M. T. Nardi
Instituto Adolfo Lutz, São José do Rio Preto, Brazil
e-mail: susilene.nardi@ial.sp.gov.br

P. D. Deps (ed.), *Hansen's Disease*, https://doi.org/10.1007/978-3-031-30893-2_14

CAPTION – DISABILITY GRADE			
Disability Grade	**Eyes** Signs and symptoms	**Hands** Signs and symptoms	**Feet** Signs and symptoms
0	**Normal muscle strength (eyelid)** • Can close eyes tightly; symmetrical eyelid folds; resists eyelid opening forced by the examiner. ***AND*** **Preserved corneal sensation.** ***AND*** **Visual acuity ≥ 0,1** (Logarithmic table) at **3 meters** or Can count fingers at 6 meters.	**Normal muscle strength (hand)** ***AND*** **Sensitivity preserved: touch is felt on the palm of the hand (2g** monofilament - **purple).**	**Normal muscle strength (foot)** ***AND*** **Sensitivity preserved: touch is felt on the sole of foot (2g** monofilament - **purple).**
1	**Muscle weakness (eyelids) is present on testing but there is no visible impairment** • Inability to hold the eyelids closed against moderate force to open them. ***AND/OR*** **Decreased or loss of blink reflex:** • Delayed or absent response to corneal stimulation or decreased/loss of blink reflex	**Muscle weakness is present (on testing) but there is no visible impairment.** ***AND/OR*** **Altered sensitivity: inability to feel the 2g monofilament (purple).**	**Muscle weakness is present (on testing) but there is no visible impairment.** ***AND/OR*** **Altered sensitivity: inability to feel the 4g monofilament (dark red).**
2	**Visible impairment due to Hansen's disease, for exemple:** • Lagophthalmos • Ectropion • Trichiasis • Corneal opacity ***AND/OR*** **Severe visual impairment** (cannot count fingers at 6 meters, visual acuity less than 6:60 regardless of cause.)	**Visible impairment due to Hansen's disease, for exemple:** • Claw finger(s) • Bone resorption • Muscle wastage • Wrist drop • Wound(s)/Ulcer(s) • Deep cracks	**Visible impairment due to Hansen's disease, for exemple:** • Claw toe(s) • Bone resorption • Muscle wastage • Foot drop • Wound(s)/Ulcer(s) • Deep cracks

RESULTS OF THE DISABILITY GRADE AND EHF SCORE								
Date	**Eyes**		**Hands**		**Feet**		**Disability Grade (Maximum Grade)**	**EHF Score Eye-Hand-Foot (a+b+c+d+e+f)**
	R (a)	**L (b)**	**R (c)**	**L (d)**	**R (e)**	**L (f)**		
/ /							G0D [　] G1D [　] G2D [　]	

Fig 1 Disability Grade and Eye-Hand-Foot Score Source: Adapted from the Brazilian Ministry of Health [6] and American Leprosy Missions [7]

2 Nerve Function Assessment Form

The "Global Leprosy (Hansen's disease) Strategy 2021-2030" has set the goal of achieving "zero leprosy" or "zero Hansen's disease" by 2030: zero infection and disease, zero disability and zero stigma, and discrimination [1]. Recent WHO guidelines have mandated that health programmes and services should incorporate regular nerve function assessment and monitoring in all patients into their routine. Use of the Nerve Function Assessment Form (NFA) helps to: identify physical impairments; correctly classify DG; detect acute nerve inflammation; monitor nerve function; support the diagnosis of HD, guide treatment of neuritis and leprosy reactions

(LR); record clinical findings and case progression; analyse the results of interventions and indicate therapies [4].

Nerve damage compromises the function of the nose, eyes, upper and lower limbs. As a result, these problems can lead to severe disabilities and permanent deformities [2, 7]. Accordingly, this chapter presents an NFA form, adapted from models adopted by the Brazilian Ministry of Health [6] and WHO [4]. For the NFA, see appendices 1, 2, and 3. It includes personal data and examination of the nose, eyes, upper and lower limbs. In sequence, the most frequent impairments are presented, as well as the suggested disability prevention and rehabilitation measures.

Ideally, the NFA should be performed at diagnosis; every 3 months during multidrug therapy (MDT); when there are complaints such as neuropathic pain, decreased sensitivity and or muscle strength, ocular or nasal discomfort; every 15 days, minimally, in cases on corticoid use, in reaction states and neuritis; in postoperative follow-up of neural decompression, at 15, 45, 90, and 180 days; at the conclusion of MDT [4]; and after completion of MDT [4, 8].

2.1 Facial Assessment, Treatment, and Care

2.1.1 Nose

Complaints: Nasal dryness, hypersecretion, obstruction, presence of crusts, and deformity are frequently reported.

Inspection: Examine external nasal and internal structures of each nostril.

Management of Disability: Self-inspection and daily self-care measures are essential.

Nasal mucosa dryness and crusting: Nasal washing with saline solution 2–3 times daily and application of 1–2 drops of glycerin/mineral oil in each nostril promote hydration and lubrication of the nasal mucosa [5, 9].

2.1.2 Eyes

Complaints: The most frequent are lagophthalmos, corneal hypoesthesia/anesthesia, ectropion, trichiasis, impaired visual acuity, itching, burning, constant tearing, irritation, photophobia, presence of foreign bodies, dry eye sensation.

Inspection: Investigate for conjunctival hyperemia, madarosis, blepharochalasis, corneal opacity, ectropion, entropion, trichiasis and presence of foreign bodies, leproma, secretion [9].

Visual acuity: Measure with the Snellen table and consider as valid the last line in which the person can correctly read 2/3 of the optotypes. If the subject cannot read the largest symbol, "finger counting", "hand movement" and "light perception" can be used [5].

Management of Disability: Visual function demands assessment and monitoring. Measures such as self-inspection and daily self-care should be part of every patients' routine.

Corneal insensitivity: Conscious blinking promotes natural ocular lubrication. Artificial lubrication (eye drops), if necessary. Daytime sunglasses protect the eye. In cases of decreased corneal sensitivity associated with lagophthalmos, indicate use of night-time eye protection [5, 9].

Muscle strength reduction /lagophthalmos: Paresis of the eye orbicularis requires strengthening exercises by closing the eyes gently and then with maximum strength, holding for 5 s and relaxing. Repeat 20 exercises, three times a day. Inability to blink requires use of eye protection and evaluation by ophthalmology as to whether surgery is indicated [5, 7, 9].

Trichiasis: Using tweezers, health care professional should remove inverted lashes.

Ectropion: Use of lubricating eye drops three times a day, sunglasses during the day and night eye protection.

Central corneal opacity: Use of lubricating eye drops three times daily [5, 9].

2.1.3 Upper and Lower Limbs Assessment, Treatment and Care

Complaints: Frequent complaints are alterations in sensory functions (light touch, pressure, heat and cold, pain, etc.), motor (decreased strength, paralysis, deformities) and autonomic (dry skin, wounds, ulcers, among others).

Inspection: Analyse the conditions of the skin and annexes (pigmentation, hydration, calluses, trophic and/or traumatic lesions, plantar ulceration, scars, among others), muscles (trophism), joints (mobility, deformities), gait abnormalities (foot drop) and other alterations such as absorptions, amputations, and signs of infection. Palpation complements the examination. A "mobile claw" is when the flexion of the fingers has a range of movement (ROM) above 25% and a "rigid claw", when it is equal to or less than 25%.

Nerve palpation: Evaluate and compare symmetrically the thickness, shape, adherences to deeper planes, nodules and occurrence of pain or shock (to the touch) [4, 10, 11].

Ulnar Nerve: Support and position the patient's elbow at 120° extension. Palpate the nerve in the epitrochlear groove and slide the fingers following its path (approximately 6 cm) in search of alterations.

Median Nerve: With the patient's wrist turned upwards and in flexion of 10–20°, percutate the anterior surface of the wrist between the flexor tendons of the fingers and evaluate the occurrence of pain or "shock" (positive Tinel).

Radial Nerve: With the patient's elbow (in 90° flexion) supported on the examiner's limb, palpate the posteroinferior region, approximately two fingers behind the deltoid muscle insertion region [9, 11].

Common Fibular Nerve: Patient seated, knee flexed (90°). Palpate the posterior surface of the fibula, at the junction between the head and body of the fibula. Move the fingers along the nerve pathway in search for alterations.

Posterior Tibial Nerve: Sitting patient, with the leg hanging down or in knee extension, palpate behind and just below the medial malleolus, on an imaginary line between it and the calcaneus tendon [4, 11].

Voluntary muscle testing: Measure according to the modified Medical Research Council—MRC scale (5-0) [12]. Alternatively, the simplified scale ("S—strong", "D—decreased" and "P—paralysed") may be used. The movements assessed are: wrist extension (radial nerve); fifth finger abduction (ulnar nerve); thumb abduction (median nerve) [4]. For operational reasons, in lower limbs, only hallux extension movements and dorsiflexion (peroneal nerve) [4, 6].

Sensory testing: The use of Semmes-Weinstein monofilaments (0.07 g, 0.2 g, 2 g, 4 g, 10 g and 300 g) is recommended [4]. The test requires a calm environment, without distractions, previous demonstration in an area of healthy skin and that the examined person should not see the area being tested. Apply the stimuli to the skin areas innervated by the radial, ulnar, median, common peroneal and posterior tibial nerves (6).

Technique:

- Apply the monofilament perpendicular to the skin (1–1.5 s) until it bends (without touching another point on the skin).
- Apply the 0.07 g and 0.2 g monofilaments up to 3 times per point, the others, only once each.
- Start the test with the lightest monofilament (0.07 g) at each examined point. If there is no response, apply the stimulus with the next heavier filament (in the sequence of 0.07 g, 0.2 g, 2 g, 4 g, 10 g up to 300 g).
- For each point tested, record the lightest monofilament that is felt, according to the standardization (Fig. 2) [4, 11, 13]. The use of monofilaments is more sensitive; however, if health services do not have them, the stimulus may alternatively be applied with the tip of a ballpoint pen [4].

Management of Disability: All patients should receive guidance on hygiene, skin care and daily hand/foot inspection [1, 4]. Worsening of chronic damage or acute events, such as LR, may accentuate the impairment of nerve function and require multi-professional interventions. For this reason, it is essential to provide periodic assessments and monitoring of nerve function, increase health education actions and stimulate self-care group activities.

Xerosis and hyperkeratosis: Indicate hydration. After washing hands, leave them immersed in clean water, at room temperature or up to 36 °C, for 10–15 min. After rinsing, massage the skin with moisturizing lotion/cream or emollient solution. For calluses, after hydratation, gently sand the callus and apply moisturizer.

Sensory loss: Provide guidance on daily hand and foot self-examination, self-care. Consider prescribing self-help devices if required, hand protection, inspection of footwear before use, appropriate footwear or simple insole [5, 9].

Aesthesiometer (Semmes-Weinstein Monofilament)*			Light Touch with Ballpoint pen (2 g)**
Lightest filament whose touch can be felt:	**Interpretação**	**Caption***	**Caption****
Green: 0,07 g	Sensation within normal limits for the hand and foot.	Green filled circle ●	Feels touch ✓
Blue: 0,2 g	Diminished light touch sensation in the hand with difficulty in fine tactile discrimination. Within normal limits for the foot.	Blue filled circle ●	Feels Touch ✓
Purple: 2 g	Diminished protective sensation in the hand but sufficient to prevent injury. Gross tactile discrimination, shape and temperature discrimination are difficult.	Purple filled circle ●	Loss of sensation X
Dark Red: 4 g	Loss of protective sensation for the hand; in some cases, for the foot. Hands particularly vulnerable to injuries. Usually, loss of temperature discrimination.	Red filled circle ●	Loss of sensation X
Orange: 10 g	Definite loss of protective sensation for the foot. Pressure and pain may still be felt in hands and feet.	Red cross ⊗	Loss of sensation X
Light red/Pink 300 g	Still able to feel deep pressure and pain.	Red circle ○	Loss of sensation X
No response	Loss of deep pressure sensation. Usually does not feel pain. Proprioceptive function may persist.	Black filled circle ●	Loss of sensation X

Fig. 2 Sensory testing with monofilaments and ballpoint pen (Source: Adapted from the Brazilian Ministry of Health [6] and SORRI [13])

Clawed fingers /clawed toes: After moisturising the skin, perform stretching exercises when there are mobile claws. Avoid if there are wounds, cracks, signs of infection and mycoses [5, 7, 9]. Devices that help an individual accomplish a task must be indicated and manufactured according to functional demands (musculo-skeletal conditions and sensory impairments) [7].

Muscle weakness: Recommend active exercises (resisted, active-free and active-assisted). For paralysis, indicate passive mobilization and stretching.

Deformity: Referral to physiotherapy, occupational therapy and rehabilitation services. Prescribe exercises; dynamic or static orthoses to correct deformities or maintain the joint in the ideal position; gait-assistive devices; appropriate footwear; AT and devices adapted for daily living, work and leisure activities [5, 7, 9].

Abnormal gait: Gait re-education therapy.

Ulcer, wound: Indicate rest; refer to medical, physiotherapy and nursing services to assess specific therapies [5, 14].

3 Assistive Technology

Assistive Technology (AT) devices contribute to increase functional abilities of people with some kind of disability and to provide assistance or rehabilitation [7, 15], providing autonomy, independence in performing activities of daily living (ADV) as well as of work, in leisure-related activities and favoring social inclusion [15]. Figures 3 and 4 show some examples of AT devices indicated for Hansen's disease disabilities.

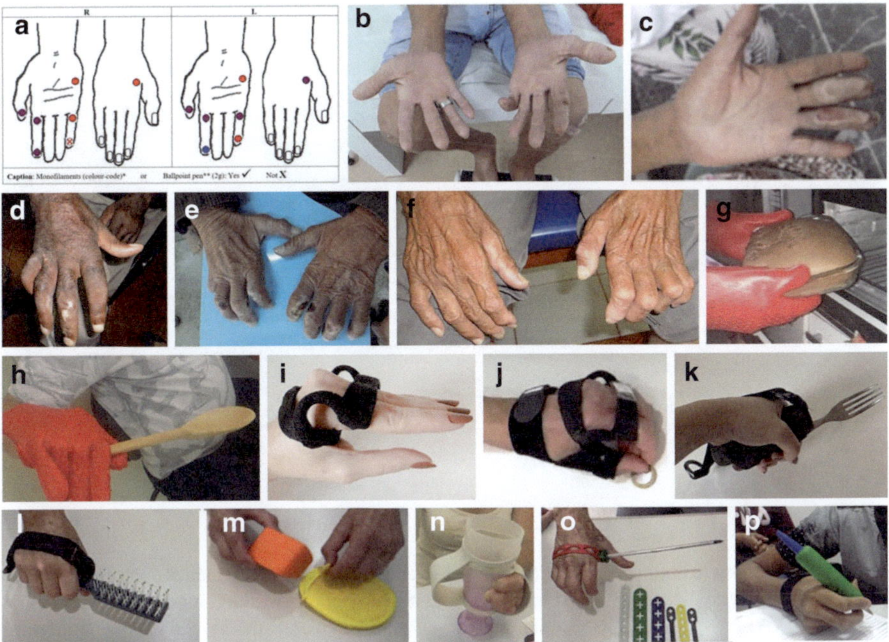

Fig. 3 (**a**) Sensory testing (Hands), i.e.; (**b**) Claw, dry skin, wound, callus and hypothenar region muscle atrophy (L hand); (**c**) Insensitive palm of the hand, burn lesions; (**d**) Dry skin, claw (ulnar nerve), wound scar; (**e**) Wounds, hand sequelae with leprosy reaction (R, L), atrophy interosseous muscles of hands, especially R, R hand fifth finger amputee; (**f**) Claws (L), atrophy interosseous muscles of hands, especially L; (**g**) Using gloves for hot domestic utensils; (**h**) Using gloves for hot domestic utensils and long wooden spoon; (**i**) Orthosis for metacarpal positioning; (**j**) Thumb abductor and orthosis for metacarpal positioning (positioning of metacarpals and thumb); (**k**) Universal adapter and object thickener; (**l**) Universal adapter and object thickener; (**m**) Multipurpose silicone sponge; (**n**) Double strap fixer; (**o**) Object fixer in strips; (**p**) Multipurpose thickener

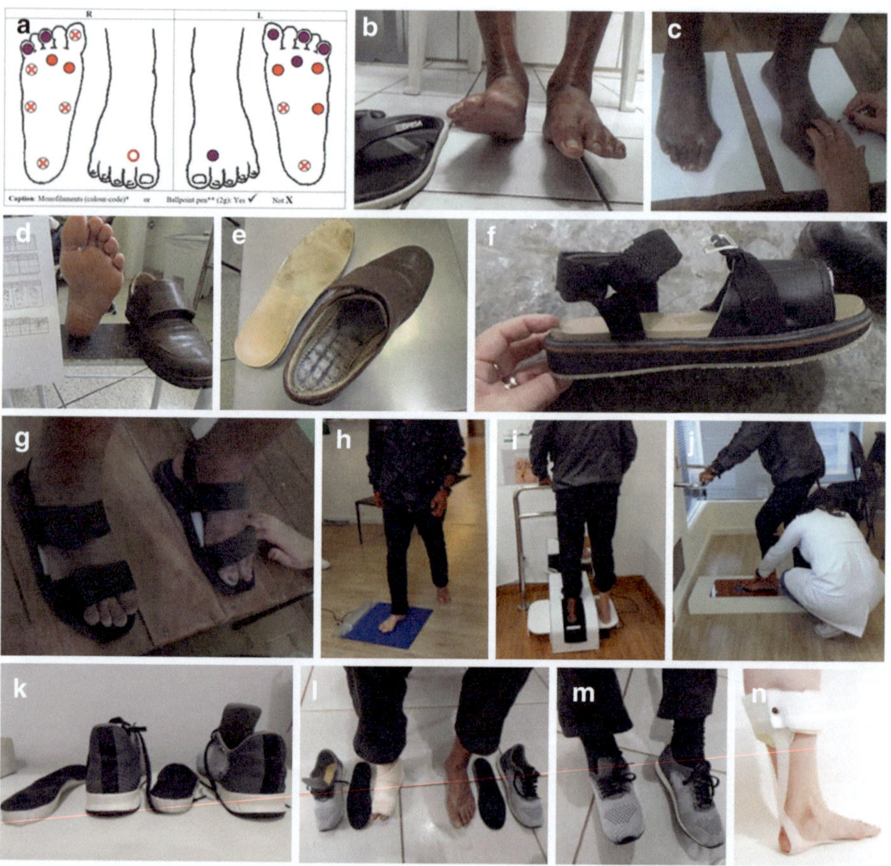

Fig. 4 (**a**) Sensory testing (Feet) i.e.; (**b**) Drop foot; (**c**) The shape of the shoe must fit the shape of the foot; (**d**) Person with sensory loss to the sole of the foot; (**e**) Molded insole (Ethylene Vinyl Acetate—EVA) for specific footwear; (**f**) Protective footwear custom-made with elastic band adaptation for ankle dorsiflexion; (**g**) Custom-made insole inserted into the patient's shoe; (**h**) Baropodometry (Measurement of pressure walking); (**i**) Foot scanning 3D; (**j**) Foot scanning; (**k**) Custom-made footwear and insoles (3 D technology); (**l**) Right foot deformity, custom-made protective footwear (3D technology); (**m**) Person wearing custom-made shoes (3D technology); (**n**) Suropodalic orthosis

4 Community-Based Rehabilitation

Community-Based Rehabilitation (CBR) was developed by WHO as a strategy that prioritizes the collective needs of people with disabilities. It consists of five components: health, education, livelihood, empowerment and social [16]. For CBR to be comprehensive, it is necessary to strengthen its principles: empowerment, equity, awareness, self-advocacy, facilitation, attention to gender issues and special needs, partnerships and sustainability [16, 17].

The needs of people with disabilities are individual and can be understood through the application of validated instruments (e.g. Screening of Activity Limit and Safety Awareness 'SALSA'; Participation Scale 'P-scale'; WHO Disability Assessment Schedule 'WHODAS'; 5-Question Stigma Indicator-community stigma '5-QSI-CS', and other tools [3, 18]. The use of several resources such as ATs and multisectoral interventions [15], based on a multi-professional approach incorporating physical rehabilitation, health education and self-care groups enables people to play their roles in civil, political, social and economic structures.

In the interventions proposed by professionals who promote CBR, it is essential that the active involvement of the person with disability, the development of self-confidence and motivation, in addition to the support and participation of the community for the inclusion to be effective and lasting [16, 17].

In this context, considering that "Global Leprosy (Hansen's disease) Strategy 2021–2030"includes Assistive Technology, inclusive approach in CBR and reduction of stigma in the set of research priorities [1], the focus of CBR actions and interventions aims to overcome activity limitations, promote social participation and improve quality of life [17].

5 Complications Requiring Immediate Intervention and/or Medical Referral

Acute decrease in visual acuity, iridocyclitis, glaucoma, lagophthalmos associated with corneal lesion [9] LR, acute neuritis [4, 19, 20], infectious wounds and/or ulcerations [3, 20], joint involvement and compressive syndromes require referral to reference services [1].

6 Conclusions

Given the relevance of nerve damage and its impact on disability at the individual and collective level, the adoption of a "Neurological Assessment Form in Hansen's Disease (NFA)" guides the clinical approach and data recording as an essential component of routine care and for the proper management of persons affected by HD (Figs. 5, 6 and 7). It also provides tools for the application of correct WHO Disability Grade classification, definition of strategic actions and public health policies.

<table>
<tr><td colspan="5" align="center">IDENTIFICATION DATA</td></tr>
<tr><td colspan="4">Patient name:</td><td>Date of birth:
 /   /</td></tr>
<tr><td colspan="2">Gender:
Male [   ]   Female [   ]</td><td colspan="2">Profession /Current occupation</td><td>Medical chart:</td></tr>
<tr><td colspan="4">Address:</td><td>Telephone:</td></tr>
<tr><td colspan="4">Health Service:</td><td>Examiner:</td></tr>
<tr><td colspan="3">Operational Classification: PB [   ]   MB [   ]
Clinical forms:
I [   ]   T [   ]   B [   ]   L [   ]   Undefined [   ]</td><td>Start   date   of MDT:

 /   /</td><td>MDT completion date:

 /   /</td></tr>
</table>

NOSE				
Chief complaint			**R**	**L**
Dryness	Y / N			
Wound	Y / N			
Nasal septal perforation	Y / N			
Caption: **Y** = Yes **N** = No				
Treatment:				

EYES				
Chief complaint			**R**	**L**
Diminished corneal sensation	Y / N			
Orbicularis oculi weakness	Y / N			
Closes eyes – gentle closure tested (Lagophthalmos)	Write 0 mm or "XX" mm			
Closes eyes – strong closure tested (Lagophthalmos)	Write 0 mm or "XX" mm			
Trichiasis	Y / N			
Ectropion	Y / N			
Corneal opacity	Y / N			
Visual acuity (use Snellen Chart).	Technique used: ( ) Snellen Chart ( ) Counting fingers ( ) Hand Movement ( ) Light perception			

Caption: —— = Without specific complaints.   **Y** = Yes   **N** = No.
Lagophthalmos: The distance between the upper and lower eyelid edges is measured with a millimeter ruler and recorded in **millimeters (mm)**. If normal closure of the eyelids, **0 (zero)**.
Visual Acuity: If the person wears corrective eyeglasses, it is recommended to perform the test: with eyeglasses **(W/E)**; no eyeglasses **(N/E)**. If the patient is unable to read the biggest optotype on the chart, it is reasonable to use "counting fingers", "hand movement" or "light perception".
Treatment:

Fig. 5 Nerve function assessment form: identification, nose, eyes. Source: Adapted from the Brazilian Ministry of Health [6] and WHO [4]

UPPER LIMBS		
Chief complaint	R	L
Inspection	R	L
Caption:	Mobile Claw = **M** · Rigid Claw = **R** · Bone Resorption ▨ · Wound/Ulcer ☐ · Scar/Callus △	

Nerve Palpation	Nerves	R	L
	Radial		
	Ulnar		
	Median		

Caption: **N** = Normal   **T** = Thickened   **P** = Pain   **S** = Tinel Sign (+)

Voluntary muscle test	Movements	R	L
	Movement: Wrist Extension. Muscle/muscle group: Wrist Extensors. (**Radial N.**)		
	Movement: Litte finger abduction. Muscle: Abductor digiti minimum (**Ulnar N.**)		
	Movement: Thumb abduction. Muscle: Abductor pollicis brevis. (**Median N.**)		

Caption: *Muscle power* - **S** = Strong; **W** = Weak; **P** = Paralyzed   *OR*
Medical Research Council - **5** = Muscle activation against examiner's full resistance, full range of motion (ROM); **4** = Muscle activation against some resistance, full ROM; **3** = Muscle activation against gravity, full ROM; **2** = Muscle activation with gravity eliminated, achieving full ROM; **1** = Trace muscle activation, such as a twitch, without achieving full ROM; **0** = No muscle activation.

Sensory testing	R	L

Caption: Monofilaments (colour-code)*   or   Ballpoint pen** (2g): Yes ✓   Not **X**

Treatment:

Fig. 6 Nerve function assessment form: upper limbs. Source: Adapted from the Brazilian Ministry of Health [6] and WHO [4]

LOWER LIMBS		
Chief complaint:	**R**	**L**
Inspection	**R**	**L**
	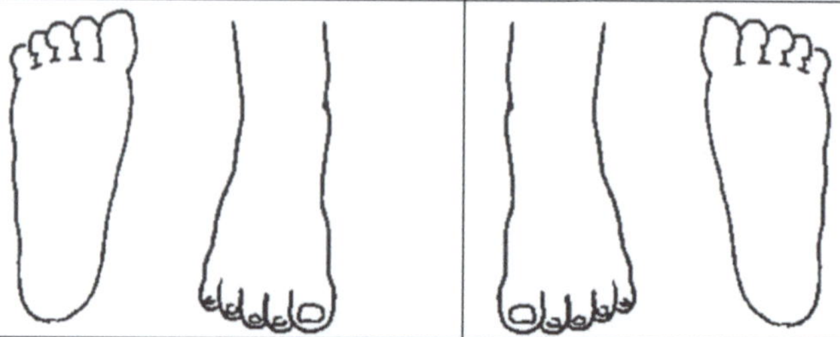 (foot diagrams)	(foot diagrams)
Caption:	Mobile Claw = **M** Rigid Claw = **R** Bone Resorption ▨ Wound/Ulcer ▭ Scar/Callus △	

Nerve palpation	**Nerves**	**R**	**L**
	Common Fibular		
	Posterior Tibial		

Caption: **N** = Normal   **T** = Thickened   **P** = Pain   **S** = Tinel Sign (+)

Voluntary muscle test	**Movements**		**R**	**L**
	Movement: Hallux Extension. Muscle: Extensor hallucis longus. **(Fibular Nerve)**	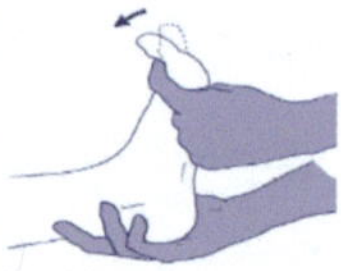 (illustration)		
	Movement: Foot Dorsiflexion. Muscle: Foot dorsiflexors. **(Fibular Nerve)**	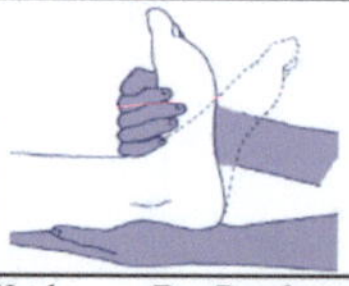 (illustration)		

Caption: *Muscle power* - **S** = Strong   **W** = Weak   **P** = Paralyzed   *OR*
Medical Research Council - **5** = Muscle activation against examiner's full resistance, full range of motion (ROM); **4** = Muscle activation against some resistance, full ROM; **3** = Muscle activation against gravity, full ROM; **2** = Muscle activation with gravity eliminated, achieving full ROM; **1** = Trace muscle activation, such as a twitch, without achieving full ROM; **0** = No muscle activation.

Sensory testing	**R**	**L**
	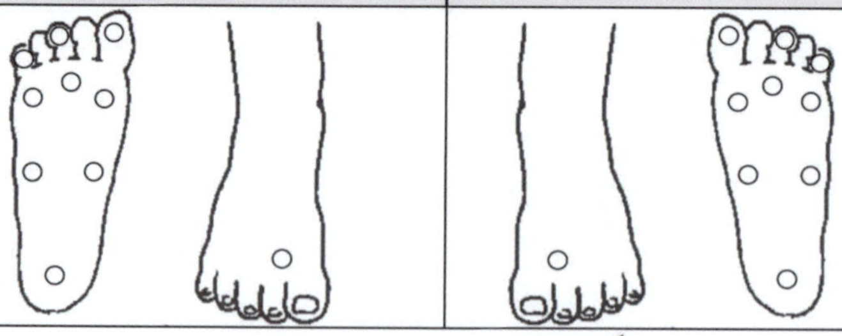 (foot diagrams with sensory test points)	(foot diagrams with sensory test points)

Caption: Monofilaments (colour-code)*   or   Ballpoint pen** (2g): Yes ✔   Not **X**

Treatment:

Fig. 7 Nerve function assessment form: lower limbs. Source: Adapted from the Brazilian Ministry of Health [6] and WHO [4]

References

1. World Health Organization. Towards zero leprosy. Global leprosy (Hansen's disease) strategy 2021–2030. New Delhi: WHO Regional Office for South-East Asia; 2021. https://apps.who.int/iris/handle/10665/340774. Accessed 11 May 2022
2. Lockwood DN, Saunderson PR. Nerve damage in leprosy: a continuing challenge to scientists, clinicians and service providers. Int Health. 2012;4(2):77–85. https://doi.org/10.1016/j.inhe.2011.09.006.
3. World Health Organization. Global leprosy strategy 2016–2020. Accelerating towards a leprosy-free world. Monitoring and evaluation guide. New Delhi: WHO Regional Office for South-East Asia; 2017. https://apps.who.int/iris/handle/10665/254907. Accessed 4 May 2022
4. World Health Organization. Leprosy/Hansen disease: management of reactions and prevention of disabilities: technical guidance. New. Delhi: WHO Regional Office for South-East Asia; 2020. https://apps.who.int/iris/handle/10665/332022. Accessed 8 May 2022
5. Brasil Ministério da Saúde. Guia prático sobre a Hanseníase. Brasília, DF: Ministério da Saúde; 2017. https://bvsms.saude.gov.br/bvs/publicacoes/guia_pratico_hanseniase.pdf. Accessed 20 Mar 2022
6. Brasil. Ministério da Saúde. Secretaria de Vigilância em Saúde. Ofício circular No 11/2021/CGDE/DCCI/SVS/MS. Brasília, DF: Ministério da Saúde; 2021. Assunto: Atualização do Formulário para avaliação neurológica simplificada e classificação do grau de incapacidade física. Modificado em 23/11/2021. http://www.aids.gov.br/pt-br/pub/2021/formulario-para-avaliacao-neurologica-simplificada-e-classificacao-do-grau-de-incapacidade. Accessed 10 May 2022
7. Lehman LF, Geryer MJ, Bolton L. Ten steps: a guide for health promotion and empowerment of people affected by neglected tropical diseases. Greenville: American Leprosy Missions; 2015. https://leprosy.org/ten-steps/. Accessed 29 Mar 2022
8. Raposo MT, Reis MC, AVDQ C, Heukelbach J, Parker LA, Pastor-Valero M, et al. Grade 2 disabilities in leprosy patients from Brazil: Need for follow-up after completion of multidrug therapy. PLoS Negl Trop Dis. 2018;12(7):e0006645. https://doi.org/10.1371/journal.pntd.0006645. Accessed 03 Jun 2022
9. Brasil. Ministério da Saúde. Manual de Prevenção de Incapacidades. Brasília: Editora MS; 2008. https://bvsms.saude.gov.br/bvs/publicacoes/manual_prevencao_incapacidades.pdf. Accessed 20 Mar 2022
10. van Brakel WH, Saunderson P, Shetty V, Brandsma JW, Post E, Jellema R, et al. International workshop on neuropathology in leprosy–consensus report. Lepr Rev. 2007;78(4):416–33.
11. Lehman LF, Orsini MBP, Fuzikawa PL, Lima RC, Gonçalves SD. Avaliação neurológica simplificada. Belo Horizonte: ALM International; 2009. https://www.sbd.org.br/mm/cms/2020/12/23/avaliacao-neurol-simplificada.pdf. Accessed 03 Mar 2022
12. Medical Research Council. Aids to examination of the peripheral nervous system. Memorandum no. 45 (superseding War Memorandum no. 7). London: Her Majesty's Stationery Office; 1976. https://www.ukri.org/wp-content/uploads/2021/12/MRC-011221-AidsToTheExaminationOfThePeripheralNervousSystem.pdf. Accessed 14 Apr 2022
13. SORRI. Monofilament Aesthesiometer. Touch sensitivity testing KIT–user's manual. Bauru: Sorri; 2020. https://sorribauru.com.br/custom/678/uploads/manusengl30.pdf. Accessed 30 May 2022
14. Alves ED, Ferreira TL, Ferreira IN. Hanseníase: avanços e desafios. Brasília: NESPROM; 2014. p. 492. http://www.morhan.org.br/views/upload/hanseniaseavancoes.pdf. Accessed 18 Feb 2022
15. Maia FB, Teixeira ER, Silva GV, Gomes MK. The use of assistive technology to promote Care of the Self and Social Inclusion in patients with sequels of leprosy. PLoS Negl Trop Dis. 2016;10(4):e0004644.
16. Khasnabis C, Heinicke Motsch K, Achu K, et al. Community-based rehabilitation: CBR guidelines. Geneva: World Health Organization; 2010. https://www.ncbi.nlm.nih.gov/books/NBK310952/. Accessed 14 Aug 2022

17. World Health Organization. WHO/ILEP technical guide on community-based rehabilitation and leprosy: meeting the rehabilitation needs of people affected by leprosy and promoting quality of life. Geneva: World Health Organization; 2007. https://apps.who.int/iris/handle/10665/43748. Accessed 28 Jul 2022
18. van Brakel WH, Officer A. Approaches and tools for measuring disability in low and middle-income countries. Lepr Rev. 2008;79(1):50–64.
19. Walker SL, Lockwood DN. Leprosy type 1 (reversal) reactions and their management. Lepr Rev. 2008;79(4):372–86.
20. World Health Organization. Global leprosy strategy 2016–2020. Accelerating towards a leprosy-free world. Operational Manual, vol. 2016. New Delhi: WHO Regional Office for South-East Asia. https://apps.who.int/iris/handle/10665/254907. Accessed 18 March 2022

Ophthalmological Alterations in Hansen's Disease

Adriana Vieira Cardozo

1 Introduction

Hansen's disease (HD) is the systemic infectious disease with the highest incidence of ocular involvement [1]. Ocular lesions triggered by *M. leprae* and *M. lepromatosis* can occur before, during or after multidrug therapy (MDT) [2–4], and present variable severity, related not only to the organic component of the disease, but also to its social determinants.

Blindness is the most serious ophthalmologic complication and reflects the impact of HD on the lives of those affected: while the rate of blindness in the general population ranges from 0.5–2% [5], in HD these figures vary from 2–11%, depending not only on disease progression and individual inflammatory response, but also on social and geographical factors, such as difficult access to specialized treatment with delayed diagnosis [5–9]. Even if *M. leprae* does not cause complete blindness, it can cause ocular symptoms in 70–75% of those affected, with 10–50% suffering severe ocular symptoms, which may be sufficient to impair quality of life [6, 7].

2 Mechanisms of Ocular Involvement

The damage caused by *M. leprae* can be didactically divided into two pathways: a direct pathway, in which the damage is caused by the bacillus' ability to invade and replicate in the host's cells; and an indirect pathway, in which the damage to the host is a consequence of its own immune response. These pathways can be synergistic or occur in isolation.

A. V. Cardozo (✉)
Secretaria Estadual de Saúde, Vitória, Brazil

P. D. Deps (ed.), *Hansen's Disease*, https://doi.org/10.1007/978-3-031-30893-2_15

The topography in which the bacillus settles also plays an important role in the development of the lesion. It is known that *M. leprae* has a predilection for temperatures below 37 °C, and experimental studies suggest that the eye has a temperature up to 3 °C lower than ambient [10], so the anterior segment of the eye would be the ideal site of primary infection [11]. Dispersion of the bacilli population begins in the anterior structures (such as the sclera and cornea) and progresses to the more posterior structures (such as the iris and ciliary body) [6, 12]. Scleral nodules, superficial punctate keratitis, conjunctivitis, uveitis, and corneal nerve involvement may be observed and become prominent [6, 11, 13].

As a result of the neurotropism of *M. leprae*, much of the ocular damage is due to the involvement of nerve bundles around the eyes. Involvement of the trigeminal and facial nerves, responsible for corneal sensitivity and eyelid motility, respectively, can lead to indirect ocular changes, such as prolonged exposure of the ocular surface [5–7].

In addition to the mechanisms of ocular involvement already mentioned, type 1 and type 2 reaction episodes can also cause ocular alterations, the most common being lagophthalmos and uveitis, respectively [6, 14, 15].

3 Clinical Manifestations

HD is a disease with a wide range of ocular manifestations and the main manifestations are listed below, which will be topographically organized from the more superficial structures in the ocular region to the deeper ones for didactic purposes (Table 1).

Table 1 Table of ocular clinical manifestations associated with HD [2, 4, 16–19]

Manifestation site	Clinical manifestations
Eyelids	Lagophthalmos; entropion; ectropion; Hansenoma
Eyelashes and eyebrows	Trichiasis; ptosis of eyelashes; Madarosis
Lacrimal system	Lacrimal hyposecretion; Dacryocystitis
Sclera and Episclera	Scleritis; Episcleritis; vascular changes in the sclerocorneal limbus; Hansenoma
Cornea	Diminished sensitivity; spotty keratitis; nerve thickening; ulceration; opacification; staphyloma; vascular changes in the sclerocorneal limbus
Uveal tract	Acute or chronic iridocyclitis, Irian atrophy, Iris nodules, Irian pearls, pupillary abnormalities
Pupil	Pupil posterior synechiae with consequent pupillary deformity
Lens	Cataract with decreased visual acuity
Ocular bulb	Pathophthalmitis; phthisis bulbi

The three most important causes of visual impairment and blindness in HD are secondary to direct invasion of the anterior segment by *M. leprae*, or as a result of neural damage to the eyelids. These include [13, 16]: Corneal opacification and scarring

- damage to the structures of the uveal tract
- secondary cataract

4 Structures External to the Eye: Eyelids

Lagophthalmos—incomplete palpebral occlusion. It is due to dysfunction of the orbicular eyelid muscle, which is responsible for eyelid occlusion, resulting from its invasion by bacilli, or by damage to the facial nerve, and/or its occipitotemporal and zygomatic branches (Fig. 1d).

This condition prolongs the exposure of the eyes to the environment, making them more susceptible to damage from foreign bodies, and the cornea tends to dry out, given the difficulty of lubricating it in the absence of blinking [13]. Its diagnosis

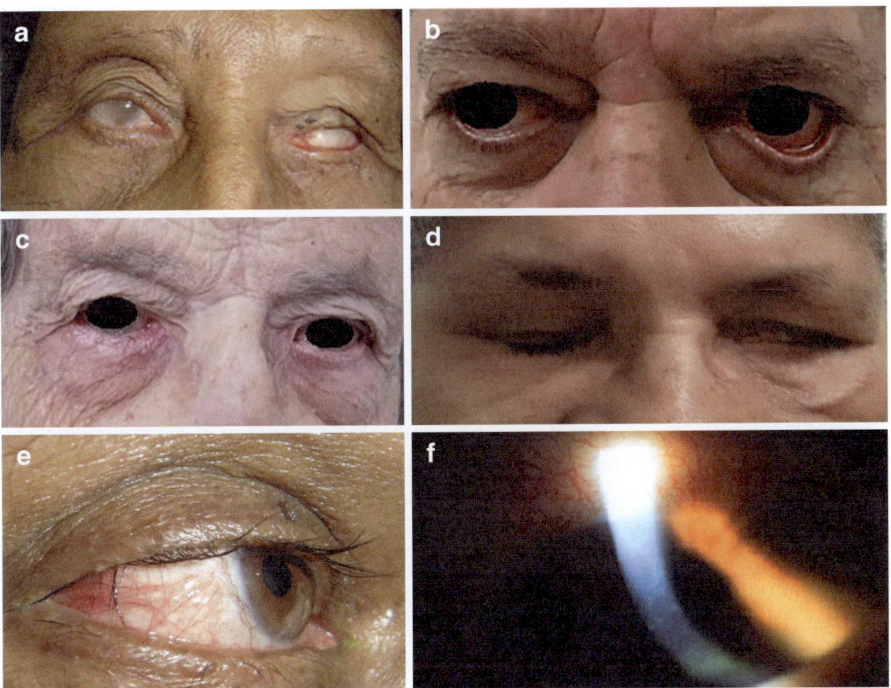

Fig. 1 (**a**) Bilateral blindness, lash, and eyebrow amaurosis. (**b**) ectropion left lower eyelid. (**c**) entropion right lower eyelid. (**d**) lagophthalmos left upper eyelid. (**e**) Trichiasis. (**f**) Superficial keratitis puntata (fluorescein stained and highlighted by cobalt blue light)

is made by observing the ocular surface during execution of the command to close the eyes gently: if the sclera or cornea are visible even in the patient with "eyes closed," lagophthalmos is confirmed [5, 13, 20].

Treatment of lagophthalmos can be pharmacological with systemic steroids, usually resolutive when its recognition is early (before 6 months). Physiotherapy can also help, but more severe cases usually require surgical intervention [13, 21, 22].

Ectropion (Fig. 1b) is an outward turning of the eyelid from the globe, his leaves the inner eyelid surface exposed and prone to irritation, having the same clinical repercussions as lagophthalmos [4, 7].

In the occurrence of inadequate eyelid occlusion, such as lagophthalmos and ectropion, it is important to investigate Bell's physiological phenomenon, which is characterized by the elevation of the eye bulb during eye closure. It protects the cornea from prolonged exposure since it is hidden by the upper eyelid [5]. A weak Bell's phenomenon increases the risk of corneal complications such as opacifications, ulcerations, and perforations with loss of intraocular content and blindness.

Entropion (Fig. 1c), characterized by the inversion of the palpebral border, which turns toward the surface of the eye bulb, causing greater friction of the eyelid and eyelashes on the corneal surface, which may cause ulcerations and/or staphyloma (protrusion or ectasia of the cornea or sclera resulting from trauma or inflammation, through which herniation of the uvea may occur). Such lesions may generate solutions of continuity between the interior of the ocular bulb and the environment, making it more susceptible to pathogen invasion [5, 20].

4.1 Eyelashes and Eyebrows

Eyelash ptosis refers to the lowering of the eyelashes secondary to loss of anterior lamella tonus, a consequence of hypotonia of the orbicular muscle of the eye.

Trichiasis—refers to ingrowth or introversion of the eyelashes, coming into contact with the surface of the eye bulb (Fig. 1e).

Trichiasis and ciliary ptosis may also contribute to corneal damage, since in these two situations, the lashes that turn toward the eye bulb may rub against the cornea. If corneal ulceration is not treated promptly, perforation of the ocular structures may occur, causing blindness [7, 20].

Madarosis is the loss of hair from the eyelashes and/or eyebrows. It is a common manifestation in HD patients, which can occur on the eyebrow and/or eyelid [5, 20, 23] (Fig. 1a).

5 Eye Structures

5.1 Cornea

As previously mentioned, most ocular damage in HD is not caused by the bacillary invasion, but as a consequence of other repercussions, such as nerve damage. In addition to the eyelid alterations already mentioned, the cornea can also suffer damage due to a decrease in its sensitivity as a consequence of the fifth cranial nerve lesion, which is responsible for its sensory innervation, and which will lead to a decrease in tear production and consequent ocular dryness, as well as a decrease in the blink reflex and in the perception of a foreign body on its surface, thus damaging the protection of the eye. Such circumstances may lead to a process of corneal opacification [13, 21], which may be potentiated by ulcerations (more frequent due to infectious keratitis) [16, 24, 25]. In the treatment of ulcerations, steroid-free eye drops and/or antibiotic ointments may be used in order to prevent complications, remembering that these cases constitute an ophthalmological emergency. The use of glasses and ocular lubricants can also be prophylactic, making it difficult for foreign bodies to enter the eyes and avoiding dryness, respectively [5, 13].

Superficial keratitis puntata. Caused by exacerbated proliferation of *M. leprae* in the cornea leading to the death of some cell groups [5], or by trauma to the corneal surface, either by ciliary touch or even corneal dryness (Fig. 1f).

5.2 Uveal Tract

Complications in the uvea are one of the most serious causes of blindness in patients. It may be asymptomatic and accompanied by small nodules in the iris. Bacillary invasion into the structures of the eye is followed by vascular spread of *M. leprae*, which follows with bilateral eye damage, manifested by conjunctival nodules and involvement of the cornea and anterior uvea [5, 20, 25]. **Irian pearls**, a pathognomonic sign of leprosy, are formed from dead bacteria. They grow slowly and coalesce, become pedunculated, and fall into the anterior chamber of the eye, where they eventually disappear [26, 27] **Anterior uveitis** is inflammation of the anterior uveal tract, which is composed of the iris and the ciliary body and may lead to **iridocyclitis**: a severe and silent condition that may be acute or chronic, caused especially when Hansen's bacilli start multiplying in the ciliary body, making the ciliary body and the iris vulnerable to inflammatory reactions. These reactions can also occur despite the presence of bacilli, during episodes of hypersensitivity [5].

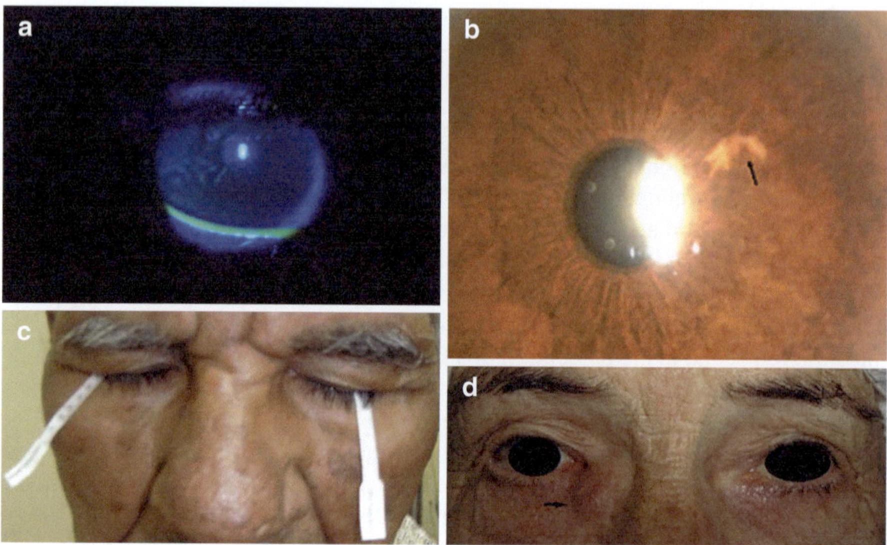

Fig. 2 (a)Tear film breakup time test- BUT. Areas not stained by fluorescein demonstrate where the cornea is dry. (b) iris atrophy (arrow). (c) Shirmer test. (d) Dacryocystitis (arrow- enlarged lacrimal sac)

The acute and subacute forms of iridocyclitis may go unnoticed or may be associated with eye pain and redness [13, 20], which may evolve into gradual iris atrophy, leading to pupillary irregularity and defects in iris structure [14, 27]. Some episodes may be severe enough to lead to irreversible vision loss, as in type 2 reaction episodes [13].

The **chronic iridocyclitis** is almost exclusively developed by multibacillary patients [13]. Clinical manifestations include pain, photophobia with tearing, visual blurring, perilimbal injection, pupillary seclusion, and aqueous clouding with inflammatory exudates [5, 6]. The inflammatory process may course with anterior synechiae (Irian tissue adheres to the corneal tissue) and/or posterior synechiae (Irian tissue adheres to the lens), which may restrict the aqueous humor flow and cause glaucoma [4, 5, 18]. Some patients may develop ocular hypotension if adrenergic control is dysregulated, a situation that occurs due to impairment of autonomic nervous system fibers. This condition also influences the ciliary body and the trabecular meshwork [28, 29]. The use of topical and mydriatic corticosteroids may be useful in an attempt to reduce the sequelae in intraocular inflammatory reactions [5, 13], but it is worth noting that both topical and systemic corticosteroids may cause increased intraocular pressure in some patients [11, 28]. Other important changes in the uveal tract involve bacillary invasion and/or nerve damage: **iris atrophy** (Fig. 2b) may be due to muscle breakdown and destruction, caused by an inflammatory process, or secondary to muscle atrophy from damage to the iris autonomic nervous system [14].

Pupillary abnormalities, in general, are most commonly due to chronic iritis with loss of the iris stroma, miosis, decreased reaction to light, difficulty dilating in response to anticholinergic eye drops, and early presbyopia. There are reports in the literature of a tonic pupil in a patient with the lepromatous form, characterized by mydriasis, absence of reaction to light and near light, and hypersensitivity to weak concentrations of cholinergic solution [26]. In advanced stages of the disease, Irian stromal atrophy and synechia may be associated with the development of miosis [14, 28, 30], and severe forms of Irian atrophy may lead to polycoria and affect vision [3].

Over time, destruction of the ciliary body nerves may extend to the posterior ciliary nerves, beyond the posterior pole of the ocular bulb and lateral to the optic nerve, in a process of ascending axonopathy, similar to glove and boot anesthesia [31].

Involvement of the posterior segment of the eye or optic nerve is rare in HD, but some studies suggest subclinical optic nerve involvement, especially in the reactional phase of the disease.

5.3 The lens

Cataract is secondary to inflammatory processes, as demonstrated by histological examinations [11], or as a result of the use of topical or systemic corticosteroids for the treatment of reactors [32]. The treatment of patients with leprosy in these cases differs from the others only in the caution regarding chronic uveitis since these are complex cases and may have complications. Moreover, patients with iris atrophy occasionally present greater difficulties in performing surgical intervention for the treatment of cataract [33]. In children, cataract with decreased visual acuity is secondary to the inflammatory process of iridocyclitis [9].

6 Other Ocular Manifestations in HD

6.1 Dry Eye

HD patients may present with dry eye for several reasons: hyposecretion of the aqueous layer of the tear film (due to injury to the parasympathetic nerve fibers that innervate the lacrimal gland and accompany the facial nerve); hypoesthesia or corneal anesthesia (corneal sensitivity is an important stimulus for tear production) [7, 8]; dysfunction of the sebaceous Meibomian glands, causing tear film instability [7]; increased evaporation of the tear due to increased exposure of the ocular surface secondary to eyelid changes (lagophthalmos, ectropion), as previously discussed. These changes can be diagnosed by tear film breakup time test (Fig. 2a) shorter than 10 s (positive BUT) and decreased Schirmer I test (Fig. 2c) ($\leq$10 mm), which can be attributed to infection or inflammatory process resulting from *M. leprae* invasion. Patients, especially multibacillary patients, may maintain the same results after MDT, with intensification of symptoms, by the use of clofazimine [3]. Clofazimine crystals may be deposited in the periphery of the cornea, in the region of the palpebral fissure [34, 35].

6.2 *Dacryocistitis*

Dacryocystitis (Fig. 2d) in HD patients results from alterations in the nasal mucosa, which can cause a blockage in the tear duct and consequently bacterial infection with an incidence of 2.6% of purulent dacryocystitis [7, 20].

Since the ocular manifestations of HD continue to occur, even with early diagnosis and adequate treatment of the disease, health professionals and all HD patients need to be aware that new eye symptoms and signs require prompt ophthalmology review to prevent avoidable blindness, due to the life-long risk of sight-threatening ocular complications.

References

1. Joffrion VC. Ocular Leprosy. In: Hastings RC, Opromolla DVA, editors. Leprosy. 2nd ed. Edinburgh: Churchill Livingstone; 1994. p. 353–65.
2. Courtright P, Daniel E, Sundarrao RJ, Mengistu F, Belachew M, Celloria RV, Ffytche T. Eye disease in multibacillary leprosy patients at the time of their leprosy diagnosis: findings from the longitudinal study of ocular leprosy (LOSOL) in India, The Philippines an Ethiopia. Lepr Rev. 2002;73:225–38.
3. Daniel E, Ffytche TJ, Kempen JH, Rao PS, Diener-West M, Courtright P. Incidence of ocular complications in patients with multibacillary leprosy after completion of a 2 year course of multidrug therapy. Br J Ophthalmol. 2006;90(8):949–54. https://doi.org/10.1136/bjo.2006.094870. Daniel E, Ffytche TJ, Kempen JH, et al. Incidence of ocular complications in patients with multibacillary leprosy after completion of a 2 year course of multidrug therapy. Br J Ophthalmol 2006; 90:949
4. Lewallen S, Tungpakorn NC, Kim SH, Courtright P. Progression of eye disease in "cured" leprosy patients: implications for understanding the pathophysiology of ocular disease and for addressing eyecare needs. Br J Ophthalmol. 2000;84(8):817–21. https://doi.org/10.1136/bjo.84.8.817.
5. Srinivas G, Muthuvel T, Lal V, Vaikundanathan K, Schwienhorst-Stich EM, Kasang C. Risk of disability among adult leprosy cases and determinants of delay in diagnosis in five states of India: a case-control study. PLoS Negl Trop Dis. 2019;13(6):e0007495. Published 2019 Jun 27. https://doi.org/10.1371/journal.pntd.0007495.
6. Citirik M, Batman C, Aslan O, Adabag A, Ozalp S, Zilelioglu O. Lepromatous iridocyclitis. Ocul Immunol Inflamm. 2005;13(1):95–9. https://doi.org/10.1080/09273940490912380.
7. Daniel E, Koshy S, Rao GS, Sundar Rao PS. Ocular complications in newly diagnosed borderline lepromatous and lepromatous leprosy patients: baseline profile of the Indian cohort. Br J Ophthalmol. 2002;86:1336–40.

8. Chen X, Zha S, Shui TJ. Presenting symptoms of leprosy at diagnosis: clinical evidence from a cross-sectional, population-based study. PLoS Negl Trop Dis. 2021;15(11):e0009913. Published 2021 Nov 23. https://doi.org/10.1371/journal.pntd.0009913.

9. Waddell KM, Saunderson PR. Is leprosy blindness avoidable? The effect of disease type, duration, and treatment on eye damage from leprosy in Uganda. Br J Ophthalmol. 1995;79(3):250–6. https://doi.org/10.1136/bjo.79.3.250.

10. Nunzi E, Massone C. Leprosy: a practical guide. Milano: Spinger; 2012.

11. Shamsi FA, Chaudhry IA, Moraes MO, Martinez AN, Riley FC. Detection of mycobacterium leprae in ocular tissues by histopathology and real-time polymerase chain reaction. Ophthalmic Res. 2007;39(2):63–8. https://doi.org/10.1159/000099375.

12. Cardozo AV, Deps P, Antunes JM, Belone Ade F, Rosa PS. Mycobacterium leprae in ocular tissues: histopathological findings in experimental leprosy. Indian J Dermatol Venereol Leprol. 2011;77(2):252–3. https://doi.org/10.4103/0378-6323.77490.

13. Malik AN, Morris RW, Ffytche TJ. The prevalence of ocular complications in leprosy patients seen in the United Kingdom over a period of 21 years. Eye (Lond). 2011;25(6):740–5. https://doi.org/10.1038/eye.2011.43.

14. Daniel E, Sundar Rao PS, Ffytche TJ, Chacko S, Prasanth HR, Courtright P. Iris atrophy in patients with newly diagnosed multibacillary leprosy: at diagnosis, during and after completion of multidrug treatment. Br J Ophthalmol. 2007;91(8):1019–22. Epub 2006 Nov 15

15. Rathinam SR, Khazaei HM, Job CK. Histopathological study of ocular erythema nodosum leprosum and post-therapeutic scleral perforation: a case report. Indian J Ophthalmol. 2008;56(5):417–9. https://doi.org/10.4103/0301-4738.42421.

16. Iraha S, Kondo S, Yamaguchi T, Inoue T. Bilateral corneal perforation caused by neurotrophic keratopathy associated with leprosy: a case report. BMC Ophthalmol. 2022;22(1):42.

17. Soomro FR, Pathan GM. Ocular disabilities in leprosy, Larkana District, Sindh, Pakistan. J Pak Assoc Dermatol. 2007;17:11–3.

18. Roldan-Vasquez A, Roldan-Vasquez E, Vasquez AM. Uveitic glaucoma and Hansen's disease, a case report. Am J Ophthalmol Case Rep. 2021;22:101096.

19. Wroblewski KJ, Hidayat A, Neafie R, Meyers W. The AFIP history of ocular leprosy. Saudi J Ophthalmol. 2019;33(3):255–9. https://doi.org/10.1016/j.sjopt.2019.09.003.

20. Mvogo CE, Bella-Hiag AL, Ellong A, Achu JH, Nkeng PF. Ocular complications of leprosy in Cameroon. Acta Ophthalmol Scand. 2001;79(1):31–3. https://doi.org/10.1034/j.1600-0420.2001.079001031.x.

21. El Toukhy E. Gold weight implants in the management of lagophthalmos in leprosy patients. Lepr Rev. 2010;81(1):79–81. PMID: 20496572

22. Wagenaar I, Post E, Brandsma W, Bowers B, Alam K, Shetty V, et al. Effectiveness of 32 versus 20 weeks of prednisolone in leprosy patients with recent nerve function impairment: A randomized controlled trial. PLoS Negl Trop Dis. 2017;11(10):e0005952. Published 2017 Oct 4. https://doi.org/10.1371/journal.pntd.0005952.

23. Pavezzi PD, do Prado RB, Boin Filho PÂ, AdS G, Tuma B, Fornazieri MA, et al. Evaluation of ocular involvement in patients with Hansen's disease. PLoS Negl Trop Dis. 2020;14(9):e0008585. https://doi.org/10.1371/journal.pntd.0008585.

24. Mukhopadhyay S, Sen S, Datta H. Comparative role of 20% cord blood serum and 20% autologous serum in dry eye associated with Hansen's disease: a tear proteomic study. Br J Ophthalmol. 2014;99(1):108–12. added to CENTRAL: 28 February 2015|2015 Issue

25. Kaushik J, Jain VK, Parihar JKS, Dhar S, Agarwal S. Leprosy presenting with Iridocyclitis: a diagnostic dilemma. J Ophthalmic Vis Res. 2017;12(4):437–9. https://doi.org/10.4103/jovr.jovr_155_15.

26. Lana-Peixoto MA, Campos WR, Reis PA, Campos CM, Rodrigues CA. Tonic pupil in leprosy. Arq Bras Oftalmol. 2014;77(6):395–6. https://doi.org/10.5935/0004-2749.20140098.

27. Morais LNA, David JPF, Peres Lima JV, Demachki S, Diniz DG, Almeida EF. Acquired acoria and iris pearls in leprosy: Case report. Eur J Ophthalmol. 2021;32(6):NP36–40. https://doi.org/10.1177/11206721211024057.

28. Lewallen S, Courtright P, Lee HS. Ocular autonomic dysfunction and intraocular pressure in leprosy. Br J Ophthalmol. 1989;73(12):946–9. https://doi.org/10.1136/bjo.73.12.946.
29. Brandt F, Malla OK, Anten JG. Influence of untreated chronic plastic iridocyclitis on intraocular pressure in leprous patients. Br J Ophthalmol. 1981;65(4):240–2. https://doi.org/10.1136/bjo.65.4.240.
30. Choyce DP. The diagnosis and management of ocular leprosy. Br J Ophthalmol. 1969;53(4):217–23.
31. Ebenezer GJ, Daniel E. Expression of protein gene product 9.5 in lepromatous eyes showing ciliary body nerve damage and a "dying back" phenomenon in the posterior ciliary nerves. Br J Ophthalmol. 2004;88(2):178–81. https://doi.org/10.1136/bjo.2003.027276.
32. Manabe S, Bucala R, Cerami A. Nonenzymatic addition of glucocorticoids to lens proteins in steroid-induced cataracts. J Clin Invest. 1984;74(1):803.
33. Chen HS, Wu ZM, Chen Y, He MS, Lin ZD. Clinical research of phacoemulsification with intraocular lens implantation in the treatment of cataract in leprosy patients. Int J Ophthalmol. 2015;15(10):1814–6. added to CENTRAL: 31 January 2016|2016 Issue 1
34. Barot RK, Viswanath V, Pattiwar MS, Torsekar RG. Crystalline deposition in the cornea and conjunctiva secondary to long-term clofazimine therapy in a leprosy patient. Indian J Ophthalmol. 2011;59:328–9.
35. Font RL, Sobol W, Matoba A. Polychromatic corneal and conjunctival crystals secondary to clofazimine therapy in leper. Ophthalmology. 1989;96:311–5.

Ear, Nose, Throat, and Mouth Alterations in Hansen's Disease

Marilda A. Milanez Morgado de Abreu and Patrícia D. Deps

1 Introduction

Hansen's disease mainly affects the peripheral nervous system and the skin; however, the causative mycobacteria enter the human body via the mucosa of the upper respiratory tract. In many cases, clinical manifestations of Hansen's disease may be limited to the head, particularly complaints and alterations associated with the nose. Mucosal lesions often occur with long-term evolution of the virchowian (lepromatous) form of Hansen's disease in untreated patients. At the tuberculoid pole, mucosal lesions are uncommon. Lesions in the mucous membranes of the upper airways serve as sources of infection in people with Hansen's disease, who can expel large numbers of bacilli when they spit, sneeze, cough, or talk [1, 2].

2 Mouth

The frequency of oral Hansen's disease lesions has dropped dramatically since the institution of multidrug therapy although the reported prevalence of specific oral mucosal involvement is highly variable, ranging from 0 to 70% [1–3]. Similarly, there is lack of consensus regarding the bacillus's preferred site of involvement—hard palate or soft palate [4–8]. Both these areas have lower

M. A. Milanez Morgado de Abreu (✉)
Universidade do Oeste Paulista (UNOESTE), Presidente Prudente, São Paulo, Brazil
e-mail: marilda@morgadoeabreu.com.br

P. D. Deps
Universidade Federal do Espírito Santo, Vitória, Brazil
e-mail: patricia.deps@ufes.br

P. D. Deps (ed.), *Hansen's Disease*, https://doi.org/10.1007/978-3-031-30893-2_16

temperatures because of the airflow and are therefore preferred by *M. leprae* [6, 7]. Bacilli can be found on the uvula, pharyngeal walls, palatine tonsils, tongue, gums, and lips, but the buccal mucosa is not usually affected except in the most severe cases [4, 6, 9]. However, histopathological involvement may exist, even without visible lesions [10]. Although there is no oral lesion pathognomonic of Hansen's disease [2], bilateral ulcers with symmetrical distribution, located on the palate, are indicative [7]. These are typically asymptomatic and contain a large number of bacilli [1].

Several classifications have been proposed for Hansen's disease lesions in the oral cavity, the most recent of which classifies lesions as specific or non-specific according to the presence or absence, respectively, of acid-fast bacilli (AFB). This classification is as follows [1, 2, 11]:

2.1   Specific Mouth Lesions in Virchowian Hansen's Disease

Palate: Lesions begin with a change in the color of the mucosa, which becomes pale or erythematous, and progress to infiltrations, papules, plaques, tubercles, and nodules that ulcerate and, upon healing, leave scars, atrophy, and deformities (Figs. 1 and 2) [4–6, 9]. Hard palate injuries can result in bone perforation, albeit a rare complication in the modern era. In the soft palate, they can result in reduced function [5].

Tongue: The dorsal surface is the most commonly affected area, especially the anterior two-thirds [6, 12, 13]. Glossitis, geographic tongue, leukoplakia, papillary hypertrophy, coating, plaques, nodules—sometimes separated by fissures (cobblestone appearance)—fissures, infiltration, erosions, ulcerations, macroglossia, fibrosis, and granulations are described (Fig. 3) [2, 5, 6, 10, 12–14].

Fig. 1 Soft palate infiltration

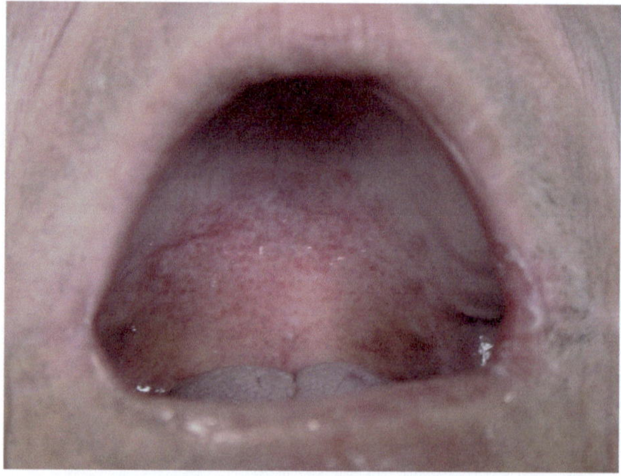

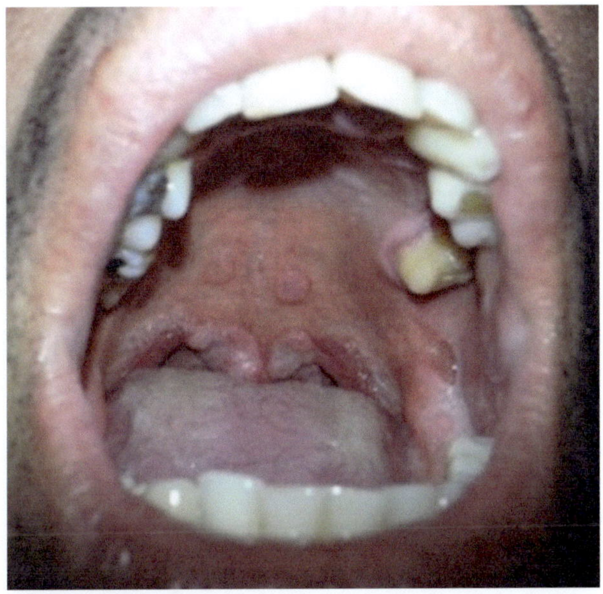

Fig. 2 Nodules on the soft palate and uvula

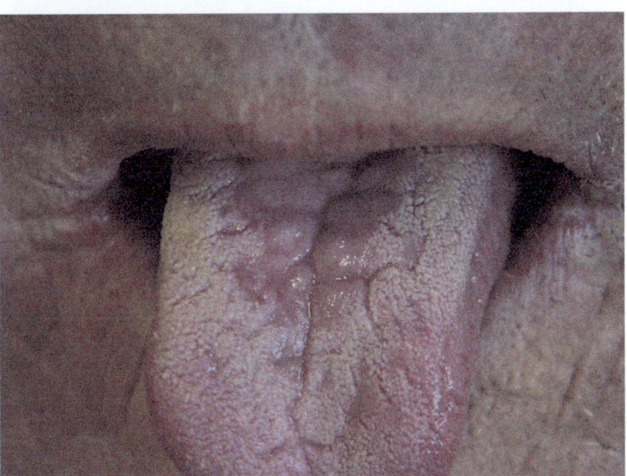

Fig. 3 Nodular infiltration on the surface of the tongue

Gums: There is a high incidence of gingivitis and periodontitis [4, 5], with halitosis as a consequence (Fig. 4) [15]. Infiltration, retraction, atrophy of the maxillary process, and nodules are also observed [5, 6]. In most cases, lesions on the gums are an extension of those on the hard palate [6].

Uvula: The uvula may present with nodules or with atrophy and destruction (Fig. 2) [5, 9].

Buccal mucosa: The buccal mucosa is not usually affected [4, 6].

Lips: Nodules can be observed, blurring delineation with the skin, infiltrations and ulcerations with crusts (Fig. 5). When lesions compromise the orbicularis-oris muscle, the mouth aperture can be reduced after healing, resulting in a "fish mouth" aspect [4, 5].

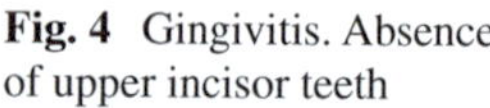

Fig. 4 Gingivitis. Absence of upper incisor teeth

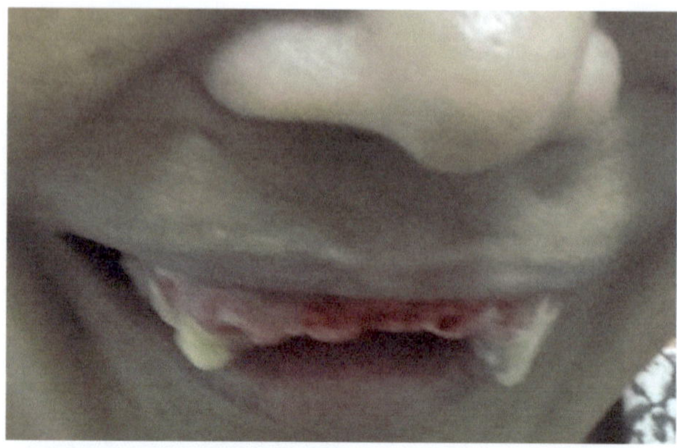

Fig. 5 Lip nodules

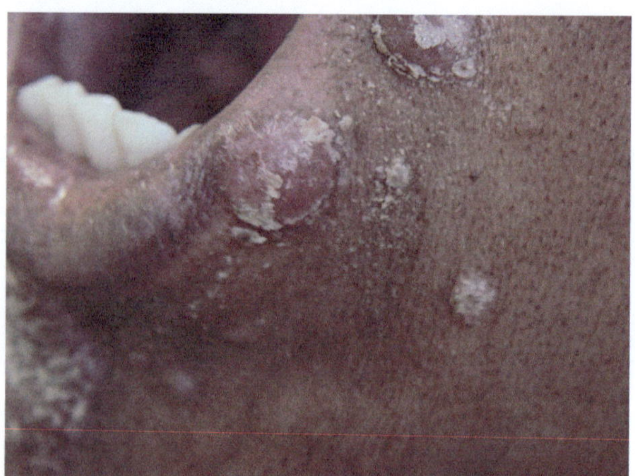

2.2 Specific Mouth Lesions in Tuberculoid Hansen's Disease

Lesions in the tuberculoid form of Hansen's disease are rare (Fig. 6). Usually are caused by nerve involvement. Lesions manifest as trophic ulcers and/or partial or complete paralysis of the lips, face, and soft palate muscles; the muscles of mastication are spared [4, 9]. Mucosal sensitivity can be affected and taste may be reduced or preserved [13, 14].

2.3 Specific Mouth Lesions in Hansen's Disease Reactions

In reactional outbreaks, existing lesions become edematous, painful, and ulcerated, leading to scarring and atrophy [5, 16]; the uvula can be destroyed [16]. Deformities, macrocheilia, and pseudoparalysis may occur due to edema or paralysis of the

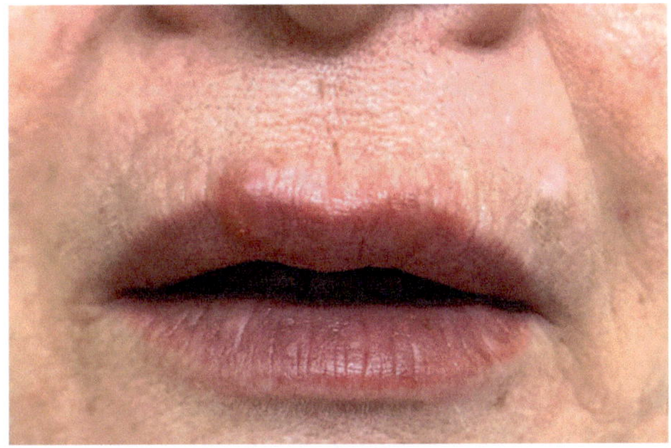

Fig. 6 Erythemato-edematous papules on the upper lip in Type 1 reaction

palate muscles [7, 9]. In the borderline-tuberculoid form of Hansen's disease, enanthema, infiltration, edema, papules and, less frequently, plaques and ulceration have been described (Fig. 6) [17].

2.4 Non-specific Lesions

Non-specific lesions are those that can also be found in individuals without Hansen's disease [2]. The importance of distinguishing non-specific lesions from specific lesions is because non-specific lesions are not a source of contagion, as they do not present AFB [1, 2]. These are also more frequent in multibacillary Hansen's disease, especially in virchowian patients. Non-specific lesions include [2, 8]:

Palate: papules and plaques.

Buccal mucosa: erythematous, hypochromic or hyperchromic macules, enanthema, and pallor.

Tongue: fissured tongue (the alteration most frequently observed), edema, infiltration, atrophy, and geographic tongue.

Gums: gingivitis.

3 Dental Changes

The most common occurrences of dental change are periodontal disease, present in 81% of Hansen's disease patients, and gingival bleeding (92%) [3]. In one study in Brazil, 73% of Hansen's disease patients had decayed teeth and at least 71% had lost at least one tooth; the average number of lost teeth among the patients was nine [18]. Maxillary central incisors are involved, especially in advanced virchowian Hansen's disease (Fig. 4). Radiological analysis of the alveolar bone shows an extensive interdental bone loss, sometimes followed by premature exfoliation of the upper anterior teeth [18]. This can be explained by the infection of the nasal mucosa that spreads, invading the anterior nasal spine and, further down, the maxillary incisor region.

4 Nose

Hansen's disease most frequently affects the nasal mucosa, and this can occur before neurocutaneous alterations. The involvement occurs in 97% of patients with virchowian Hansen's disease. Nasal discharge in these patients contains millions of potentially infectious bacilli, and it is therefore likely that it is mainly by this route that infection is spread [19, 20].

The most common complaint is nasal obstruction, with secretion and formation of crusts, either unilateral or bilateral [18]. More rarely, epistaxis occurs. Hyposmia is common and may occur in more than 40% of patients with virchowian Hansen's disease [19, 20]. In clinical examination, anterior rhinoscopy should always be performed, and nasofibroscopy may be necessary [18].

The anatomical site typically involved first is the anterior end of the inferior turbinate and next the nasal septum. Initially, the nasal mucosa presents hyperemia and congestion. The earliest recognizable sign of virchowian Hansen's disease is a pale nodular or plaque-like thickening of nasal mucosa. With progression, diffuse infiltration occurs and nodules appear with inflammation and severe obstruction. Subsequently, there is development of ulcers in the nasal septum, followed by involvement of the lower turbinate bone, which is covered with granulation tissue and crusts (Fig. 7).

Secondary infection and ischemia of the perichondrium can cause perforation of the cartilaginous nasal septum (Fig. 8). The bony part of the septum is rarely affected. Perichondritis and periostitis of the nasal cartilages, inferior turbinates,

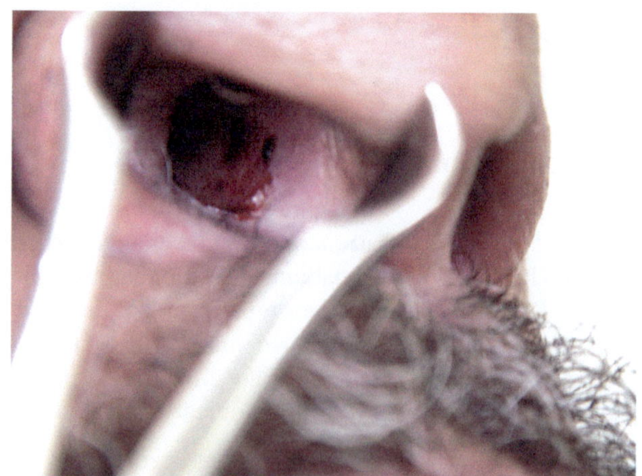

Fig. 7 Nasal septum ulceration

Fig. 8 Nasal septum perforation

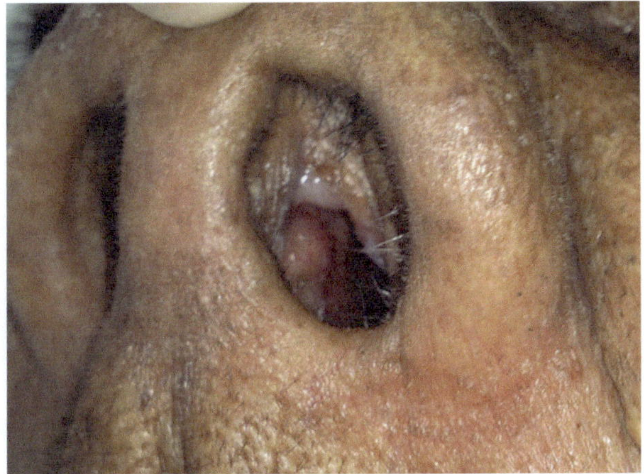

Fig. 9 Saddle nose

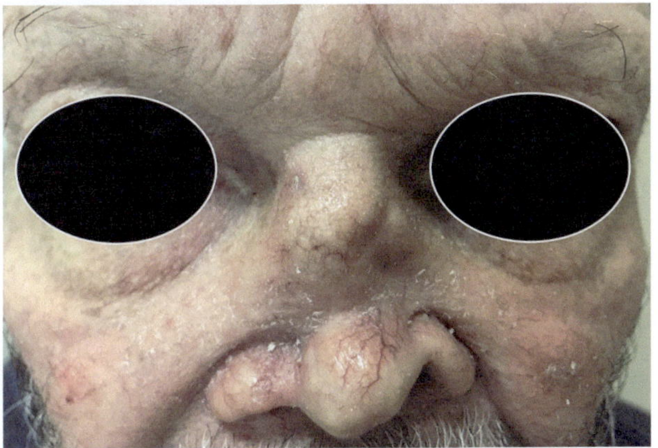

and anterior nasal spine cause the collapse of the nose (saddle-shaped nose) and atrophic rhinitis with pallor, drying, and loss of nasal hair with alteration of sensitivity (Fig. 9). The skin and alar cartilages are generally preserved. Perforation of the external nose with fistulization occurs rarely. Occasionally, atresia or stenosis of the airways can occur [19, 21, 22].

Rhinomaxillary syndrome is a set of seven maxillofacial bone alteration and manifests clinically with saddle nose, sunken (retracted) nose, reduced maxillary projection (maxillary retrognathia), and inverted upper lip [23–25].

5   Ear

Ear involvement in Hansen's disease is reported in 38–73% of patients, seeming to affect only its external part. This involvement may be minimal or extensive, typically affecting the ear lobes and helices. Initially, diffuse infiltrations or discrete

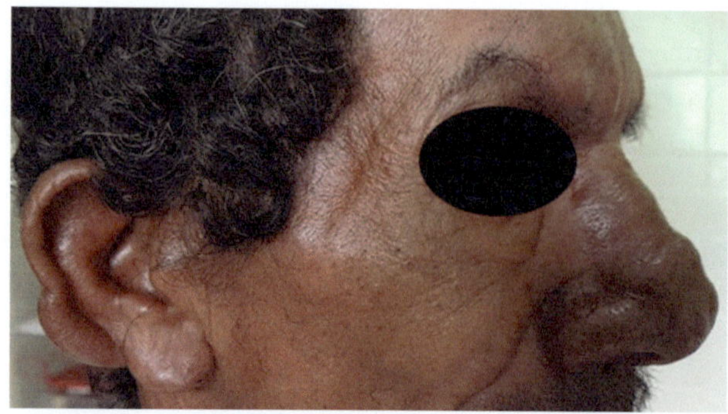

Fig. 10 Nose and ear lobe infiltration

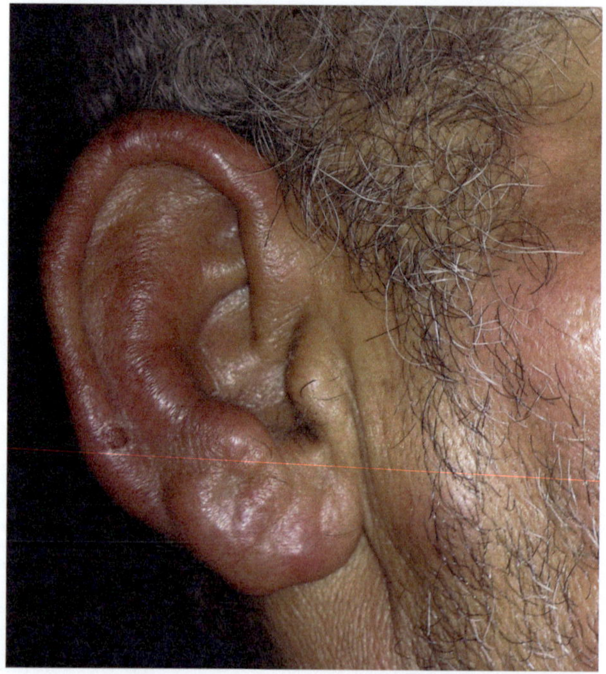

Fig. 11 Erythema and edema of the auricular pavilion in Type 1 reaction

nodules occur (Figs. 10 and 11). In severe cases, ulceration takes place followed by scarring of tissue. Later, the earlobe may be enlarged due to distention by infiltration and may remain stretched, elongated, and pendulous. A rare deformity of the ear is caused by reabsorption of cartilage leading to obstruction of the external auditory canal by prolapsed soft tissue [9, 26].

Inspissated cerumen is common and otological evaluation should include otoscopy. The membrana tympani may be estar retracted. It is common to see crusts and debris hanging over and around the auditory tuba opening [9].

Otologic alterations such as ear pain, hypoacusis, tinnitus, and vertigo are uncommon.

Edema of the external hearing duct and hearing loss have been described. When it occurs, the pathophysiology of hearing loss in Hansen's disease is considered to be attributable to involvement of cochlear, involvement of VIII cranial nerve (vestibulocochlear nerve) or problems in the middle ear secondary to rhinopharyngeal processes. Complementary exams such as audiometry and immitanciometry may be required [9, 19]. Slit skin smear should be taken from ear lobes for demonstration of AFB [26].

6   Throat

Lesions of the oropharynx and nasopharynx are extension, respectively, from the oral and nasal mucosa, and are present only in the long-term development of untreated virchowian Hansen's disease. Infiltration and nodules followed by atrophy and pallor are observed [9].

Laryngeal involvement in Hansen's disease was quite frequent in the pre-sulfone era [26], with most reports being based on autopsy findings. Laryngeal stricture was found to be the cause of death in 1.3% of necropsies, and laryngeal lesions were observed in 65% of virchowian Hansen's disease cases; involvement of the larynx in 31% of early virchowian Hansen's disease cases was reported [27].

The epiglottis is the site of predilection for *M. leprae* in the larynx because the stream of inspired air flows over the epiglottis before entering into the larynx and the temperature of the air at this point is approximately 2 °C cooler than body temperature, creating favorable conditions for *M. leprae* [27]. Lesions develop gradually and may be asymptomatic; the most common symptom is chronic cough and hoarseness [27].

Direct laryngoscopy or video laryngoscopy may be required to give a good view of the entire larynx. In the early stage, only the anterior parts of the larynx are affected. In the later stages, the entire larynx may be filled with grayish nodular tissue [27].

Laryngeal lesions can appear in two forms: fibrotic, with immobilization of vocal folds giving rise to hoarseness; or ulcerous, leading to hoarseness, pain, and dyspnea. The edema that occurs makes breathing difficult, but tracheotomy is not usually required until stenosis occurs. These lesions have not been observed under early multidrug therapy [19, 27].

References

1. de Abreu MAMM, Michalany NS, Weckx LLM, et al. The oral mucosa in leprosy: a clinical and histopathological study. Braz J Otorhinolaryngol. 2006;72:312–6. https://doi.org/10.1016/s1808-8694(15)30962-9.
2. de Abreu MAMM, de Avelar Alchorne MM, Michalany NS, et al. The oral mucosa in paucibacillary leprosy: a clinical and histopathological study. Oral Surg Oral Med Oral Pathol Oral Radiol Endod. 2007;103:e48–52. https://doi.org/10.1016/j.tripleo.2006.10.002.

3. Souza VA, Emmerich A, Coutinho EM, et al. Dental and oral condition in leprosy patients from Serra, Brazil. Lepr Rev. 2009;80:156–63.
4. Lighterman I, Watanabe Y, Hidaka T. Leprosy of the oral cavity and adnexa. Oral Surg Oral Med Oral Pathol. 1962;15:1178–94. https://doi.org/10.1016/0030-4220(62):90153-6.
5. Reichart P. Facial and oral manifestations in leprosy. An evaluation of seventy cases. Oral Surg Oral Med Oral Pathol. 1976;41:385–99. https://doi.org/10.1016/0030-4220(76):90152-3.
6. Girdhar BK, Desikan KV. A clinical study of the mouth in untreated lepromatous patients. Lepr Rev. 1979;50:25–35. https://doi.org/10.5935/0305-7518.19790004.
7. Scheepers A, Lemmer J, Lownie JF. Oral manifestations of leprosy. Lepr Rev. 1993;64:37–43. https://doi.org/10.5935/0305-7518.19930005.
8. Costa A, Nery J, Oliveira M, et al. Oral lesions in leprosy. Indian J Dermatol Venereol Leprol. 2003;69:381–5.
9. Pinkerton FJ. Leprosy of the ear, nose and throat: observations on more than two hundred cases in Hawaii. Arch Otolaryngol. 1932;16:469–87. https://doi.org/10.1001/archotol.1932.00630040481001.
10. Kumar B, Yande R, Kaur I, et al. Involvement of palate and cheek in leprosy. Indian J Lepr. 1988;60:280–4.
11. dos Santos GG, Marcucci G, Marchese LM, Guimarães Jr. J (2000) Aspectos estomatológicos das lesões específicas e não-específicas em pacientes portadores da moléstia de Hansen. Pesqui Odontol Bras 14:268–272. doi:https://doi.org/10.1590/S1517-74912000000300014.
12. Mukherjee A, Girdhar BK, Desikan KV. The histopathology of tongue lesions in leprosy. Lepr Rev. 1979;50:37–43. https://doi.org/10.5935/0305-7518.19790005.
13. Soni NK. Leprosy of the tongue. Indian J Lepr. 1992;64:325–30.
14. Sharma VK, Kaur S, Radotra BD, Kaur I. Tongue involvement in lepromatous leprosy. Int J Dermatol. 1993;32:27–9. https://doi.org/10.1111/j.1365-4362.1993.tb00957.x.
15. Matos FZ, Aranha AMF, Borges ÁH, et al. Can different stages of leprosy treatment influence the profile of Oral health? Oral status in leprosy. Med Oral Patol Oral Cir Bucal. 2018;23:e376–83. https://doi.org/10.4317/medoral.22220.
16. Scheepers A, Lemmer J. Erythema nodosum leprosum: a possible cause of oral destruction in leprosy. Int J Lepr Other Mycobact Dis. 1992;60:641–3.
17. Alfieri N, Fleury RN, Opromolla DV, et al. Oral lesions in borderline and reactional tuberculoid leprosy. Oral Surg Oral Med Oral Pathol. 1983;55:52–7. https://doi.org/10.1016/0030-4220(83)90305-5.
18. Deps P, do Espírito Santo RB, Charlier P, Collin SM. Rhinomaxillary syndrome in Hansen's disease: a clinical perspective. Int J Dermatol. 2020;59(11):e404–6. https://doi.org/10.1111/ijd.15202.
19. da Silva GM, Patrocinio LG, Patrocinio JA, Goulart IMB. Otorhinolaryngologic evaluation of leprosy patients protocol of a National Reference Center Giselle Mateus da Silva 1, Lucas Gomes Patrocinio 2, José Antonio Patrocinio 3, Isabela Maria Bernardes Goulart 4. Intl Arch Otorhinolaryngol. 2008;12:77–81.
20. Barton RP, Davey TF. Early leprosy of the nose and throat. J Laryngol Otol. 1976;90:953–61. https://doi.org/10.1017/s0022215100082967.
21. Serafim RA, Espírito Santo RB, Mello RAF, et al. Case report: nasal Myiasis in an elderly patient with atrophic rhinitis and facial sequelae of leprosy. Am J Trop Med Hyg. 2020;102:448–50. https://doi.org/10.4269/ajtmh.19-0708.
22. Yassin A, el Shennawy M, el Enany G, et al. Leprosy of the upper respiratory tract. A clinical bacteriological, histopathological and histochemical study of twenty cases. J Laryngol Otol. 1975;89:505–11. https://doi.org/10.1017/s0022215100080671.
23. do Espírito Santo RB, Serafim RA, Loureiro RM, et al. Clinical and radiological assessment of rhinomaxillary syndrome in Hansen's disease. Indian J Dermatol Venereol Leprol. 2021;88:1–11. https://doi.org/10.25259/IJDVL_1203_20.
24. do Espírito Santo RB, DVC G, Serafim RA, et al. Evaluation of proposed cranial and maxillary bone alteration parameters in persons affected by Hansen's disease. PLoS Negl Trop Dis. 2021;15:e0009694. https://doi.org/10.1371/journal.pntd.0009694.

25. Pollack JD, Pincus RL, Lucente FE. Leprosy of the head and neck. Otolaryngol Head Neck Surg. 1987;97:93–6. https://doi.org/10.1177/019459988709700120.
26. Soni NK. Leprosy of the larynx. J Laryngol Otol. 1992;106:518–20. https://doi.org/10.1017/s002221510012002x.
27. Gupta OP, Jain RK, Tripathi PP, Gupta S. Leprosy of the larynx: a clinicopathological study. Int J Lepr Other Mycobact Dis. 1984;52:171–5.

Osteoarticular Alterations in Hansen's Disease

Rachel Bertolani do Espírito Santo and Patrícia D. Deps

In addition to affecting the skin and peripheral nerves, Hansen's disease may also compromise nasal tissues and bones [1]. Facial and extremity skeletal deformities are historical markers and part of the stigma of this disease [2]. Patients with multibacillary (lepromatous) Hansen's disease are at increased risk of developing physical disabilities, which are also found in paucibacillary patients [3].

The etiologic agents of Hansen's disease, are an obligate intracellular pathogen capable of invading the peripheral nervous system, where it is predominantly found within the Schwann cells. It can also be found in the bone marrow, where it sometimes remains viable even after specific treatment [4]. Despite being one of the oldest diseases recorded by humankind, the underlying mechanisms of Hansen's disease-induced bone damage are not completely known.

1 Pathogenesis of Bone Lesion

Bone lesion may be caused by direct invasion of causative agents into bone tissue and may be a consequence of peripheral nerve involvement.

It has also been described that *M. leprae* inhibits the expression of the PHEX gene (phosphate-regulating gene with homologies to endopeptidase on the X chromosome) in osteoblasts and this can lead to bone resorption. Therefore, defects of bone mineralization may also be involved in the pathogenesis [2].

Visible bone changes usually occur in long-term disease and are more pronounced in the bacillary borderline and lepromatous presentations; however,

R. B. do Espírito Santo (✉) · P. D. Deps
Universidade Federal do Espírito Santo, Vitória, Brazil
e-mail: patricia.deps@ufes.br

P. D. Deps (ed.), *Hansen's Disease*, https://doi.org/10.1007/978-3-031-30893-2_17

increased bone resorption has been demonstrated in both pauci and multibacillary forms of the disease, independent of duration and bacterial load [1, 5, 6].

The nasal mucosa is involved in transmission and is considered an important entry and elimination route for *M. leprae*. Over the years, the nose has been confirmed as the initial site of lesions in Hansen's disease [7, 8]. Ninety-five percent of patients with the virchowian (lepromatous) form and about 80% of patients with bacilliferous borderline forms have involvement of the nasal mucosa [9, 10]. Mucosal lesions comprise granulomatous infiltration, nodules (lepromas), ulceration, vasculitis, secondary infection, and atrophy. From the mucosa the bacilliferous granulomas invade the cartilage. These alterations, associated with the decrease of blood flow in the perichondrium, may generate perforation of the nasal septum cartilage, whose extension may increase, evolving to the destruction of the entire cartilage and extending to the bony portion [10]. Bacilliferous granulomas probably also cause discrete shallow erosions in the bone and reach the bone marrow [11, 12].

The anterior nasal spine may also be affected by the bacillus [13]. Osteoclasia is the main pathogenic factor for resorption of the anterior nasal spine, but secondary infections in the cartilage and bony portion of the nasal septum also aggravate the destruction of these tissues [14].

Oral lesions in Hansen's disease are secondary to nasal involvement and occur more frequently in multibacillary patients. *M. leprae* has an affinity for cooler regions of the body. Mouth breathing due to nasal obstruction observed in patients with the lepromatous form, favors the decrease of the mean temperature in the anterior structures of the oral cavity. The hard palate has been described as the most frequent site of involvement. A particularly favorable site for the development of the bacillus is the incisive papilla, situated just behind the upper central incisors, where the mean temperature remains around 27.4 °C. Nodular submucosal infiltrate, ulceration, and even perforation of the hard palate can be observed [9, 14, 15].

Hansen's disease reactions may intensify the nasal and palatal bone resorptive process due to the increase in pro-inflammatory cytokines that participate in the induction of osteoclasia [14]. Erythema nodosum (reaction type 2) is postulated to be an important cause of destruction, perforation, and deformation of the palate [9, 15, 16].

The gums are usually affected in the posterior region of the maxillary central incisors, often by contiguity of lesions of the hard palate. Microscopic lepromatous infiltration has been described in the gingiva, periodontal membrane, alveolar bone, and bone marrow. Bacilli in osteoblasts disrupt the reorganization of the alveolar bone with resulting fibrosis, osteoporosis, and local bone loss [11]. The changes described are chronic gingivitis, periodontitis, and periodontoclasia [15].

The resorption of the maxillary alveolar bone is carried out by osteoclasts and is independent of the occurrence of inflammatory periodontal disease in the upper incisor teeth but may be intensified by the presence of *M. leprae* in the vicinity.

The pathogenesis of maxillary deformities in Hansen's disease is likely to be multifactorial; caused by the chronic inflammatory process in the adjacent connective tissue, by reactive bone changes, by loss of neurotrophic stimuli, and by the involvement of the nasopalatine nerve, which originates from the sphenopalatine nerve in the nasal cavity and penetrates the incisive canal until it exits into the incisive fossa [14].

When invading the peripheral nerves, the Hansen's bacillus causes inflammation, culminating in progressive loss of nerve function, known as primary nerve damage [2]. It is also important to mention that Hansen's disease reactions (type 1 and type 2) may cause neuritis, potentiating the primary nerve damage [17].

The peripheral neuropathy of Hansen's disease is mixed, involving sensory, motor, and autonomic nerve fibers. It generally affects one or more nerves [18], generating paresis, loss of sensation, autonomic alterations such as dry skin, contributing to the appearance of a sequence of events such as cracks and ulcerations in the skin, secondary soft-tissue infection, osteitis, osteomyelitis, and bone resorption, finally causing bone deformities [19–21].

These deformities include "claw" hands and feet, bone resorption and loss of distal, middle and proximal phalanges of the chiro and pododactyles [22–25]. Arthritis secondary to Hansen's disease can lead to deformities in the hands known as "boutonnière" and "swan" neck fingers and in the feet "hammer" toes [26]. The feet may also present with neuropathic osteoarthropathy or Charcot deformity [27]. On the face, patients may present with a "saddle" nose due to the involvement of nasal cartilaginous and bony structures [9].

Bone changes in Hansen's disease are divided into specific, non-specific, and osteoporotic.

2   Specific Bone Changes

Specific alterations are seen in patients with virchowian form of Hansen's disease, and their frequency varies from 3 to 5% [28]. They are due to bone invasion by the bacillus and affect mainly bones of the face, hands, and feet (Fig. 1). Initially, there is the involvement of the periosteum, and later of the cortex, cancellous bone, and medullary canal. The bone trabeculae are invaded by granulation tissue containing macrophages with large numbers of bacilli. Fragmentation, necrosis, and gradual destruction of the trabeculae occur [29].

2.1   *Specific Bone Changes in the Face*

The "saddle nose" deformity corresponds to the loss of dorsal nasal height due to cartilaginous and/or bony collapse. It also includes features such as: loss of nasal tip support and definition, columellar retrusion, shortened vertical nasal length, and retrusion of the anterior bony nasal spine and caudal septum [30, 31] (Fig. 2).

Fig. 1 Bones frequently affected by specific changes

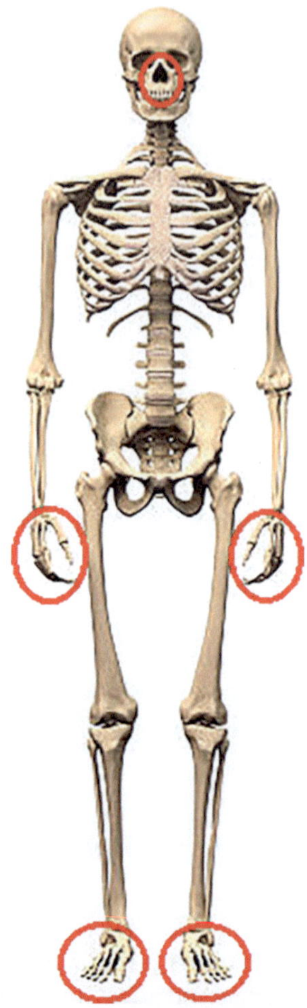

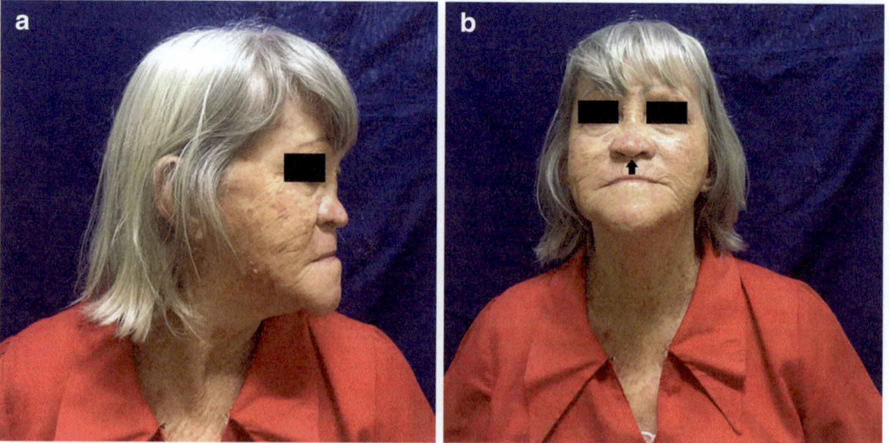

Fig. 2 (**a**) Saddle nose, loss of nasal dorsal height, decreased support and projection of the nose tip. (**b**) Arrow: retrusion of the columella [32]

Fig. 3 Bones of the face

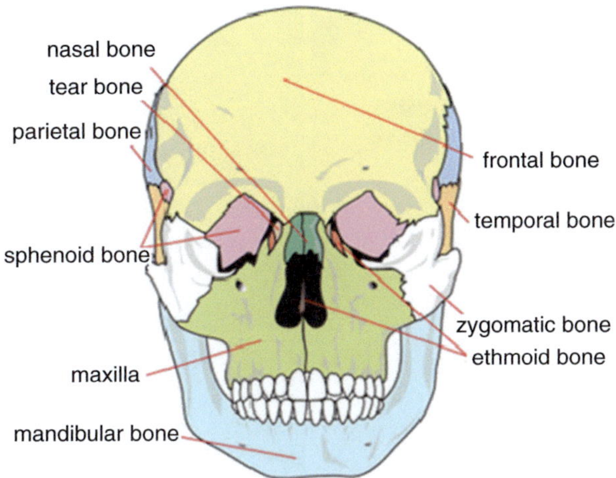

Direct bone invasion by *M. leprae* causes granulomatous lesion seen as a focal area of rarefaction on radiograph. The nasal lesion has been described as bone change specific, with destruction of the nasal bone associated with destruction of the septal cartilage, the alar cartilages, and the perpendicular lamina of the ethmoid and vomer bones (Fig. 3) [28, 33, 34].

2.2 *Rhinomaxillary Syndrome*

The rhinomaxillary syndrome was first described by Andersen and Manchester in 1992 [12], based on paleopathological studies. However, this terminology should also be adopted in the clinic [32, 35], and may present varying degrees of involvement of the following structures:

(a) Anterior nasal spine—partial or total resorption.
(b) Alveolar processes (anterior) of the maxilla—partial bilateral and symmetrical absorption, starting at the prosthion and culminating with the loss of the upper incisor teeth.
(c) Posterior alveolar margins of the maxilla—much less affected than the anterior portion, resorption can occur in the region of the molar teeth.
(d) Nasal and oral surface of the palatine process of the maxilla—inflammation, localized bone destruction, definitive perforation of the palate.
(e) Nasal turbinates and septum—inflammation, partial or total destruction.
(f) Nasal aperture—progressive resorption of the margins leading to widening and loss of the piriform shape (pear shape).

These bone changes above reflect a clinical picture with the following characteristics (Fig. 4) [32]:

(a) Saddle nose (loss of nasal dorsal height and shortened length of nose).

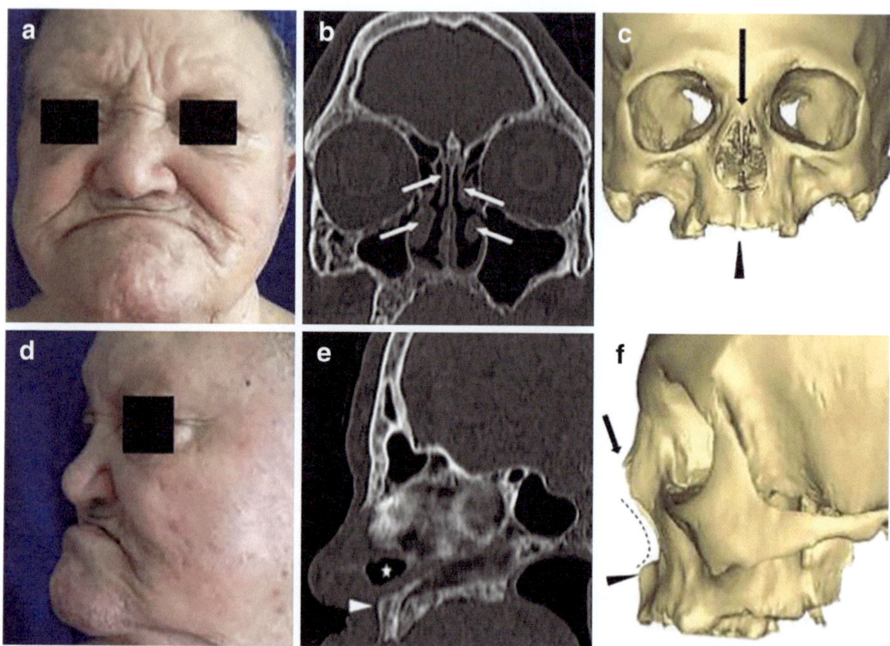

Fig. 4 Patient with rhinomaxillary syndrome. Frontal (**a**) and lateral (**d**) facial aspect showing facial profile changes including moderate saddle nose which was sunken in concave middle third of face, and reduced maxillary projection with inverted upper lip. Coronal (**b**) and sagittal (**e**) CT images showing variable atrophy of the middle and inferior nasal turbinates (arrows) and marked resorption of the anterior nasal spine (arrowhead) and a perforation in the nasal septum (star). Frontal (**c**) and lateral (**f**) three-dimensional reconstruction CT images showing (**c**) resorption of the nasal bones (arrow) and alveolar process of the maxilla (arrowhead); (**f**) marked resorption of the anterior nasal spine (arrowhead) and nasal bones (arrow), as well loss of sharpness of the pyriform aperture (dashed line) [32]

(b) Concave middle third of the face with sunken (retracted) nose, caused by erosion of the zygomatic process and enlargement and loss of the pyriform shape of the nasal aperture (pear shape).
(c) Reduced maxillary projection (maxillary retrognathia).
(d) Inverted upper lip because of reduced maxillary height.

For the evaluation of the rhinomaxillary syndrome, computed tomography (CT) is more recommended than plain sinus radiography. Images without overlapping structures allow a 3D reconstruction and are better for identifying soft tissue and bony anatomical variations [32, 36].

2.3 Specific Bone Changes in Hands and Feet

Upon reaching the medullary cavity, *M. leprae* can multiply in the bones of hands and feet [37]. This involvement can trigger several events such as bone rarefaction, cysts, widening of the nourishing foramen, necrosis, periostitis, osteitis, and osteomyelitis. Eventually, the damage becomes irreversible. Pathological fracture and epiphyseal collapse may occur [38, 39].

3   Non-specific Bone Changes

Non-specific bone lesions are the most common. They arise from peripheral nerve involvement, with subsequent denervation and loss of proprioception leading to neuropathic osteoarthropathy. Vascular changes, trauma, and secondary infections may also contribute to the non-specific changes [28].

They can occur in all clinical forms of Hansen's disease. The hands and feet are the most commonly affected sites (Fig. 5) [38].

Bone resorption thins and/or shortens the phalanges, metacarpals, and metatarsals. Distal resorption reduces bone length, while resorption of trabecular bone, also

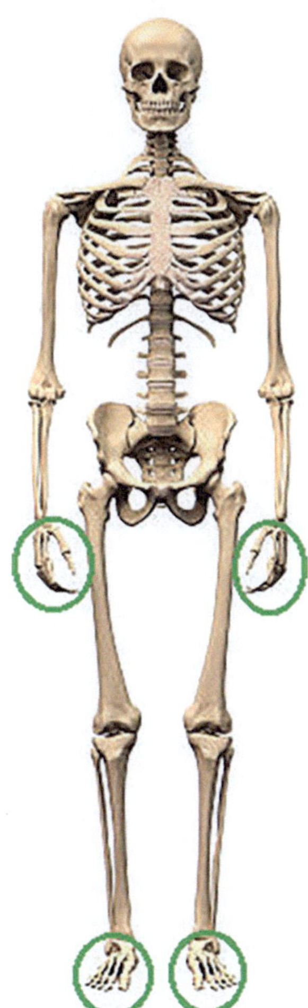

Fig. 5 Bones often affected by non-specific changes

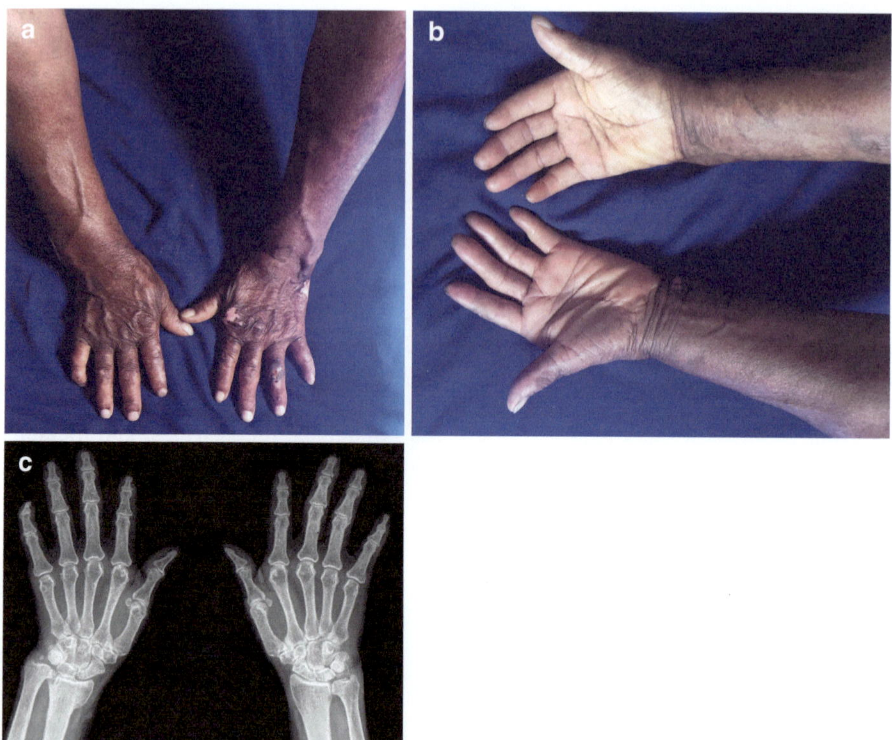

Fig. 6 (**a**) Right ulnar claw, ulceration on dorsum of left fourth finger. (**b**) Apparent reduction in the length of the distal phalanges of the second and fifth right fingers. (**c**) Radiography of the hands shows resorption of the second and fifth right distal phalanges, the latter with a "licked candy stick" appearance

called concentric bone atrophy, reduces width. The combination of the changes gives the bone a "pencil" appearance, also called "licked candy stick" [40].

In the hands, bone resorption starts at the ends of the distal phalanges, the areas most subject to trauma, with subsequent involvement of the middle and proximal phalanges and, more rarely, of the metacarpal, carpal joint, and radiocarpal bones [41–44].

Concentric bone atrophy of the diaphyses of the phalanges makes them gradually diminished, and with gradual erosion of the cortical portion of the bones, a frequent end result is the complete disappearance of the affected bone (Figs. 6 and 7) [45].

A neuropathic foot is defined as a foot in which there is loss of at least one of the peripheral nerve functions (motor, sensory, or autonomic). The loss of protective sensation and the paralytic lesions favor trauma. Since pain sensation is compromised, the patient may not notice the trauma and continue walking, causing further damage to the affected area.

Abnormal load distribution on the plantar surface also leads to trauma at the site of greatest pressure, causing ulceration, bone resorption, or secondary osteoarthritic

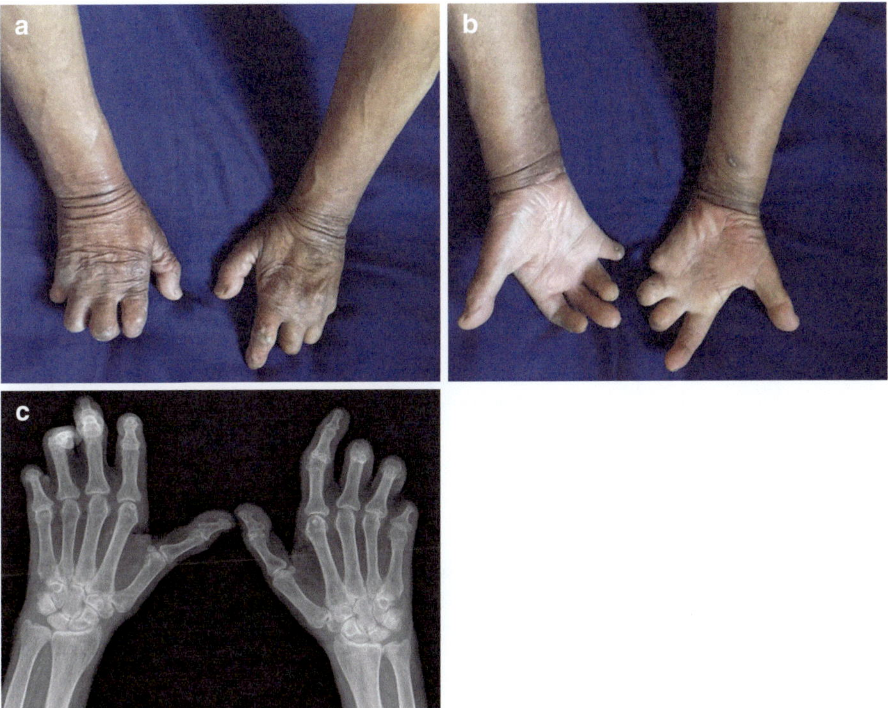

Fig. 7 (**a**) Cubitomedian claw and amyotrophy. (**b**) Resorption of phalanges. (**c**) Radiography of the hands shows resorption of multiple phalanges, most marked on the left hand. The proximal phalanx of the left fifth digit has a "licked candy stick" appearance

changes. Plantar ulceration, especially on the metatarsal heads, is a frequent complication of Hansen's disease neuropathy and secondary infection leads to cellulitis and osteomyelitis. Besides the phalanges, the distal end of the metatarsals can also be affected.

The neuropathic changes described facilitate the onset of fractures, which can also be triggered by osteoporosis. Thus, the combination of neural impairment, changes in biomechanical forces and osteoporosis may result in a neuro-osteoarthropathic change called "active Charcot foot." This foot, if inadequately treated, may progress to an irreversible sequela, the "Charcot deformity" [22, 27, 38–42, 46–52]. The most commonly observed radiological image of neuro-osteoarthropathy is the disintegration of the tarsal bones [42, 53]. The bones of the feet can be seen in Fig. 8.

Five radiological patterns of disintegration of the tarsal bones are described:

1. Posterior pillar: involvement of the calcaneus and subtalar joint.
2. Central pillar: involvement of the talus and subtalar joint.
3. Anterior pillar medial arch: involvement of the talus-navicular and cuneiform area. This is the most frequently seen pattern.

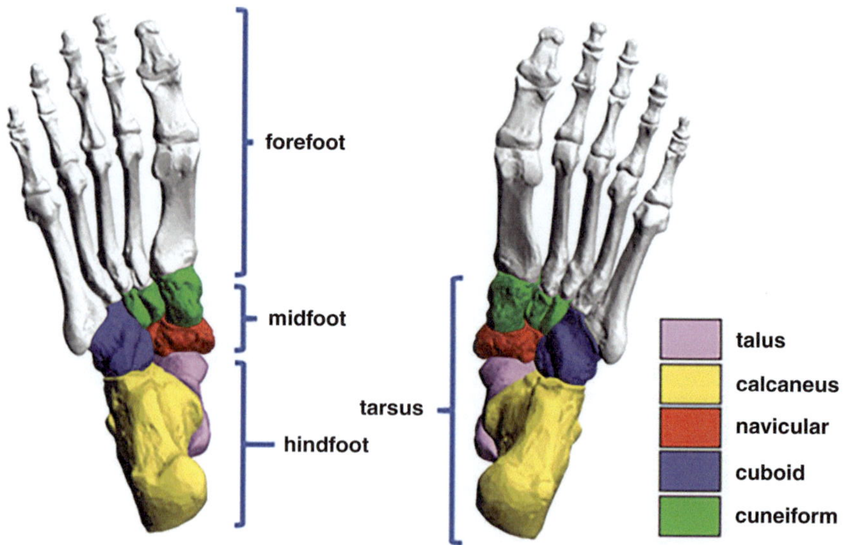

Fonte: BodyParts3D, © the Database Center for Life Science licensed under CC Attribution·Share Alike 2.1 Japan.

Fig. 8 Bones and regions of the foot

4. Anterior pillar lateral arch: the cuboid and cuboid-metatarsal joint are involved.
5. Cuneiform-metatarsal region.

Figure 9 illustrates the osteoarticular changes in the feet

Radiological changes in the midfoot bones of persons affected by Hansen's disease may be found without any clinical symptoms of neuro-osteoarthropathy and with normal or nearly normal foot shape [42, 54, 55].

Osteomyelitis can also be triggered by trauma that predisposes to infection of the affected bones. Less frequently, the bone marrow infection can be caused by *M. leprae* itself. Osteomyelitis is mainly seen, therefore, as a complication of a neuropathic hand or foot with an ulcer and may lead to amputation of the involved limb [20, 38, 39, 42, 56, 57].

The diagnosis of osteomyelitis involves clinical, laboratory, and radiological examination [42, 57, 58]. Early radiological features may be soft-tissue edema, periosteal thickening, and osteopenia. Late cortical destruction appears as small holes that coalesce, become larger lesions, and finally progress to completely involve a region of the cortex.

During the follow-up and evaluation of patients with neuropathic foot, plain radiology is often the first examination of choice. However, when clinical signs of inflammation appear, it is often complicated to distinguish between cellulitis, osteomyelitis, and neuro-osteoarthropathy, both clinically and radiographically. MRI has been shown to be the method of choice, enabling differentiation between soft-tissue infection and osteomyelitis [40, 42, 59, 60].

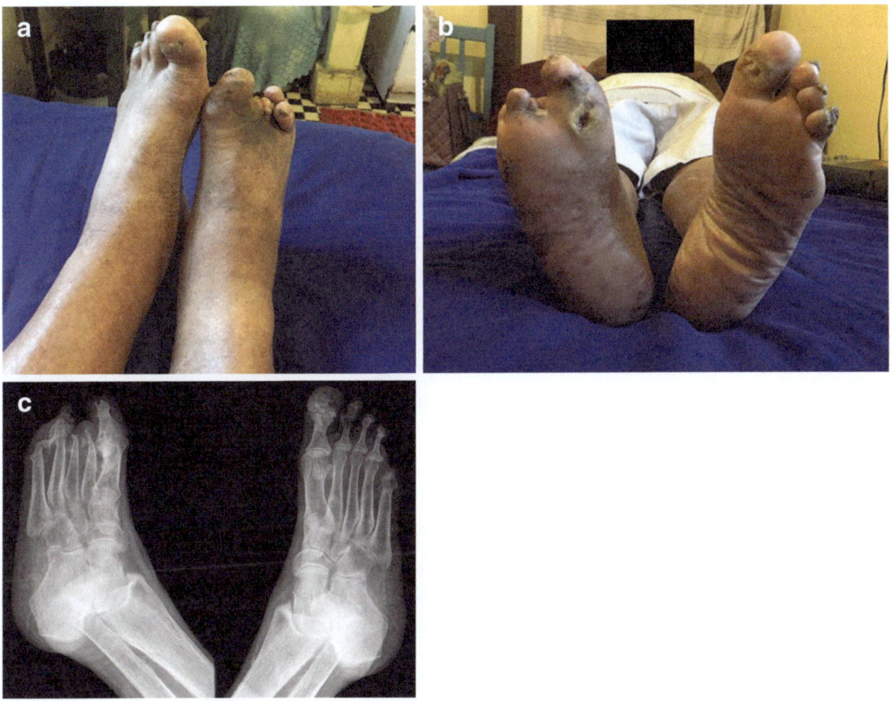

Fig. 9 (**a**) Phalangeal resorption. (**b**) Plantar ulcer on the head of the first right metatarsal and on the proximal phalanx of the first left finger. (**c**) Radiography of the feet shows resorption of multiple phalanges, more marked on the right foot, where metatarsal resorption is also observed. There is ankylosis of the right first metatarsophalangeal and bilateral first to third tarsometatarsal joints. Soft-tissue calcifications are also observed

3.1 Osteoporosis

Osteoporosis in women is characterized by marked bone loss after menopause, while in men it is usually associated with diseases and medications that threaten bone mass [61].

Osteoporosis triggered by Hansen's disease may manifest in a localized manner, due to immobilization or disuse of a paralyzed extremity; or it may manifest in a diffuse manner, resulting from high bacillary load, testicular atrophy with low testosterone level in males, and chronic use of systemic corticosteroids in the therapy of Hansen's disease reactions.

Bone mass loss in male patients with Hansen's disease is directly related to age, occurring in about 33% in the 50–59 age group, increasing progressively, reaching 75% in patients aged 80–89 years [62, 63].

Its detection and treatment is very important since osteoporosis increases the risk of bone fractures, which are also recognized as a common cause of disability and can lead to death [42, 61, 64].

3.2 Joint Changes in Hansen's Disease

Although there is no formal classification to date, arthritis in Hansen's disease can be divided into five groups:

1. Neuropathic osteoarthropathy or "active Charcot foot." This is a neuropathic foot with complications ("warm and diffuse" edema of all or part of the foot, osteoporotic changes, with or without fractures on X-ray). It is also described as non-infectious destruction of bone and joint associated with neuropathy [24, 27].
2. Septic arthritis. Secondary infections can trigger septic arthritis.
3. Specific arthritis. *M. leprae*-specific arthritis is rare and results from localized infectious focus extension into bone or periarticular tissue, or less commonly by hematogenous dissemination. Occasionally, bacilli are detected in synovial fluid [65].
4. Acute polyarthritis of Hansen's disease reaction. Reaction arthritis is acute at onset, evolving into a symmetrical inflammatory polyarthritis affecting small joints of the hands and feet, similar to rheumatoid arthritis (RA).
5. Chronic arthritis of Hansen's disease [26, 66]. In patients with Hansen's disease, chronic symmetric polyarthritis, identical to RA and not associated with reactions, has also been described. Permanent joint damage occurs, especially in the hands, leading to "boutonnière" finger deformities and "swan-neck" finger deformities as well as ulnar deviation and "hammertoe" fingers: highly suggestive of RA [26, 66–68] (Figs. 10 and 11). The clinical symptoms of arthritis are pain and swelling with joint effusion. In patients presenting with inflammatory joint involvement, the most common radiological changes are fusiform soft-tissue swelling, juxta-articular porosis, erosions and joint space reduction. The chronic polyarthritis of Hansen's disease must be differentiated from RA. Frequently, the radiographic changes in RA are more pronounced than those seen in Hansen's disease [26, 39, 40].

World Health Organization multidrug therapy, consisting of rifampicin, dapsone, and clofazimine, is used as the main treatment for Hansen's disease. This therapy appears to have limited impact on bone loss, which can persist and progress even several years after treatment has ended. Dental and otorhinolaryngological follow-up, the institution of therapies that prevent bone resorption in the early stages of the disease, prevention, and treatment of osteoporosis and other osteoarticular changes are important measures [69]. This emphasizes the need for a multidisciplinary approach to the treatment of Hansen's disease.

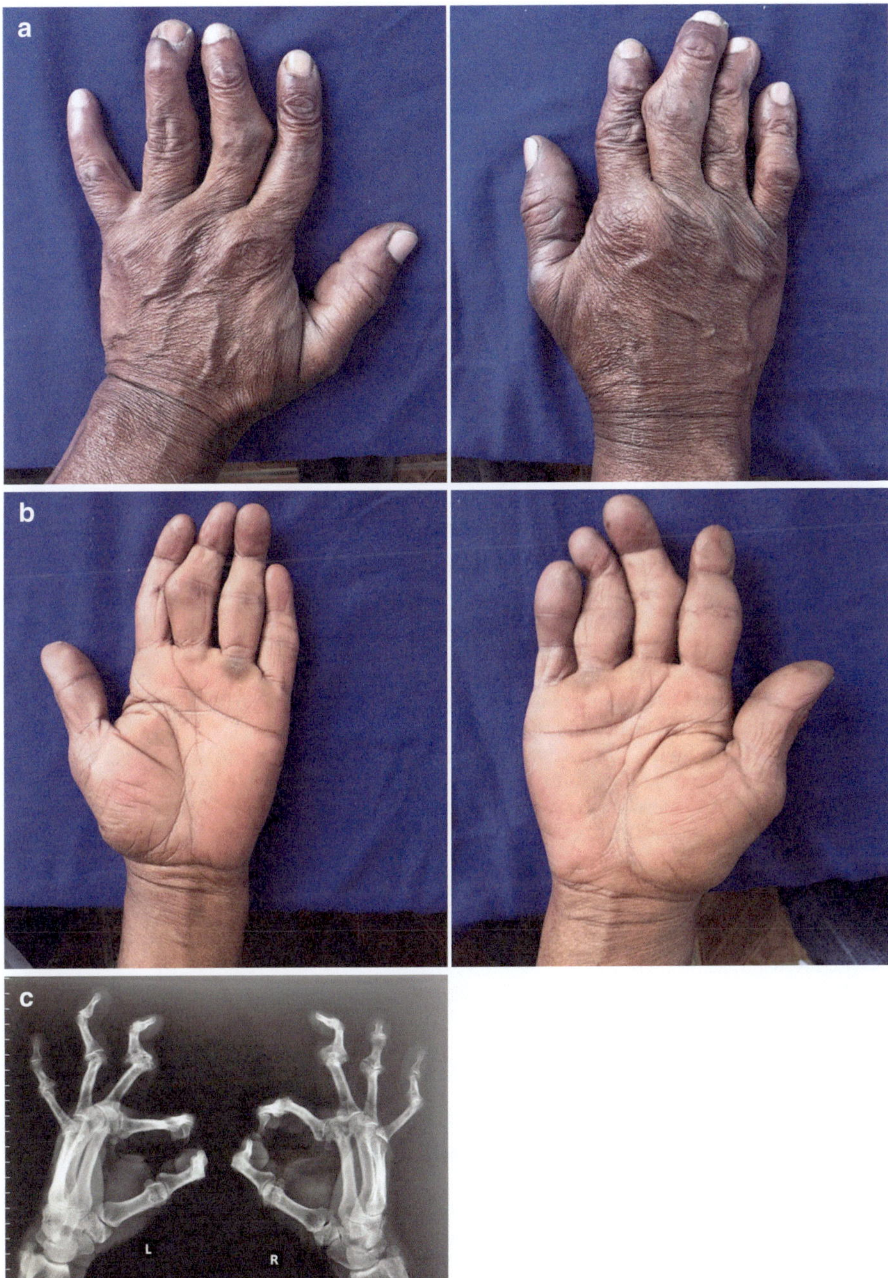

Fig. 10 (**a** and **b**) Right and left hands showing joint deformities of Hansen's disease mimicking rheumatoid arthritis (RA), with synovitis of the proximal interphalangeal and metacarpophalangeal joints. (**c**) Radiography of the hands shows "Boutonnière" deformity (fifth right finger) and "swan neck" deformity (third right finger, and third, fourth, and fifth left fingers)

                                               R. B. do Espírito Santo and P. D. Deps

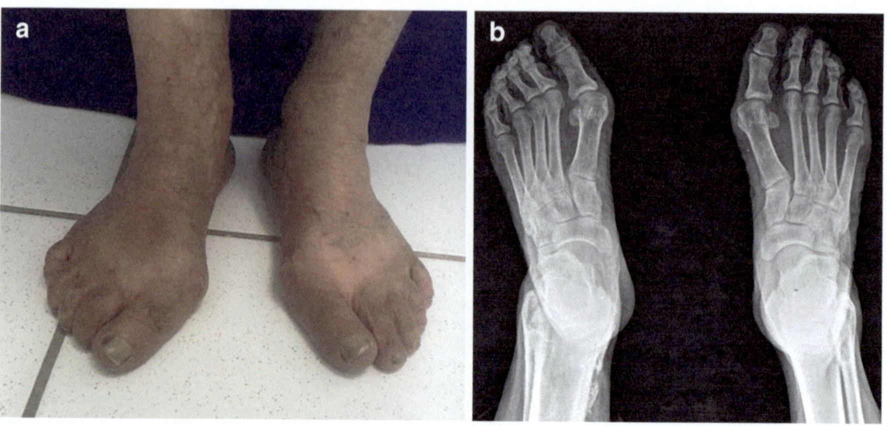

Fig. 11 (**a**) Right foot: hammer toes. (**b**) Radiography of the feet shows bilateral hallux valgus

References

1. Swathi M, Raio R, Silvia WD. Evaluation of bone resorption markers in leprosy. Intl J Clin Diag Res. 2014;2(2: II).
2. Silva SRB, Tempone AJ, Silva TP, Costa MRSN, Pereira GMB, Lara FA, Pessolani MCV, Esquenazi D. Mycobacterium leprae downregulates the expression of PHEX in Schwann cells and osteoblasts. Mem Inst Oswaldo Cruz. 2010;105(5):627–3.
3. de Paula HL, de Souza CDF, Silva SR, Martins-Filho PRS, Barreto JG, Gurgel RQ, et al. Risk factors for physical disability in patients with leprosy: a systematic review and meta-analysis. JAMA dermatol. 2019;155(10):1120–8. https://doi.org/10.1001/jamadermatol.2019.1768. Epub 2019/08/08. PubMed PMID: 31389998; PubMed Central PMCID: PMCPMC6686771
4. Somanath P, Vijay KC. Bone marrow evaluation in leprosy: clinical implications. Lepr Rev. 2016;87:122–3.
5. Kumar WR, Kothari SY, Swamy MKS. Deformities and bony changes in leprosy. Ind J Phys Med Rehabil. 2014;25(1):13–7.
6. Freitas JAS, Santos WM. Alterações ósseas da face na hanseníase virchowiana. Hansen Int. 1986;11(l/2):24–43.
7. Martins AC, Castro E, JD, Moreira JS. A ten-year historic study of paranasal cavity endoscopy in patients with leprosy. Braz J Otorhinolaryngol. 2005;71:609–15.
8. Sun W-H, Li Y-R. Leprosy manifesting as nasal obstruction and epistaxis. J Formos Med Assoc. 2018;117:1032e1033.
9. Bhat R, Sharma VK, Deka RC. Otorhinolaryngologic manifestations of leprosy. Int J Dermatol. 2007;46:600–6.
10. Rebello PFB, Pennini SN, Souza RT, Talhari AC, Talhari S. Manifestações otorrinolaringológiocas. In: Talhari S, editor. Hanseníase. Manaus: DiLivros; 2015. p. 101–9.
11. Reichart P, Ananatasan T, Reznik G. Gingiva and periodontium in lepromatous leprosy. A clinical, radiological, and microscopical study. J Periodontol. 1976;47(8):455–60. https://doi.org/10.1902/jop.1976.47.8.455.
12. Andersen J, Manchester K. The rhinomaxillary syndrome in leprosy: a clinical, radiological and palaeopathological study. Int J Osteoarchaeol. 1992;2(2):121–9.
13. Pfaltzgraff RE, Bryceson A. Clinical leprosy. In: Hastings RC, editor. Leprosy. Hong Kong: Longman Group (FE); 1985. p. 134–76.

14. Costa MRSN. Considerações sobre o envolvimento da cavidade bucal na hanseníase. Hansen Int. 2008;33(1):41–4.
15. Pallagatti S, Sheikh S, Kaur A, Aggarwal A, Singh R. Oral cavity and leprosy. Indian Dermatol Online J. 2012;3(2):101–4. https://doi.org/10.4103/2229-5178.96700. PMID: 23130281; PMCID: PMC3481884
16. Costa A, Nery J, Oliveira M, Cuzzi T, Silva M. Oral lesions in leprosy. Indian J Dermatol Venereol Leprol. 2003;69(6):381–5.
17. Illarramendi X, Carregal E, Nery JA, Sarno EN. Progression of acral bone resorption in multibacillary leprosy. Acta Leprol. 2000;12:29–37.
18. Agrawal A, Pandit L, Dalal M, Shetty JP. Neurological manifestations of Hansen's disease and their management. Clin Neurol Neurosurg. 2005;107:445–54.
19. Garbino JA. O paciente com suspeita de hanseníase primariamente neural. Hansen Int. 2007;32:203–6.
20. Brandsma JW, et al. Report from the workshop on the neurologically impaired foot: 5-9 June 2000, green pastures hospital, Pokhara, Nepal Assessment and examination of the neurologically impaired foot. Lepr Rev. 2001;72:254–62.
21. Van Brakel WH. Peripheral neuropathy in leprosy and its consequences. Lepr Rev. 2000;71(Suppl):S146–53.
22. Moonot P, Ashwood N, Lockwood D. Orthopaedic complications of leprosy. J Bone Joint Surg (Br). 2005;87:1328–32.
23. Mohammad W, Malhotra SK, Garg PK. Clinico-radiological correlation of bone changes in leprosy patients presenting with disabilities/deformities. Indian J Lepr. 2016;88:83–95.
24. Kothari SY, Kumar WR, Swamy MKS. Deformities and bony changes in leprosy. Ind J Phys Med Rehabil. 2014;25:13–7.
25. Botou A, Bangeas A, Alexiou I, Sakkas LI. Acro-osteolysis. Clin Rheumatol. 2017;36:9–14.
26. Do Espírito Santo RB, Serafim RA, Bitran JBG, Collin SM, Deps P. Case report: leprosy osteoarticular alterations mimicking rheumatoid arthritis. Am J Trop Med Hyg. 2020;102:1316–8.
27. Faber WR, Dutch Neuropathic Foot Society. Comment on reports from the workshop on the neurologically impaired foot. Lepr Rev. 2003;74:84–5.; author reply 86.
28. Job CK. Pathology of leprosy. In: Hastings RC, editor. Leprosy. London: Churchill Livingstone; 1994.
29. Paterson DE, Rad M. Bone changes in leprosy, their incidence, progress, prevention and arrest. Int J Lepr. 1961;29:393–422.
30. Daniel RK, Brenner KA. Saddle nose deformity: a new classification and treatment. Facial Plast Surg Clin North Am. 2006;14:301–12.
31. Durbec M, Disant F. Saddle nose: classification and therapeutic management. Eur Ann Otorhinolaryngol Head Neck Dis. 2014;131:99–106.
32. do Espírito Santo RB, Serafim RA, Loureiro RM, Sumi DV, de Mello RAF, Nascimento IF, AFJM L, Collin JD, Collin SM, Deps P. Clinical and radiological assessment of rhinomaxillary syndrome in Hansen's disease. Indian J Dermatol Venereol Leprol. 2021;7:1–11. https://doi.org/10.25259/IJDVL_1203_20. Epub ahead of print
33. Job, C. K., Selvapandian, A. J. & Kurian, P. V. Leprosy: diagnosis and management. 1975.
34. Job CK. Pathology of leprous osteomyelitis. Int J Lepr. 1963;31:26–33.
35. Deps P, do Espírito Santo RB, Charlier P, Collin SM. Rhinomaxillary syndrome in Hansen's disease: a clinical perspective. Int J Dermatol. 2020;59:e404. https://doi.org/10.1111/ijd.15202.
36. Serafim RA Craniofacial and tomographic changes in leprosy patients from Leprosy control programme and leprosy colony Pedro Fontes, Cariacica (ES). 2017. http://doencasinfecciosas.ufes.br/pt-br/pos-graduacao/PPGDI/detalhes-da-tese?id=11989. (Universidade Federal do Espírito Santo, Vitória, Brasil).
37. Faget GH, Mayoral A. Bone changes in leprosy: a clinical and Roentgenologic study of 505 cases. Radiology. 1944;42:1–13.
38. Resnick D, Niwayama G. Osteomyelitis, septic arthritis and soft tissue infection: the organisms. In: Diagnosis of bone and joint disorders. Philadelphia: Saunders; 1988.

39. Pereira HLA, Ribeiro SLE, Ciconelli RM, Fernandes AD. Avaliação por imagem do comprometimento osteoarticular e de nervos periféricos na hanseníase. Rev Bras Reumatol. 2006;46:30–5.
40. Slim FJ, Faber WR, Maas M. The role of radiology in nerve function impairment and its musculoskeletal complications in leprosy. Lepr Rev. 2009;80:373–87.
41. Harverson G, Warren AG. Tarsal bone disintegration in leprosy. Clin Radiol. 1979;30:317–22.
42. Carpintero P, García-Frasquet A, Pradilla P, García J, Mesa M. Wrist involvement in Hansen's disease. J Bone Joint Surg (Br). 1997;79:753–7.
43. Enna CD, Jacobson RR, Rausch RO. Bone changes in leprosy: a correlation of clinical and radiographic features. Radiology. 1971;100:295–306.
44. Nagano J, Tada K, Masatomi T, Horibe S. Arthropathy of the wrist in leprosy—what changes are caused by long-standing peripheral nerve palsy? Arch Orthop Trauma Surg. 1989;108:210–7.
45. Chamberlain WE, Wayson NE, Garland LH. The bone and joint changes of leprosy: a Roentgenologic study. Radiology. 1931;17:930–9.
46. MacMoran JW, Brand PW. Bone loss in limbs with decreased or absent sensation: ten year follow-up of the hands in leprosy. Skelet Radiol. 1987;16:452–9.
47. Duerksen F. Desintegração do tarso. In: Duerksen F, Virmond M, editors. Cirurgia Reparadora e Reabilitação Em Hanseníase. Santa Catarina: ALM International; 1997. p. 329–39.
48. Warren, G. Neuropathic feet. In Surgical reconstruction & rehabilitation in leprosy and other neuropathies Schwarz, R. J. & Brandsma, J. W. Ekta Books, Kathmandu. 2004.
49. Onvlee GJ. The Charcot foot: a critical review and an observational study of a group of 60 patients. Leiden: University of Leiden; 1998.
50. Karat S, Karat AB, Foster R. Radiological changes in bones of the limbs in leprosy. Lepr Rev. 1968;39:147–69.
51. Kulkarni VN, Mehta JM. Tarsal disintegration (T.D.) in leprosy. Lepr India. 1983;55:338–70.
52. Thappa DM, Sharma VK, Kaur S, Suri S. Radiological changes in hands and feet in disabled leprosy patients: a clinico-radiological correlation. Indian J Lepr. 1992;64:58–66.
53. Horibe S, Tada K, Nagano J. Neuroarthropathy of the foot in leprosy. J Bone Joint Surg (Br). 1988;70:481–5.
54. Harris JR, Brand PW. Patterns of disintegration of the tarsus in the anaesthetic foot. J Bone Joint Surg (Br). 1966;48:4–16.
55. Maas M, Slim EJ, Akkerman EM, Faber WR. MRI in clinically asymptomatic neuropathic leprosy feet: a baseline study. Int J Lepr Other Mycobact Dis. 2001;69:219–24.
56. Macdonald MR, et al. Report from the workshop on the neurologically impaired foot: 5–9 June 2000, green pastures hospital, Pokhara, Nepal Complications and management of the neurologically impaired foot. Lepr Rev. 2001;72:263–75.
57. Slim FJ, Hoeksma AF, Maas M, Faber WR. A clinical and radiological follow-up study in leprosy patients with asymptomatic neuropathic feet. Lepr Rev. 2008;79:183–92.
58. Riordan DC. The hand in leprosy. A seven-year clinical study. J Bone Joint Surg Am. 1960;42-A:661–82.
59. Berendt AR, Lipsky B. Is this bone infected or not? Differentiating neuro-osteoarthropathy from osteomyelitis in the diabetic foot. Curr Diab Rep. 2004;4:424–9.
60. Maas M, et al. MR imaging of neuropathic feet in leprosy patients with suspected osteomyelitis. Int J Lepr Other Mycobact Dis. 2002;70:97–103.
61. Kanaji A, Higashi M, Namisato M, Nishio M, Ando K, Yamada H. Effects of risedronate on lumbar bone mineral density, bone resorption, and incidence of vertebral fracture in elderly male patients with leprosy. Lepr Rev. 2006 Jun;77(2):147–53.
62. Ishikawa A, Ishikawa S, Hirakawa M. Osteoporosis, bone turnover and hypogonadism in elderly men with treated leprosy. Lepr Rev. 2001;72:322–9.
63. Ishikawa S, Ishikawa A, Yoh K, Tanaka H, Fujiwara M. Osteoporosis in male and female leprosy patients. Calcif Tissue Int. 1999;64:144–7.
64. Kanaji A, et al. Trochanteric hip fracture in an elderly patient with leprosy during osteoporosis treatment with risedronate and alfacalcidol. J Bone Miner Metab. 2005;23:90–4.

65. Louie JS, Kornasky JR, Cohen AH. Lepra cells in synovial fluid of a patient with erythema nodosum leprosum. N Engl J Med. 1973;289:1410–1.
66. Chauhan S, Wakhlu A, Agarwal V. Arthritis in leprosy. Rheumatology (Oxford). 2010;49:2237–42.
67. Atkin SL, et al. Clinical and laboratory studies of inflammatory polyarthritis in patients with leprosy in Papua New Guinea. Ann Rheum Dis. 1987;46:688–90.
68. Cossermelli-Messina W, Festa Neto C, Cossermelli W. Articular inflammatory manifestations in patients with different forms of leprosy. J Rheumatol. 1998;25:111–9.
69. Eichelmann K, González González SE, Salas-Alanis JC, Ocampo-Candiani J. Leprosy. An update: definition, pathogenesis, classification, diagnosis, and treatment. Actas Dermosifiliogr. 2013;104:554–63.

Diagnostic Imaging in Hansen's Disease: Conventional Radiography, Computed Tomography, Magnetic Resonance Imaging, and Dual-Energy X-Ray Absorptiometry

Rafael Maffei Loureiro, Rachel Bertolani do Espirito Santo, and Patrícia D. Deps

Imaging plays a pivotal role in the diagnosis of Hansen's disease (HD)-related abnormalities in multiple organs, primarily involving the bones, joints, and peripheral nerves. Each imaging modality has its advantages, drawbacks, and indications. In this chapter, conventional radiography, computed tomography (CT), magnetic resonance imaging (MRI), and dual-energy X-ray absorptiometry are discussed. Ultrasonography (US) is covered in another chapter.

1 Conventional Radiography

HD typically involves the bones of the face, hands, and feet. The bone changes are classified as specific (caused by bacillary invasion or direct action) and non-specific (caused by trauma and infection imposed upon denervated tissues). Plain radiographs are frequently used as an initial imaging modality to assess the bone changes in the hands and feet, due to their high availability, low cost, and good accuracy [1, 2]

The radiographic findings of specific bone changes include bone rarefaction, osteolytic granulomas (appearing as punched-out areas), endosteal thinning, widening of the nutritional foramen, and fusiform swelling of the surrounding soft tissues. The distal aspects of the proximal and middle phalanges are more commonly affected in the hands. In the feet, the metatarsal heads are more commonly

R. M. Loureiro (✉)
Hospital Israelita Albert Einstein, São Paulo, Brazil
e-mail: rafael.loureiro@einstein.br

R. B. do Espirito Santo (✉) · P. D. Deps
Universidade Federal do Espírito Santo, Vitória, Brazil
e-mail: patricia.deps@ufes.br

P. D. Deps (ed.), *Hansen's Disease*, https://doi.org/10.1007/978-3-031-30893-2_18

affected. As the disease progresses, imaging reveals bone destruction with a cystic or honeycombed appearance. Pathological fractures frequently occur in later stages [1].

A rare form of direct bone involvement in HD is virchowian (leprous) osteomyelitis, which leads to rapid bone resorption, pathologic fractures, and deforming joint infection [3]. Periostitis and osteitis can occur in the long bones, such as the tibia, fibula, and ulna, and are considered manifestations of acute HD reactions [1].

Primary arthritis caused by the infiltration of *M. leprae* into a joint is uncommon in HD patients [2]. Possible presentations of HD-related arthritis include acute polyarthritis of HD (lepra) reactions (which may rarely have chronic or relapsing-remitting course) and chronic symmetrical polyarthritis; both presentations can resemble rheumatoid arthritis. Radiological findings of HD-related arthritis include juxta-articular erosion, bone rarefaction, swelling of the surrounding soft tissues, joint space narrowing, and joint subluxation [4–6].

Non-specific bone lesions are much more common and often occur following the loss of sensation and motor changes due to peripheral nerve involvement, leading to repetitive trauma and infection. Imaging findings include fractures, varying degrees of bone erosion, osteitis, and bone resorption [1, 2].

Bone resorption can be visualized as a decrease in bone width (also called concentric resorption) and/or length; the combination of decreases in the length and width results in a tapered appearance of the bone, also called the "licked candy stick" appearance. Partial or total loss of one or more phalanges typically occurs as resorption progresses, possibly extending to the proximal bones (Fig. 1). Secondary infection and pathological fractures may further increase the resorption and gradual disappearance of multiple bones [3, 7].

Neuropathic osteoarthropathy represents a spectrum of destructive bone and joint processes associated with neurosensory deficits, occurring more frequently in the feet. HD is one among many potential causes of neuropathic osteoarthropathy, such as syringomyelia, diabetes mellitus, and syphilis. Both the hypertrophic and

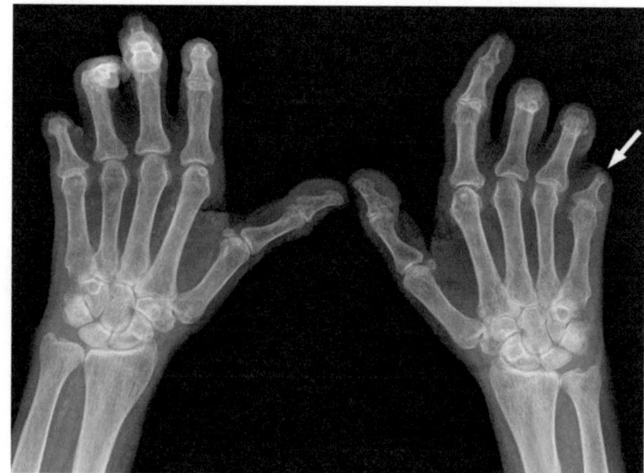

Fig. 1 Radiography of the hands shows resorption of multiple phalanges, more prominent on the left hand. The proximal phalanx of the left fifth digit has a "licked candy stick" appearance (arrow)

atrophic patterns of neuropathic osteoarthropathy are identified radiologically. The hypertrophic form manifests as joint destruction and fragmentation, osseous sclerosis, and osteophyte formation. The atrophic form, classically observed in HD, appears as bone resorption that often resembles surgical amputation. Mixed forms can also occur [7].

Neuropathic osteoarthropathy in the feet, also called Charcot foot, is a non-specific bone lesion in HD. The radiographic findings include bone resorption, joint (sub)luxation, fractures, soft-tissue swelling, ankylosis, and flattening of the longitudinal plantar arch (Fig. 2). Tarsal disintegration, characterized by fragmentation and progressive collapse of one or more tarsal bones, can occur (Fig. 3). The navicular bone is often involved, usually in combination with the talus. The calcaneus is less frequently affected, and the cuboid and cuneiform bones are rarely involved. Secondary infections such as osteomyelitis and septic arthritis can occur as a consequence of skin injury [2, 8].

If osteomyelitis is suspected, radiographs are useful as the initial screening examination because they evaluate anatomic detail and other causes of pain, such as radiopaque foreign body, fracture, and degenerative changes. However, radiographs lack sensitivity in the detection of early stages of acute osteomyelitis since early bone changes (such as bone rarefaction and destruction, endosteal scalloping, and periosteal reaction) may take 10–12 days to develop. Soft-tissue swelling precedes bone changes. After initial radiography, MRI is the modality of choice for the evaluation of superimposed osteomyelitis [9].

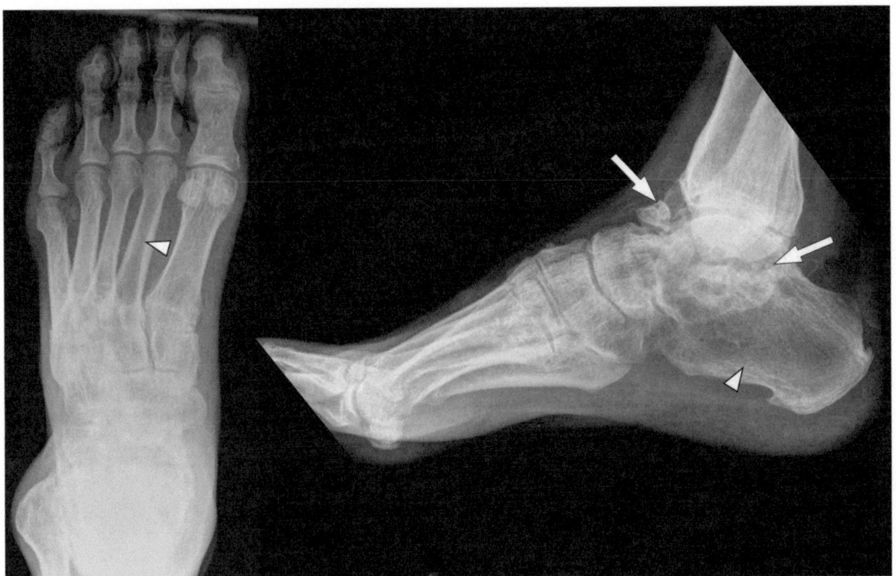

Fig. 2 Radiographs of a foot with neuropathic osteoarthropathy show fragmentation and collapse of the talus (arrows), diffuse joint space narrowing in the midfoot and hindfoot, talonavicular ankylosis, and regional bone rarefaction (more prominent in the calcaneus and metatarsal II) (arrowheads)

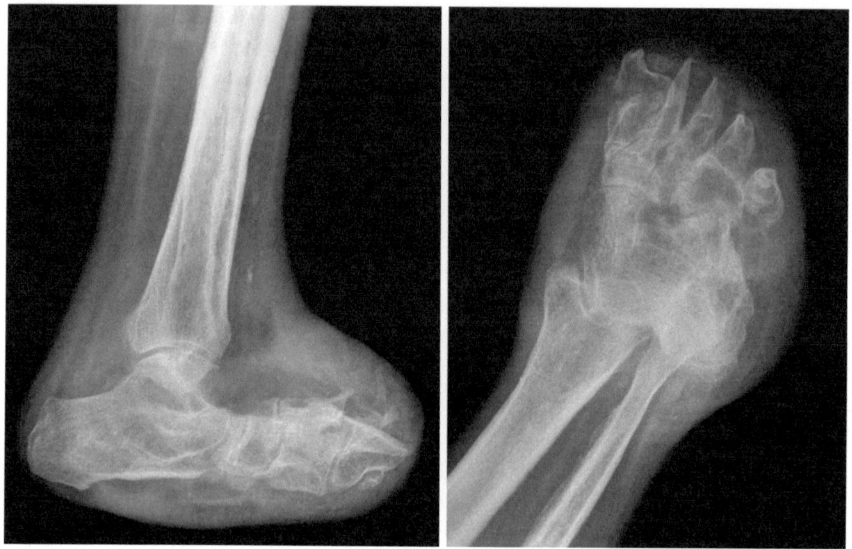

Fig. 3 Radiographs of a foot with neuropathic osteoarthropathy show marked resorption of the phalanges and metatarsal bones, diffuse bone rarefaction, tarsal disintegration, flattening of the longitudinal plantar arch, and diffuse soft-tissue swelling with scattered calcification foci

2 Computed Tomography

HD can affect the facial bones, potentially leading to bone destruction, facial changes, and disfigurement. These bone alterations have been examined in the skulls from archaeological sites, and the associated changes are known as rhino-maxillary syndrome (RMS). RMS features include collapse of the nasal bridge, resorption of the central part of the maxilla, and inflammation of the nasal cavity and the hard palate. The degree of bone alteration correlates with the type of disease at diagnosis, ranging from scarcity or absence in the tuberculoid form of HD to severe changes in the virchowian (lepromatous) form [10, 11].

Facial bone changes can be better assessed by CT of the maxillofacial region. CT aids the accurate evaluation of the maxillofacial structures with sub-millimetric spatial resolution, allowing reformation in all planes and three-dimensional reconstruction. These features overcome the limitations of radiographs, which produce two-dimensional images of three-dimensional structures, potentially leading to image superposition, magnification, and distortion. CT is also more accurate in the evaluation of bone and soft-tissue structures than radiographs. The drawbacks of CT include higher cost, less availability, and greater radiation exposure than that associated with radiographs [12].

CT findings include the resorption of the nasal bones and anterior nasal spine, the loss of sharpness of the nasal piriform aperture, nasal septum perforation, atrophy of the nasal turbinates, bone thinning and discontinuities in the hard palate, resorption of the alveolar process of the maxilla, and osteitis (Fig. 4) [10, 13].

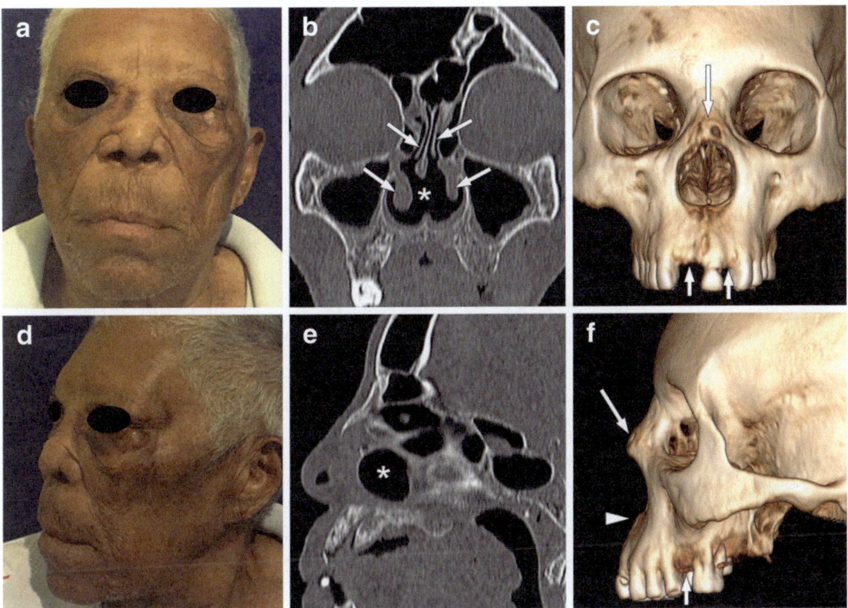

Fig. 4 A 78-year-old male patient with rhinomaxillary syndrome. Frontal (**a**) and lateral (**d**) facial aspects show saddle nose, maxillary retrognathia, inverted upper lip, and concave midface. Coronal (**b**) and sagittal (**e**) CT images show atrophy of the middle and inferior nasal turbinates (arrows) and a large nasal septum perforation (asterisks). Frontal (**c**) and lateral (**f**) three-dimensional reconstruction CT images show partial resorption and deformity of the nasal bones (long arrows), total resorption of the anterior nasal spine (arrowhead), and loss of some teeth with partial resorption of the alveolar process of the maxilla (short arrows)

CT can also be used for the evaluation of bone involvement in the hands, feet, and other joints, affording better imaging details, particularly in cases of diagnostic uncertainty on radiographs.

3   Magnetic Resonance Imaging

MRI is a useful radiation-free tool for assessing the peripheral nerve involvement in HD patients, providing optimal soft-tissue contrast. HD-related neuritis presents as a tender enlargement of the peripheral nerves at the sites of predilection and can be caused either as part of the infection course or as a result of HD reactions (types 1 and 2) [2]. The imaging features of peripheral nerve involvement include nerve thickening with a preserved fascicular architecture, disruption of the fascicular architecture, and formation of nerve abscesses (initially micro-abscesses, which may coalesce to form large abscesses that extend into the surrounding soft tissues) [14].

Martinoli et al. [15] reported that MRI and US exhibited similar results in demonstrating nerve enlargement, endoneural structural abnormalities, and compressive signs. MRI had a greater sensitivity in detecting active type 1 reactions (92%) than that observed with US (74%); active type 1 reactions appear as an increased T2 signal and gadolinium-based contrast enhancement. Compared with US, MRI is also less operator-dependent. However, MRI has drawbacks, such as lower availability (particularly in HD-endemic areas) and higher cost. Conversely, US is accessible, practical, and relatively inexpensive [15, 16].

MRI is a useful technique for assessing neuropathic feet in HD patients, allowing the depiction of early bone changes and soft-tissue abnormalities, even in asymptomatic patients [17]. In acute neuropathic arthropathy, MRI shows soft-tissue edema (occurring in the absence of infection or ulceration) and bone marrow changes, possibly associated with joint effusion and trabecular microfractures [9, 18, 19].

MRI is also ideal for the assessment of suspected osteomyelitis, septic arthritis, and soft-tissue infections. Nearly all osteomyelitis result from an ulcer or abscess in contiguous soft tissue. After initial radiography, MRI is the standard modality for the evaluation of superimposed osteomyelitis. MRI is optimal for the detection of bone marrow abnormalities (particularly in early phases, when radiographs and CT reveal no bone abnormalities), observed as low signal on T1 sequence and high signal on T2/fluid-sensitive sequence. The use of gadolinium contrast is useful to determine fluid collection/abscesses, sinus tracts, and devitalized regions [9, 18, 19].

Abnormalities of the central nervous system have rarely been described in HD patients. In this setting, MRI is the most accurate imaging modality for evaluating the brain and the spinal cord [20].

4 Dual-Energy X-Ray Absorptiometry

Osteoporosis, the most common metabolic bone disease, is characterized by the generalized loss of bone mass and deterioration of bone microarchitecture, leading to increased bone fragility and fracture susceptibility. Common fracture sites include the vertebral bodies, neck and intertrochanteric region of the femur, distal radius, and tibia. Osteopenia is a milder form of bone mass loss that can progress to osteoporosis [21, 22].

Older methods of evaluating bone mineral density include conventional radiography and single- and dual-photon absorptiometry. Currently, DEXA is the standard technique for evaluating bone mass loss [23].

DEXA calculates the bone mineral density, preferentially in the lumbar vertebrae and femur, and compares it against two reference populations, providing the resultants T-score and Z-score, both expressed in terms of standard deviations.

The T-score is the comparison to a standard young adult population and is used for postmenopausal women and men aged >50 years. The T-score is classified according to the World Health Organization criteria into normal (≥-1.0), osteopenia (<-1.0 but >-2.5), osteoporosis (≤-2.5), and severe osteoporosis (≤-2.5 with a fragility fracture). The Z-score is a comparison to age- and sex-matched controls and is used for premenopausal women and men aged <50 years. A Z-score <−2.0 is classified as being below the expected range/low bone density for a given age [22, 24].

Bone mass loss may be identified as an early event in HD patients or even at diagnosis, and likely has multiple causes, including social and nutritional factors, hypogonadism in male patients (due to testicular involvement), and possible increased production of pro-inflammatory factors. Bone mass loss appears to be an occult and initially imperceptible manifestation that commonly occurs in these patients. A prompt diagnosis and effective treatment of osteoporosis can prevent bone fractures, thereby improving patient care [25, 26].

Osteoporosis may also be a local phenomenon that affects only part of the skeleton, usually the appendicular skeleton. Regional osteoporosis may have various causes, such as immobilization or disuse (commonly associated with finger contractures in HD) and inflammatory arthropathy [21, 22]

References

1. Enna CD, Jacobson RR, Rausch RO. Bone changes in leprosy: a correlation of clinical and radiographic features. Radiology. 1971;100(2):295–306.
2. Slim FJ, Faber WR, Maas M. The role of radiology in nerve function impairment and its musculoskeletal complications in leprosy. Lepr Rev. 2009;80(4):373–87.
3. MacMoran JW, Brand PW. Bone loss in limbs with decreased or absent sensation: ten year follow-up of the hands in leprosy. Skelet Radiol. 1987;16(6):452–9.
4. do Espírito Santo RB, Serafim RA, JBG B, Collin SM, Deps P. Case Report: leprosy osteoarticular alterations mimicking rheumatoid arthritis. Am J Trop Med Hyg. 2020;102(6):1316–8.
5. Chauhan S, Wakhlu A, Agarwal V. Arthritis in leprosy. Rheumatology. 2010;49(12):2237–42.
6. Pereira HLA, Ribeiro SLE, Pennini SN, Sato EI. Leprosy-related joint involvement. Clin Rheumatol. 2009;28(1):79–84.
7. Jones EA, Manaster BJ, May DA, Disler DG. Neuropathic osteoarthropathy: diagnostic dilemmas and differential diagnosis. Radiographics. 2000;20(Suppl–1):S279–93.
8. Harverson G, Warren AG. Tarsal bone disintegration in leprosy. Clin Radiol. 1979;30(3):317–22.
9. Expert Panel on Musculoskeletal Imaging, Walker EA, Beaman FD, Wessell DE, Cassidy RC, Czuczman GJ, et al. Suspected osteomyelitis of the foot in patients with diabetes mellitus. J Am Coll Radiol. 2019;16(11S):S440–50.
10. do Espírito Santo RB, Serafim RA, Loureiro RM, Sumi DV, de Mello RAF, Nascimento IF, et al. Clinical and radiological assessment of rhinomaxillary syndrome in Hansen's disease. Indian J Dermatol Venereol Leprol. 2021:1–11.
11. Deps P, do Espírito Santo RB, Charlier P, Collin SM. Rhinomaxillary syndrome in Hansen's disease: a clinical perspective. Int J Dermatol. 2020;59(11):e404–6.
12. Loureiro RM, Collin J, Sumi DV, Araújo LC, Murakoshi RW, Gomes RLE, et al. Postoperative CT findings of orthognathic surgery and its complications: a guide for radiologists. J Neuroradiol. 2022;49(1):17–32.
13. Kasai N, Kondo O, Suzuki K, Aoki Y, Ishii N, Goto M. Quantitative evaluation of maxillary bone deformation by computed tomography in patients with leprosy. PLoS Negl Trop Dis. 2018;12(3):e0006341.
14. Jabeen S, Saini J, Vengalil S, Lavania M, Singh I, Nashi S, et al. Neuroimaging in leprosy: the nerves and beyond. Radiol Infect Dis. 2020;7(1):12–21.

15. Martinoli C, Derchi LE, Bertolotto M, Gandolfo N, Bianchi S, Fiallo P, et al. US and MR imaging of peripheral nerves in leprosy. Skelet Radiol. 2000;29(3):142–50.
16. Lastória JC, de Abreu MAMM. Leprosy: a review of laboratory and therapeutic aspects–part 2. An Bras Dermatol. 2014;89(3):389–401.
17. Slim FJ, Hoeksma AF, Maas M, Faber WR. A clinical and radiological follow-up study in leprosy patients with asymptomatic neuropathic feet. Lepr Rev. 2008;79(2):183–92.
18. Baker JC, Demertzis JL, Rhodes NG, Wessell DE, Rubin DA. Diabetic musculoskeletal complications and their imaging mimics. Radiographics. 2012;32(7):1959–74.
19. Donovan A, Schweitzer ME. Use of MR imaging in diagnosing diabetes-related pedal osteomyelitis. Radiographics. 2010;30(3):723–36.
20. Polavarapu K, Preethish-Kumar V, Vengalil S, Nashi S, Lavania M, Bhattacharya K, et al. Brain and spinal cord lesions in leprosy: a magnetic resonance imaging-based study. Am J Trop Med Hyg. 2019;100(4):921–31.
21. Chang CY, Rosenthal DI, Mitchell DM, Handa A, Kattapuram SV, Huang AJ. Imaging findings of metabolic bone disease. Radiographics. 2016;36(6):1871–87.
22. Guglielmi G, Muscarella S, Bazzocchi A. Integrated imaging approach to osteoporosis: state-of-the-art review and update. Radiographics. 2011;31(5):1343–64.
23. Genant HK. Current state of bone densitometry for osteoporosis. Radiographics. 1998;18(4):913–8.
24. Knipe H. Dual-energy x-ray absorptiometry. Reference Article Radiopaedia.org [Internet]. Radiopaedia. 2022. https://radiopaedia.org/articles/dual-energy-x-ray-absorptiometry-1?lang=us.
25. Ribeiro FB, Pereira Fde A, Muller É, Foss NT, de Paula FJ. Evaluation of bone and mineral metabolism in patients recently diagnosed with leprosy. Am J Med Sci. 2007;334(5):322–6.
26. Leal AMO, Foss NT. Endocrine dysfunction in leprosy. Eur J Clin Microbiol Infect Dis. 2009;28(1):1–7.

Co-infection and Immunosuppression in Hansen's Disease

Ciro Martins Gomes, Taynah Alves Rocha Repsold, and Patrícia D. Deps

Hansen's disease follows a chronic course punctuated by episodes of immunological reactions that are treated by immunomodulatory drugs. These aspects of Hansen's disease mean that patients are susceptible to co-infections. In this chapter, we describe some of the more common infections that can co-occur with Hansen's disease in endemic countries. We also describe how immunosuppressive drugs to treat other diseases can allow Hansen's disease to manifest clinically.

1   Hansen's Disease and COVID-19

The COVID-19 pandemic created huge challenges for national Hansen's disease programs. Lockdowns, re-prioritization of services, and disruption to health systems had a major impact on new case detection rates, which fell by 40% in 2020 compared with the average over the previous 5 years [1]. Detrimental public health effects of diagnoses include sustained transmission and increased risk of disabilities due to diagnostic delay and treatment interruption [2]. The impact of the pandemic was compounded by a shortfall in the supply of multidrug therapy (MDT), which is distributed centrally to all endemic countries via the World Health Organization. Both diseases affected disproportionately the most socioeconomically deprived people [3].

C. M. Gomes (✉)
Universidade de Brasilia, Brasília, Brazil
e-mail: cirogomes@unb.br

T. A. R. Repsold · P. D. Deps
Universidade Federal do Espírito Santo, Vitória, Brazil
e-mail: patricia.deps@ufes.br

P. D. Deps (ed.), *Hansen's Disease*, https://doi.org/10.1007/978-3-031-30893-2_19

In clinical practice, concerns were raised at the start of the pandemic around a possible increased risk of SARS-CoV-2 infection or severe COVID-19 in Hansen's disease patients receiving immunosuppressants to treat Hansen's disease reactions, and the potential for Hansen's disease reactions to be triggered or exacerbated by COVID-19 [4–6].

Clinical management of patients receiving treatment for Hansen's disease who developed COVID-19 in the pre-vaccination era has been described in a small number of published studies and case reports [7–11]. These suggest that Hansen's disease and COVID-19 co-infection did not appear to change markedly the clinical picture of either disease.

Specifically, concerns about increased frequency or severity of Hansen's disease reactions or that use of corticosteroids might contribute to the evolution of severe COVID-19 did not materialize [12, 13]. Indeed, systemic corticosteroids became an effective component of treatment of severe COVID-19 [14, 15]. Conversely, no evidence emerged to support putative beneficial effects of clofazimine or dapsone against SARS-CoV-2 infection [16–18].

Two studies in Brazil demonstrated that the proportion of Hansen's disease patients with COVID-19 who experienced reactions was similar to pre-pandemic levels [11, 13]. Two of six coinfected cases described by Arora et al. in India had persistent type 1 reactions with no change in severity during their COVID-19 illness [10], while Saxena et al. reported a favorable outcome in a patient with severe type 2 Hansen's disease reaction and COVID-19 despite continued use of corticosteroids and methotrexate [9].

Consensus from the start of the pandemic that MDT for Hansen's disease should not be suspended in cases of co-infection was therefore supplemented by no changes in recommended case-by-case assessment and appropriate treatment of Hansen's disease reactions namely, corticosteroids for type I reactions and neuritis, and thalidomide for type II reactions.

2 Hansen's Disease and Leishmaniasis

Leishmaniasis is a neglected disease with systemic (visceral) and cutaneous (tegumentary) forms that occurs in tropical countries, particularly in areas of lower socioeconomic development where it can overlap with endemic Hansen's disease [19].

"Old world" cutaneous leishmaniasis, caused mainly by *Leishmania major, L. tropica, L. aethiopica, and L. infantum,* tends to heal spontaneously without dissemination to other organs, allowing the use of local and topical therapies. 'New World' or 'American' cutaneous leishmaniasis, caused by several species including *L. braziliensis and L. panamensis,* occurs mainly in Central and South America and can lead to mucocutaneous involvement resulting in destructive and disfiguring facial lesions.

Cases of leishmaniasis and Hansen's disease co-infection have been reported in Brazil [19–22], Central America [23], and India [24], but not in sufficient numbers to identify any patterns in host immune response to dual infection or interactions between drug regimens, or to provide guidance on case management other than to treat both diseases simultaneously.

3 Hansen's Disease and Chagas Disease (American Trypanosomiasis)

American trypanosomiasis is a vector-borne disease caused by *Trypanosoma cruzi*, arising from contact with feces or urine of triatomine bugs. As with leishmaniasis, this neglected tropical disease co-exists with endemic Hansen's disease in poorer regions [25], albeit with only a single published case report [26]. Chagas disease can cause inflammation of cardiac muscles, hence use of thrombogenic medications to treat Hansen's disease reactions requires close monitoring.

4 Hansen's Disease and HIV

At the beginning of the HIV epidemic, it was thought that immunodeficiency caused by HIV might increase the incidence of newly detected cases of Hansen's disease or reduce the efficacy of MDT for Hansen's disease, but neither of these effects materialized [27, 28]. Instead, the two diseases appear in most cases to follow independent courses, including occurrence of Hansen's disease reactions [29–31].

In clinical practice, the most important aspect of HIV co-infection is the onset of Hansen's disease and reactional states due to immune reconstitution syndrome (IRIS) following initiation of antiretroviral therapy (ART) [32–37].

Four classifications have been proposed for IRIS in Hansen's disease based on case reports: Type 1 if ART unmasks undiagnosed Hansen's disease; Type 2 if Hansen's disease was already diagnosed and MDT started prior to initiation of ART, with IRIS manifesting as a type 1 Hansen's disease reaction during the 6 months post-ART initiation; type 3 describing IRIS manifesting as a type 1 Hansen's disease reaction post-ART initiation in patients with undiagnosed or previously treated Hansen's disease and who are not receiving MDT; type 4 if Hansen's disease is diagnosed after ART initiation, the patient commences MDT, and subsequently develops type 1 reaction [38].

5 Hansen's Disease and Tuberculosis

The most common form of tuberculosis is pulmonary, with ten million new cases worldwide each year. Tuberculosis is curable using MDT of 6 months' duration, extending up to 24 months in resistant cases. Bacillus Calmette-Guérin (BCG) vaccine is used in some countries and is effective against severe forms of the disease.

Hansen's disease and tuberculosis share some characteristics: both are caused by obligate intracellular acid-fast bacilli of the genus Mycobacterium, with slow growth and long incubation time; both are granulomatous infectious diseases which develop along a spectrum determined by host immune response; and both are strongly associated with socioeconomic deprivation [39].

Cutaneous tuberculosis has several clinical presentations and is diagnosed by histopathological examination and culture of *M. tuberculosis* [40, 41]. Cutaneous tuberculosis accounts for only 1–2% of tuberculosis cases, and cases of co-occurrence with Hansen's disease are rare.

Tuberculosis and Hansen's disease may be treated concomitantly, adjusting drug dosages if necessary to minimize toxicity and reduce risk of resistance [42–44].

6 Hansen's Disease and Hepatitis

Hansen's disease can occur concurrently with viral hepatitis. Some studies have suggested a higher prevalence of hepatitis B virus (HBV) infection in persons with Hansen's disease [45], and vice versa [46], while others show no association [47]. It is possible that persons with Hansen's disease are more likely to be exposed to hepatitis infection, including hepatitis C virus (HCV) [48], rather than Hansen's disease co-infection increasing the risk of developing hepatitis [49, 50].

Evidence that HBV, HCV, and other viral hepatitis co-infections could be associated with Hansen's disease reactions is inconsistent, with one study in Brazil showing that groups of patients co-infected with HBV had higher rates of neuritis and impaired nerve function compared to patients not co-infected [51], another showing no association of anti-HBc or anti-HCV antibodies with type 1 or 2 reactions [47].

7 Hansen's Disease and Immunosuppression

Chronic immune-mediated diseases, organ and stem cell transplantation, and the corresponding demand for long-term or lifelong immunosuppressive treatments are increasingly common in countries where Hansen's disease is endemic [52].

There is limited evidence of possible adverse effects on Hansen's disease development of classical immunosuppressive drugs such as corticosteroids, methotrexate, cyclosporine, and azathioprine [53], or potential effects of newer biological agents and small molecules such as anti-TNF-alpha agents (infliximab, etanercept, adalimumab, certolizumab, golimumab) used to treat autoimmune diseases including rheumatoid arthritis, psoriasis, psoriatic arthritis, ankylosing spondylitis, and inflammatory bowel diseases [54].

With the exception of a population-based observational study that showed an increased risk of developing Hansen's disease among patients receiving long-term corticosteroids or anti-TNF-alpha agents for a range of dermatological and rheumatologic autoimmune diseases [55], most reports have been case studies describing onset of Hansen's disease or Hansen's disease reactions after initiation or cessation of immunosuppressive therapies [56–60]. Cases of Hansen's disease after kidney [61–63], heart [64], and liver transplants have been reported [65].

Clinical consensus in the absence of an evidence base is that patients in endemic Hansen's disease settings should be assessed and monitored for signs of Hansen's disease before, during, and after immunosuppressive treatments.

References

1. da Paz WS, do Rosário Souza M, DDS T, et al. Impact of the COVID-19 pandemic on the diagnosis of leprosy in Brazil: an ecological and population-based study. Lancet Reg Health Am. 2022;9:100181. https://doi.org/10.1016/j.lana.2021.100181.
2. Deps P, Collin SM, de Andrade VLG. Hansen's disease case detection in Brazil: a backlog of undiagnosed cases due to COVID-19 pandemic. J Eur Acad Dermatol Venereol. 2022;jdv.18307:e754. https://doi.org/10.1111/jdv.18307.
3. Mahato S, Bhattarai S, Singh R. Inequities towards leprosy-affected people: a challenge during COVID-19 pandemic. PLoS Negl Trop Dis. 2020;14:e0008537. https://doi.org/10.1371/journal.pntd.0008537.
4. Antunes DE, Goulart IMB, Goulart LR. Will cases of leprosy reaction increase with COVID-19 infection? PLoS Negl Trop Dis. 2020;14:e0008460. https://doi.org/10.1371/journal.pntd.0008460.
5. Schmitz V, Dos Santos JB. COVID-19, leprosy, and neutrophils. PLoS Negl Trop Dis. 2021;15:e0009019. https://doi.org/10.1371/journal.pntd.0009019.
6. Rathod S, Suneetha S, Narang T, et al. Management of Leprosy in the context of COVID-19 pandemic: recommendations by SIG leprosy (IADVL Academy). Indian Dermatol Online J. 2020;11:345–8. https://doi.org/10.4103/idoj.IDOJ_234_20.
7. Cerqueira SRPS, Deps PD, Cunha DV, et al. The influence of leprosy-related clinical and epidemiological variables in the occurrence and severity of COVID-19: a prospective real-world cohort study. PLoS Negl Trop Dis. 2021;15:e0009635. https://doi.org/10.1371/journal.pntd.0009635.
8. Santos VS, Quintans-Júnior LJ, Barboza WS, et al. Clinical characteristics and outcomes in patients with COVID-19 and leprosy. J Eur Acad Dermatol Venereol. 2021;35:e1–2. https://doi.org/10.1111/jdv.16899.
9. Saxena S, Khurana A, Savitha B, et al. Severe type 2 leprosy reaction with COVID-19 with a favourable outcome despite continued use of corticosteroids and methotrexate and a hypothesis on the possible immunological consequences. Int J Infect Dis. 2020;103:549–51. https://doi.org/10.1016/j.ijid.2020.12.024.
10. Arora S, Bhatnagar A, Singh GK, et al. Hansen's disease in the era of COVID-19: an observation on a series of six patients with co-infection. Dermatol Ther. 2021;34:e14827. https://doi.org/10.1111/dth.14827.
11. Santos Morais Junior G, Shu Kurizky P, Penha Silva Cerqueira SR, et al. Enhanced IL-6 and IL-12B gene expression after SARS-CoV-2 infection in leprosy patients may increase the risk of neural damage. Am J Trop Med Hyg. 2021;104:2190–4. https://doi.org/10.4269/ajtmh.21-0034.
12. Bhardwaj A, Gupta SK, Narang T, et al. Updates on Management of Leprosy in the context of COVID-19 pandemic: recommendations by IADVL SIG leprosy. Indian Dermatol Online J. 2021;12:S24–30. https://doi.org/10.4103/idoj.idoj_513_21.
13. Repsold TAR, Collin SM, Bouth RC, et al. Hansen's disease and COVID-19 co-infection in Brazil. Int J Dermatol. 2022;61(12):1506–10. https://doi.org/10.1111/ijd.16319.

14. WHO Rapid Evidence Appraisal for COVID-19 Therapies (REACT) Working Group, JAC S, Murthy S, et al. Association between administration of systemic corticosteroids and mortality among critically ill patients with COVID-19: a meta-analysis. JAMA. 2020;324:1330–41. https://doi.org/10.1001/jama.2020.17023.

15. Wagner C, Griesel M, Mikolajewska A, et al. Systemic corticosteroids for the treatment of COVID-19. Cochrane Database Syst Rev. 2021;8:CD014963. https://doi.org/10.1002/14651858.CD014963.

16. Yuan S, Yin X, Meng X, et al. Clofazimine broadly inhibits coronaviruses including SARS-CoV-2. Nature. 2021;593:418. https://doi.org/10.1038/s41586-021-03431-4.

17. Farouk A, Salman S. Dapsone and doxycycline could be potential treatment modalities for COVID-19. Med Hypotheses. 2020;140:109768.

18. Yuan S, Yin X, Meng X, et al. Clofazimine is a broad-spectrum coronavirus inhibitor that antagonizes SARS-CoV-2 replication in primary human cell culture and hamsters. Res Sq. 2020:1–17. https://doi.org/10.21203/rs.3.rs-86169/v1.

19. De Carvalho AG, Guimarães Luz JG, Leite Dias JV, et al. Hyperendemicity, heterogeneity and spatial overlap of leprosy and cutaneous leishmaniasis in the southern Amazon region of Brazil. Geospat Health. 2020;15(2) https://doi.org/10.4081/gh.2020.892.

20. Vernal S, Bueno-Filho R, Gomes CM, Roselino AM. Clinico-immunological spectrum of American tegumentary leishmaniasis and leprosy coinfection: a case series in Southeastern Brazil. Rev Soc Bras Med Trop. 2019;52:e20180172. https://doi.org/10.1590/0037-8682-0172-2018.

21. Mercadante LM, Santos MASD, Pegas ES, Kadunc BV. Leprosy and American cutaneous leishmaniasis coinfection. An Bras Dermatol. 2018;93:123–5. https://doi.org/10.1590/abd1806-4841.20186698.

22. Goulart IMB, Patrocínio LG, Nishioka SDA, et al. Concurrent leprosy and leishmaniasis with mucosal involvement. Lepr Rev. 2002;73:283–4.

23. Soto LA, Caballero N, Fuentes LR, et al. Leprosy associated with atypical cutaneous Leishmaniasis in Nicaragua and Honduras. Am J Trop Med Hyg. 2017;97:1103–10. https://doi.org/10.4269/ajtmh.16-0622.

24. Patrao NAR, Bhat RM, Dandekeri S, Kambil SM. Diffuse cutaneous leishmaniasis in coexistence with leprosy. Int J Dermatol. 2015;54:1402–6. https://doi.org/10.1111/ijd.12954.

25. van Wijk R, van Selm L, Barbosa MC, et al. Psychosocial burden of neglected tropical diseases in eastern Colombia: an explorative qualitative study in persons affected by leprosy, cutaneous leishmaniasis and Chagas disease. Glob Ment Health (Camb). 2021;8:e21. https://doi.org/10.1017/gmh.2021.18.

26. Kurizky PS, Cerqueira SRPS, Cunha DV, et al. The challenge of concomitant infections in the coronavirus disease 2019 pandemic era: severe acute respiratory syndrome coronavirus 2 infection in a patient with chronic Chagas disease and dimorphic leprosy. Rev Soc Bras Med Trop. 2020;53:e20200504. https://doi.org/10.1590/0037-8682-0504-2020.

27. Ustianowski AP, Lawn SD, Lockwood DNJ. Interactions between HIV infection and leprosy: a paradox. Lancet Infect Dis. 2006;6:350–60. https://doi.org/10.1016/S1473-3099(06)70493-5.

28. Massone C, Talhari C, Ribeiro-Rodrigues R, et al. Leprosy and HIV coinfection: a critical approach. Expert Rev Anti-Infect Ther. 2011;9:701–10. https://doi.org/10.1586/eri.11.44.

29. Pires CAA, Jucá Neto FOM, de Albuquerque NC, et al. Leprosy reactions in patients coinfected with HIV: clinical aspects and outcomes in two comparative cohorts in the Amazon region, Brazil. PLoS Negl Trop Dis. 2015;9:e0003818. https://doi.org/10.1371/journal.pntd.0003818.

30. Pereira GAS, Stefani MMA, Araújo Filho JA, et al. Human immunodeficiency virus type 1 (HIV-1) and mycobacterium leprae co-infection: HIV-1 subtypes and clinical, immunologic, and histopathologic profiles in a Brazilian cohort. Am J Trop Med Hyg. 2004;71:679–84.

31. Trindade MÂB, Miyamoto D, Benard G, et al. Leprosy and tuberculosis co-infection: clinical and immunological report of two cases and review of the literature. Am J Trop Med Hyg. 2013;88:236–40. https://doi.org/10.4269/ajtmh.2012.12-0433.

32. Deps PD, Gripp CG, Madureira BPR, Lucas EA. Immune reconstitution syndrome associated with leprosy: two cases. Int J STD AIDS. 2008;19:135–6. https://doi.org/10.1258/ijsa.2007.007163.
33. Lawn SD, Wood C, Lockwood DN. Borderline tuberculoid leprosy: an immune reconstitution phenomenon in a human immunodeficiency virus-infected person. Clin Infect Dis. 2003;36:e5–6. https://doi.org/10.1086/344446.
34. Cusini A, Günthard HF, Weber R, et al. Lepromatous leprosy with erythema nodosum leprosum as immune reconstitution inflammatory syndrome in an HIV-1 infected patient after initiation of antiretroviral therapy. BMJ Case Rep. 2009;2009:bcr0520091904. https://doi.org/10.1136/bcr.05.2009.1904.
35. Arakkal GK, Damarla SV, Chanda GM. Immune reconstitution inflammatory syndrome unmasking erythema nodosum leprosum: a rare case report. Indian J Dermatol. 2015;60:106. https://doi.org/10.4103/0019-5154.147883.
36. Deps P, Lucas S, Porro AM, et al. Clinical and histological features of leprosy and human immunodeficiency virus co-infection in Brazil. Clin Exp Dermatol. 2013;38:470–7. https://doi.org/10.1111/ced.12028.
37. Menezes VM, Sales AM, Illarramendi X, et al. Leprosy reaction as a manifestation of immune reconstitution inflammatory syndrome: a case series of a Brazilian cohort. AIDS. 2009;23:641–3. https://doi.org/10.1097/QAD.0b013e3283291405.
38. Deps P, Lockwood DNJ. Leprosy presenting as immune reconstitution inflammatory syndrome: proposed definitions and classification. Lepr Rev. 2010;81:59–68.
39. Rawson TM, Anjum V, Hodgson J, et al. Leprosy and tuberculosis concomitant infection: a poorly understood, age-old relationship. Lepr Rev. 2014;85:288–95.
40. Kaul S, Kaur I, Mehta S, Singal A. Cutaneous tuberculosis. Part I: pathogenesis, classification, and clinical features. J Am Acad Dermatol. 2022:S0190-9622(22)00202-X. https://doi.org/10.1016/j.jaad.2021.12.063.
41. Kaul S, Jakhar D, Mehta S, Singal A. Cutaneous tuberculosis. Part II: complications, diagnostic workup, histopathological features, and treatment. J Am Acad Dermatol. 2022:S0190-9622(22)00203-1. https://doi.org/10.1016/j.jaad.2021.12.064.
42. Shetty S, Umakanth S, Manandhar B, Nepali PB. Coinfection of leprosy and tuberculosis. BMJ Case Rep. 2018;2018:bcr2017222352. https://doi.org/10.1136/bcr-2017-222352.
43. Kama G, Huang GKL, Taune M, et al. Tuberculosis treatment unmasking leprosy: management of drug-resistant tuberculosis and leprosy co-infection. Public Health Action. 2019;9:S83–5. https://doi.org/10.5588/pha.18.0104.
44. Mangum L, Kilpatrick D, Stryjewska B, Sampath R. Tuberculosis and leprosy coinfection: a perspective on diagnosis and treatment. Open forum Infect Dis. 2018;5:ofy133. https://doi.org/10.1093/ofid/ofy133.
45. Leitão C, Ueda D, de Moraes Braga AC, et al. Leprosy and hepatitis B coinfection in southern Brazil. Braz J Infect Dis. 2014;18:8–12. https://doi.org/10.1016/j.bjid.2013.04.003.
46. Blumberg BS, Melartin L. Australia antigen and lepromatous leprosy studies in South India and elsewhere. Int J Lepr Mycobact Dis. 1970;38:60–7.
47. Costa JEF, Morais VMS, Gonçales JP, et al. Prevalence and risk factors for hepatitis B and C viruses in patients with leprosy. Acta Trop. 2017;172:160–3. https://doi.org/10.1016/j.actatropica.2017.04.024.
48. de Moraes Braga AC, Reason IJM, Maluf ECP, Vieira ER. Leprosy and confinement due to leprosy show high association with hepatitis C in Southern Brazil. Acta Trop. 2006;97:88–93. https://doi.org/10.1016/j.actatropica.2005.09.003.
49. Papaioannou DJ, Kaklamani EP, Parissis NG, et al. Hepatitis B virus (HBV) serum markers in Greek leprosy patients. Int J Lepr Mycobact Dis. 1986;54:245–51.
50. Ramos JMH, Costa e Silva ÁM, Martins RMB, Souto FJD. Prevalence of hepatitis B and C virus infection among leprosy patients in a leprosy-endemic region of Central Brazil. Mem Inst Oswaldo Cruz. 2011;106:632–4. https://doi.org/10.1590/s0074-02762011000500019.

51. Machado PRL, Machado LM, Shibuya M, et al. Viral co-infection and leprosy outcomes: a cohort study. PLoS Negl Trop Dis. 2015;9:e0003865. https://doi.org/10.1371/journal.pntd.0003865.
52. Shu Kurizky P, dos Santos Neto LL, Barbosa Aires R, et al. Opportunistic tropical infections in immunosuppressed patients. Best Pract Res Clin Rheumatol. 2020;34(4):101509. https://doi.org/10.1016/j.berh.2020.101509.
53. Barroso DH, Brandão JG, Andrade ESN, et al. Leprosy detection rate in patients under immunosuppression for the treatment of dermatological, rheumatological, and gastroenterological diseases: a systematic review of the literature and meta-analysis. BMC Infect Dis. 2021;21:347. https://doi.org/10.1186/s12879-021-06041-7.
54. Cogen AL, Lebas E, De Barros B, et al. Biologics in leprosy: a systematic review and case report. Am J Trop Med Hyg. 2020;102:1131–6. https://doi.org/10.4269/ajtmh.19-0616.
55. Martins Gomes C, Vicente Cesetti M, Sevilha-Santos L, et al. The risk of leprosy in patients using immunobiologics and conventional immunosuppressants for the treatment of dermatological and rheumatological diseases: a cohort study. J Eur Acad Dermatol Venereol. 2020;35:e21–4. https://doi.org/10.1111/jdv.16764.
56. Antônio JR, Soubhia RMC, Paschoal VDA, et al. Biological agents: investigation into leprosy and other infectious diseases before indication. An Bras Dermatol. 2013;88:23–5. https://doi.org/10.1590/abd1806-4841.20132187.
57. Teixeira FM, Vasconcelos LMF, de AD RC, et al. Secondary leprosy infection in a patient with psoriasis during treatment with infliximab. J Clin Rheumatol. 2011;17:269–71. https://doi.org/10.1097/RHU.0b013e3182288870.
58. Scollard DM, Joyce MP, Gillis TP. Development of leprosy and type 1 leprosy reactions after treatment with infliximab: a report of 2 cases. Clin Infect Dis. 2006;43:e19–22. https://doi.org/10.1086/505222.
59. Lydakis C, Ioannidou D, Koumpa I, et al. Development of lepromatous leprosy following etanercept treatment for arthritis. Clin Rheumatol. 2012;31:395–8. https://doi.org/10.1007/s10067-011-1903-2.
60. Camacho ID, Valencia I, Rivas MP, Burdick AE. Type 1 leprosy reaction manifesting after discontinuation of adalimumab therapy. Arch Dermatol. 2009;145:349–51. https://doi.org/10.1001/archdermatol.2009.10.
61. Aytekin S, Yaşar Ş, Göktay F, et al. Lepromatous leprosy in a renal transplant recipient. Am J Transplant. 2017;17:2224–6. https://doi.org/10.1111/ajt.14335.
62. de Rezende Dutra FA, Araújo MG, de Paula Farah K, et al. Hanseníase multibacilar em paciente transplantado renal: relato de caso. Braz J Nephrol. 2015;37:131–4. https://doi.org/10.5935/0101-2800.20150019.
63. Guditi S, Ram R, Ismal KM, et al. Leprosy in a renal transplant recipient: review of the literature. Transpl Infect Dis. 2009;11:557–62. https://doi.org/10.1111/j.1399-3062.2009.00428.x.
64. Modi K, Mancini M, Joyce MP. Lepromatous leprosy in a heart transplant recipient. Am J Transplant. 2003;3:1600–3. https://doi.org/10.1046/j.1600-6135.2003.00284.x.
65. Trindade MAB, Palermo ML, Pagliari C, et al. Leprosy in transplant recipients: report of a case after liver transplantation and review of the literature. Transpl Infect Dis. 2011;13:63–9. https://doi.org/10.1111/j.1399-3062.2010.00549.x.

Differential Diagnosis of Cutaneous Lesions of Hansen's Disease

Mecciene Mendes Rodrigues and Patrícia D. Deps

A wide range of skin diseases can be mistaken for several forms of Hansen's disease (HD) and HD reactions. The complex pathogenesis of HD accounts for the remarkable diversity of possible skin lesions caused by interaction between the agents of the disease and the host, as represented in the Ridley-Jopling classifications. Skin lesions vary in morphological appearance and color and may appear as hypochromic (hypopigmented), erythematous (reddish), erythematous-violaceous, brownish, or copper-colored. The form of HD depends on the host immune response, as do the cutaneous lesions which can evolve gradually or appear spontaneously and which can be localized or disseminated, including patches (macules), papules, plaques, nodules or tumors, swellings, infiltrations, ulcers, vesicles, and blisters.

Skin lesions with anesthesia or paresthesia, enlarged peripheral nerves and a definite loss of sensation to light touch, pinprick, or temperature are cardinal signals and symptoms of HD. Numbness, tingling, nerve pain, dryness of skin and mucous membrane, and hair loss may lead to suspicion of HD.

M. M. Rodrigues (✉)
Universidade Federal de Pernambuco, Recife, Brazil
e-mail: mecciene.silva@ufpe.br

P. D. Deps
Universidade Federal do Espírito Santo, Vitória, Brazil
e-mail: patricia.deps@ufes.br

P. D. Deps (ed.), *Hansen's Disease*, https://doi.org/10.1007/978-3-031-30893-2_20

1 Differential Diagnosis of the Indeterminate Form of Hansen's Disease

1.1 Anemic and Achromic Nevi

Characterized by hypopigmented patches. The limits are well defined, and the shape and contours have the appearance of a geographical map. In general, this nevus presents from birth although appearance during childhood is possible.

Clinical features are hypo or achromic macular lesions, usually single, varying in size, and well-delineated (Fig. 1). In the anemic nevus, the abnormality is in cutaneous vascularization, and in the achromic nevus, an absence of melanin pigment. Pressure or friction can differentiate the two types by the absence of erythema in the area of the lesion in anemic nevus. Note that, in anemic nevi, the histamine test will not be complete and should not be used in the clinical differentiation of the indeterminate form of HD.

1.2 Pityriasis Versicolor (Hypopigmented Form)

This is a superficial mycosis caused by fungi of the genus *Malassezia*. It occurs frequently in tropical and warm regions. It generally affects regions of greater sebaceous production such as the upper trunk, neck, and face. It presents as lenticular

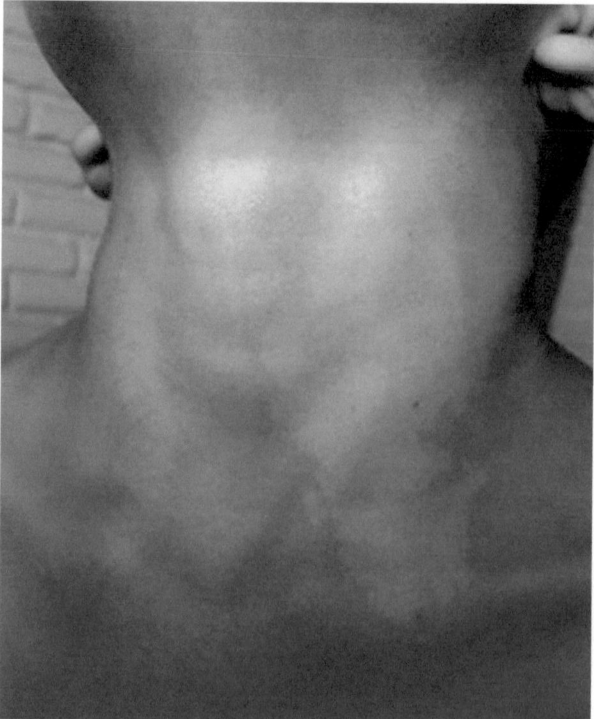

Fig. 1 Anemic nevus. Macula that does not become erythematous after rubbing

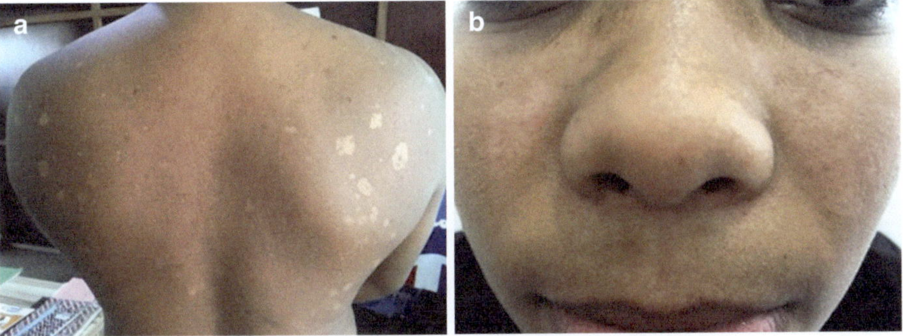

Fig. 2 Pityriasis versicolor. (**a**) Hypopigmented maculas well-defined limited and slight peeling on the trunk. (**b**) Hypopigmented and erythematous macules with fine scaling on the face

lesions with furfuraceous desquamation, and discretely erythematous and brownish lesions may also occur, hence the name versicolor, i.e., polychromic (Fig. 2). Zileri's sign (stretching of the skin) shows hypopigmented skin patch and the nail sign allows the visualization of furfuraceous scaling.

1.3 Pityriasis Alba

A common disease of unknown etiology, possibly associated with *Staphylococcus aureus* and environmental and nutritional factors, including vitamin A deficiency. It is a cutaneous manifestation of atopy and seborrheic dermatitis although not restricted to those conditions. Hypopigmented macula presenting light scaling, single or in small numbers, often found on the face (Fig. 3), upper trunk, arms, and thighs, rarely disseminated. Small follicular papules may be visualized and noticeable on palpation. It affects mainly children and may present mild pruritus. Hair loss may be present due to excoriation. Histamine test can be used to differentiate pityriasis alba from the indeterminate form of HD, especially in young children.

1.4 Post-inflammatory Hypopigmentation

This is a frequent dermatosis, common on arms and legs, which appears after several cutaneous inflammatory processes (Fig. 4). It presents as hypopigmented macules due to inflammatory, infectious, traumatic skin diseases or resulting from excoriations.

1.5 Vitiligo

Vitiligo is a common disease and occurs worldwide. It is a skin disease of multifactorial origin, with an autoimmune destruction of melanocytes. Patients with vitiligo present with one to several amelanotic macules that appear chalk- or milk-white in

Fig. 3 Pityriasis alba

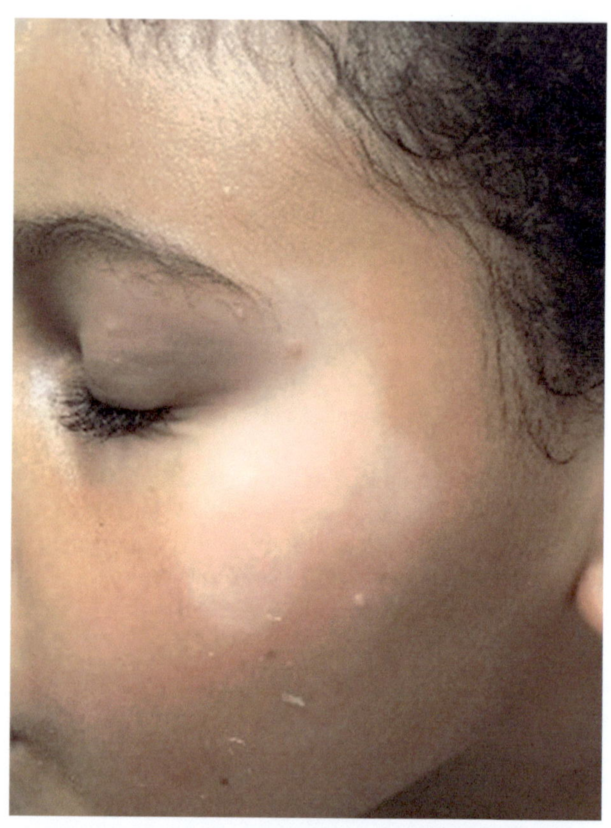

Fig. 4 Post-inflammatory hypopigmentation

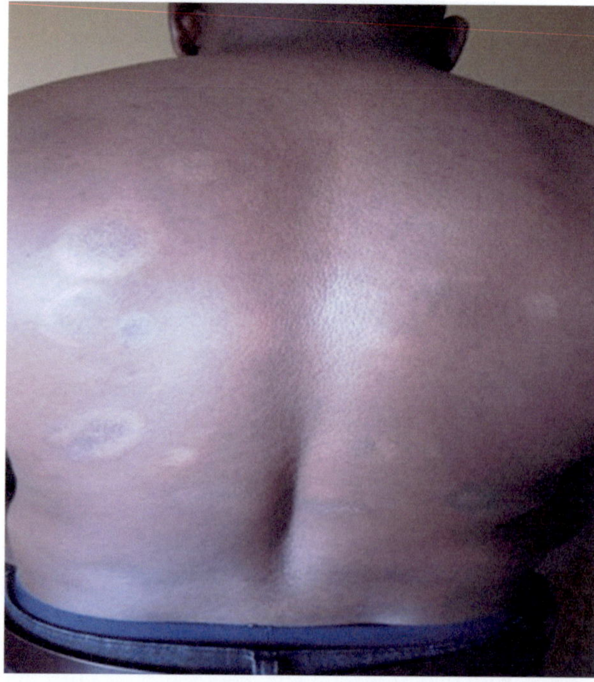

Fig. 5 Vitiligo

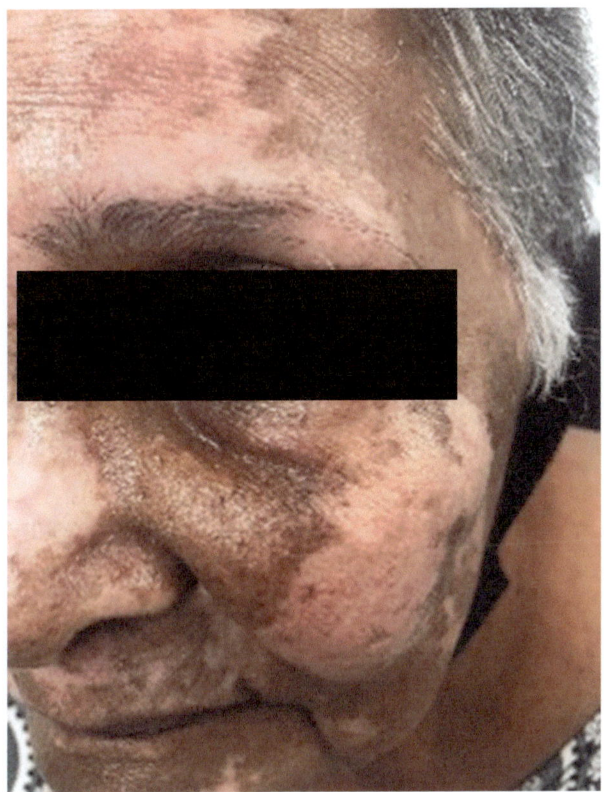

color. In general, lesions have a symmetrical distribution and can appear anywhere on the body, including mucous membranes. Initial lesions occur most frequently on the hands, forearms, feet, and face. When vitiligo occurs on the face, perioral and periocular are the most common sites (Fig. 5).

1.6 Seborrheic Dermatitis

Seborrheic dermatitis has sites of predilection such as face, ears, scalp, and upper part of the trunk (Fig. 6). In some cases, seborrheic dermatitis can be observed with hypopigmented patches similar to macular lesions of the indeterminate form of HD.

1.7 Hypopigmented Mycosis Fungoides

This is a rare presentation of cutaneous T-cell lymphoma that differs from classic mycosis fungoides because it affects younger people, with slower progression and the majority of patients remaining in stage 1 with treatment. Initially, it appears as a

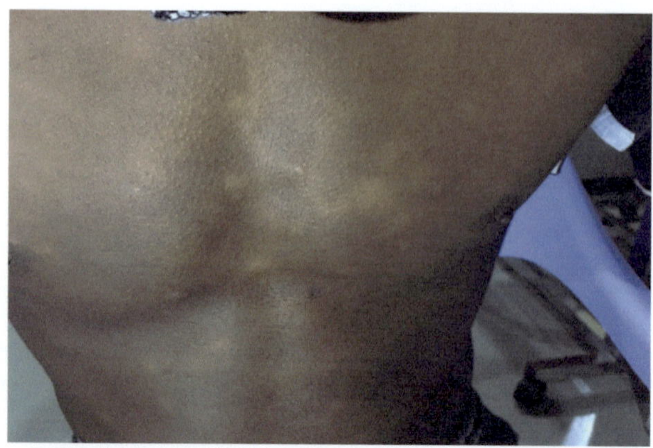

Fig. 6 Seborrheic dermatitis

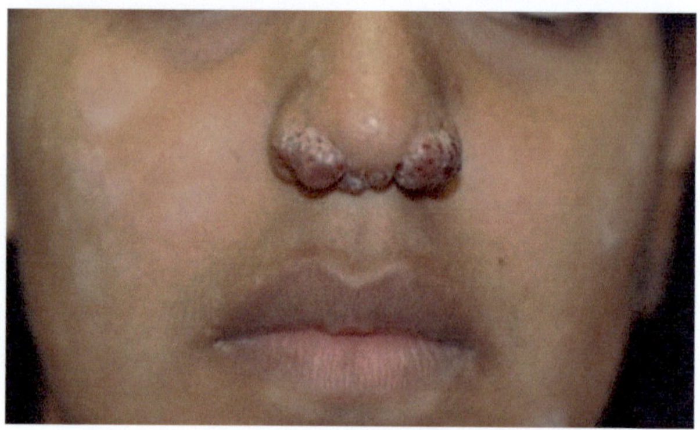

Fig. 7 Mycosis fungoides (hypopigmented macules)

hypopigmented patch (Fig. 7). Diagnosis is usually made by histopathological examination [1].

1.8 Leukoderma Punctata

These are small, asymptomatic, achromic skin lesions, located mainly on the sun-exposed areas of the upper and lower limbs (Fig. 8), and that begin in adulthood in patients who have had heavy sun exposure.

1.9 Localized Scleroderma (Morphea) and Lichen Sclerosus (et Atrophicus)

These are inflammatory diseases, with juvenile localized scleroderma (morphea) the predominant form in childhood, affecting the skin and sometimes extending to the underlying fascia, muscle, joints, and bone [2]. Hyperchromic plaques, which

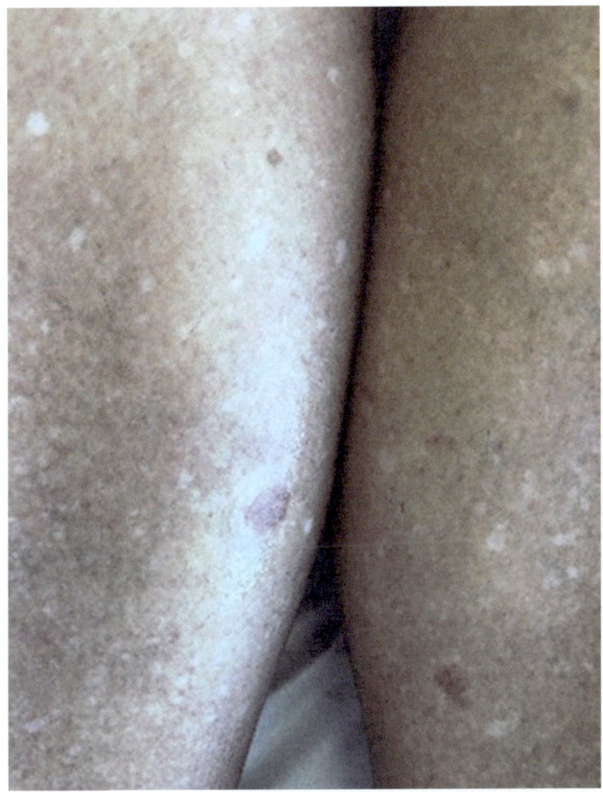

Fig. 8 Leukoderma punctata

may be surrounded by a copper halo, evolve to hypopigmentation, atrophy, and sclerosis (hardening).

Lichen sclerosus is characterized by hypopigmentation and skin atrophy. It involves most commonly genital skin. Lesions can evolve towards the destruction of anatomic structures, with functional impairment and risk of malignant evolution [3]. The Table 1 presents hypopigmented skin disease according to clinical characteristics such as external limit' itching, sensitivity, sweating and peeling.

Table 1 Skin diseases with hypopigmented lesions that are differential diagnoses of the indeterminate form of Hansen's disease

	Clinical characteristics				
	External limit	Itching	Sensitivity	Sweating	Peeling
Indeterminate form of HD	In general, poorly defined	Absent	In general, changed	Often absent	Absent
Anemic and achromic nevi	Well defined	Absent	Preserved	Preserved	Absent
Pityriasis versicolor	Well defined	Can be present	Preserved	Preserved	Generally present
Post-inflammatory hypopigmentation	Well defined	Absent	Absent	Preserved	Absent
Pityriasis alba	Poorly defined	Can be present	Absent	Preserved	Can be present
Vitiligo	Well defined	Absent	Absent	Absent	Absent
Localized scleroderma	Poorly defined	Absent	Absent	Absent	Absent

2 Differential Diagnosis of Tuberculoid and Borderline-Tuberculoid Forms of HD

2.1 *Granuloma Annulare*

This is a benign inflammatory skin disease associated with many conditions such as malignancy, trauma, thyroid disease, diabetes mellitus, and HIV infection. It can occur at any age. A localized variant occurs more commonly in children with a skin lesion characterized by a single or small number of erythematous, non-scaling plaques with raised, hardened edges, located most frequently on the extremities (Figs. 9 and 10). Spontaneous regression is observed. A generalized form presents more commonly in adult diabetic patients [4].

2.2 *Tinea Corporis*

Tinea corporis is caused by dermatophytes and is a common skin disease in tropical countries, affecting all age groups. It appears as a well-defined reddish plaque, scaling at the edges, which may occur as single lesions or in small numbers anywhere on the body (Fig. 11). Pruritus, excoriated lesions with secondary infection (impetiginization) and eczematization are frequently found [5].

2.3 *Pityriasis Rosea*

This is a disease with a probable viral etiology [6]. It presents as small, centrifugally growing papular erythematous lesions that evolve to annular lesions with discrete scaling on the inner border, distributed in an arboriform arrangement, generally on

Fig. 9 Granuloma annulare

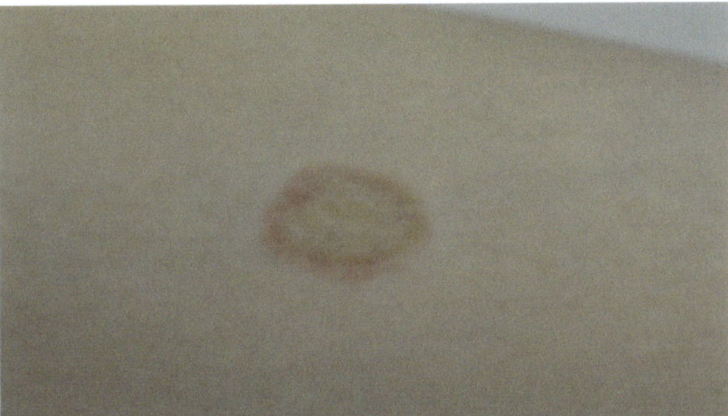

Fig. 10 Granuloma annulare

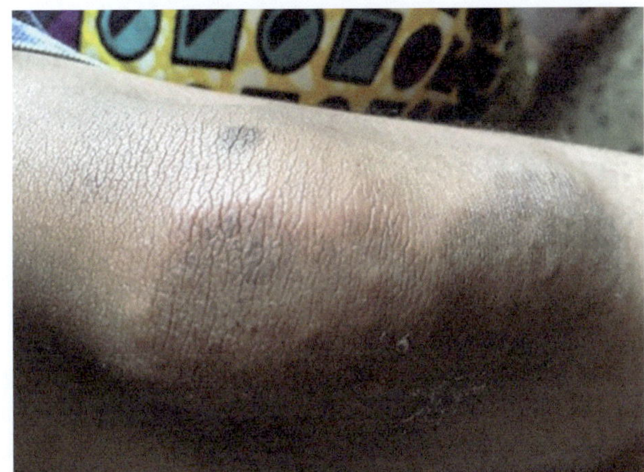

Fig. 11 Tinea corporis

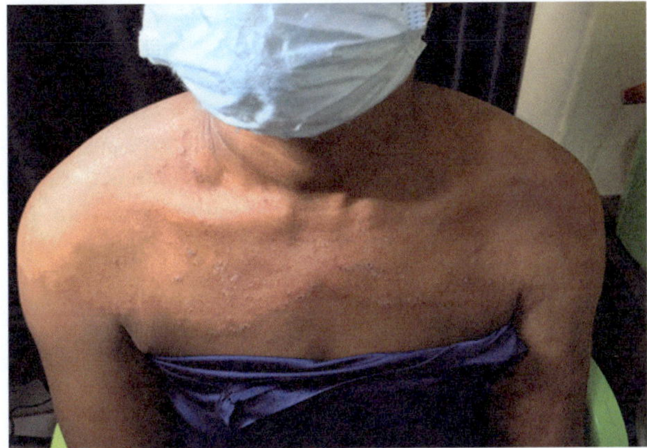

the trunk and neck (Fig. 12a). The first skin lesion is called the "herald patch" (Fig. 12b). The disease is self-limiting and lasts about 8 weeks. Lesions may be found in several stages of evolution: macules, papules, and annular lesions. Pruritus may be present.

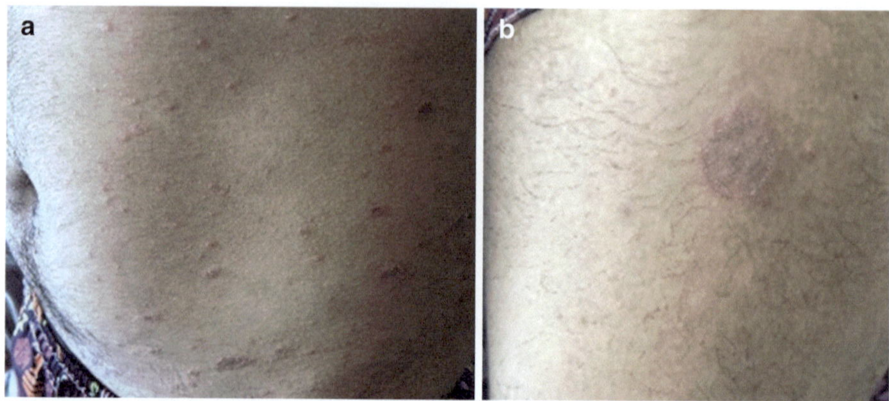

Fig. 12 Pityriasis rosea. (**a**) Erythematous plaques with collared desquamation and "Christmas tree" arrangement. (**b**) Initial lesion (herald patch)

2.4 Lupus Vulgaris (Cutaneous Tuberculosis)

Cutaneous tuberculosis (CTb) is a chronic infectious disease with several clinical presentations that are rare and difficult to diagnose. Lupus vulgaris (LV) is the most frequent form. *Mycobacterium tuberculosis* is the main causative agent of LV but, more rarely, the disease can be caused by *Mycobacterium bovis* or bacillus Calmette-Guérin (BCG). Lesions are most often located on the face, around the nose, eyelid, lips, cheeks, and ears (Fig. 13). LV is characterized by an erythematous plaque with multiple nodules that spread irregularly leading to scarring and destruction of tissue [7].

2.5 Sarcoidosis

This is a chronic multisystemic granulomatous disease of unknown etiology. It affects patients of all ages and races. The skin is the second most commonly affected organ, with a polymorphous presentation (Fig. 14a, b). Lupus pernio manifests as insidious purpuric or purplish-blue lesions localized on the nose, cheeks, lips, and ears, associated with swelling of the fingers and toes [8]. Typical erythema nodosum may be a manifestation of sarcoidosis, generally limited to the lower limbs, which is a clinical differential from ENL lesions that can occur anywhere on the body. Chest radiography and histopathology may help in the diagnosis. Histopathology reveals a non-caseating tuberculoid granuloma without the presence of lympho-cytes, also known as "naked granuloma" (Fig. 14c, d) [9].

Fig. 13 Lupus vulgaris (Cutaneous tuberculosis)

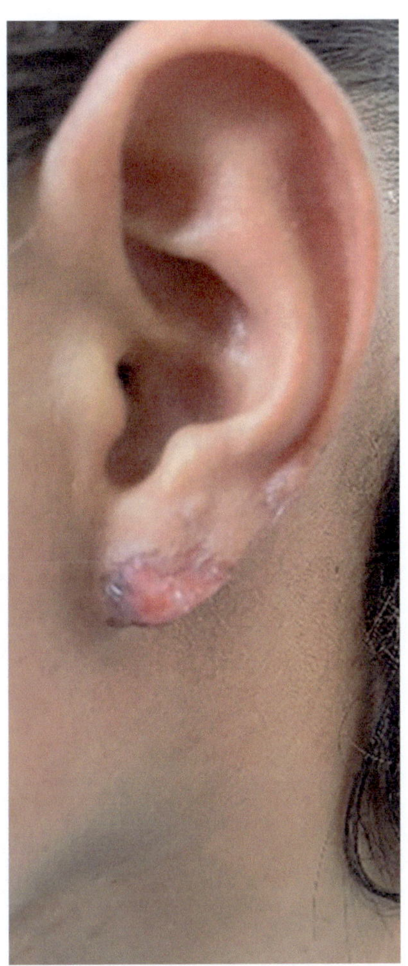

2.6 *Discoid Lupus Erythematosus*

A chronic autoimmune disease, this is the form of lupus erythematosus limited to the skin, occurring more frequently in young women. Lesions are located on photo-exposed areas, including the face, scalp, upper limbs, and, more rarely, may generalize to the whole integument. In this type of cutaneous lupus, the skin lesions are round (disk-shaped), thick, scaly, and red. They may present as atrophic, alopecic, and with erythema and edema of the borders when active. Residual lesions present as achromic and hyperchromic.

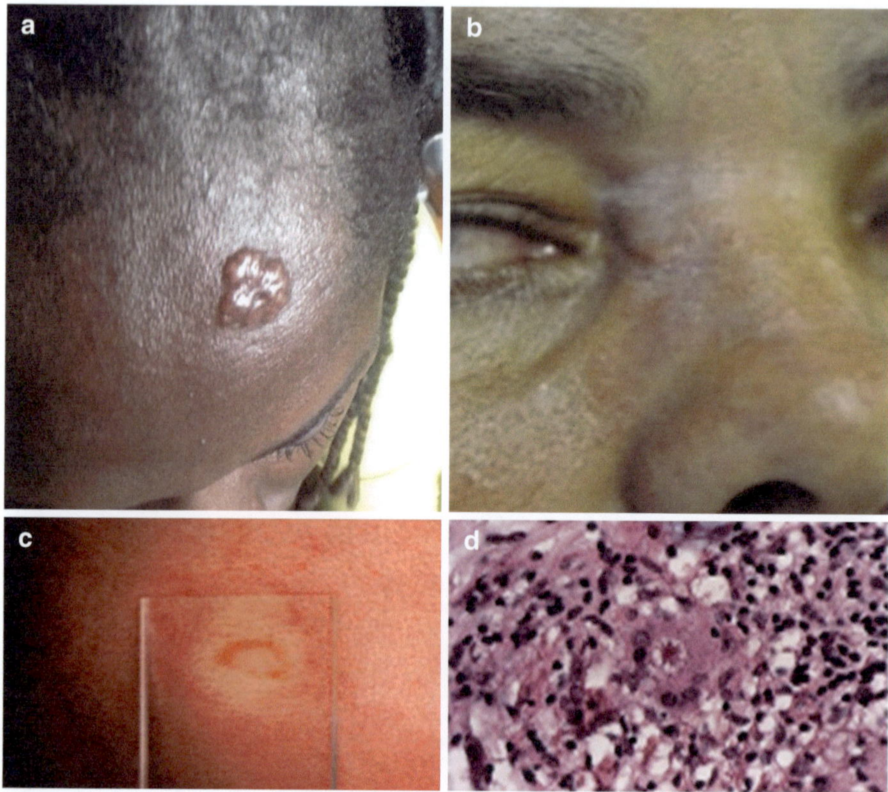

Fig. 14 Sarcoidosis. (**a**) Roughly defined erythematous-elevated nodule (**a**) and plaque (**b**). (**c**) Compression with a glass slide showing the presence of an apple-jelly aspect characteristic of sarcoidosis. (**d**) Histopathology (Hematoxylin-Eosin) with the presence of naked granuloma

2.7 Lyme Disease

A systemic disease common in the Northern Hemisphere caused by *Borrelia burgdorferi* transmitted by infected Ixodes ticks. Lesions occur as erythematous macula with migratory "bulls-eye target" appearance and may be associated with fever, headache, myalgia, and arthralgia. Diagnosis can be made by serological detection of anti-*B. burgdorferi* antibodies.

2.8 Contact Dermatitis

This is a common inflammatory skin condition characterized by erythematous and pruritic skin lesions that occur after contact with a foreign substance. There are two forms of contact dermatitis: irritant and allergic [10]. Skin lesions often occur at the site of contact and progress to erythema and scaling with visible borders (Fig. 15).

Fig. 15 Contact dermatitis

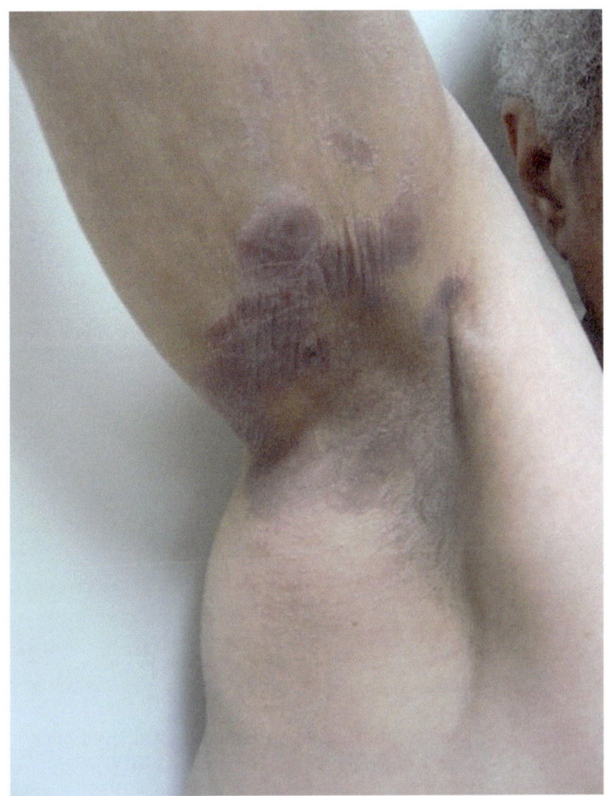

3   Differential Diagnosis of Borderline and Virchowian Forms of HD

3.1   Secondary Syphilis

This disease is caused by *Treponema pallidum*. Weeks or months after the primary infection, numerous small, oval, erythematous papules may develop, and subtle peripheral scaling (Biet's collar) may be found. It can occur on the whole integument, including the palms and soles (Fig. 16a–d). On the face, in patients with Fitzpatrick phototypes V and VI, arciform lesions with raised borders forming "drawings" may be observed, a picture known as "elegant syphilis." The lesions are asymptomatic, last for 3–4 weeks and regress spontaneously. Recurrences are possible, in a milder form, leaving residual hyperpigmented lesions with mild atrophy. The diagnosis must be confirmed by serological tests for antibodies to *T. pallidum*.

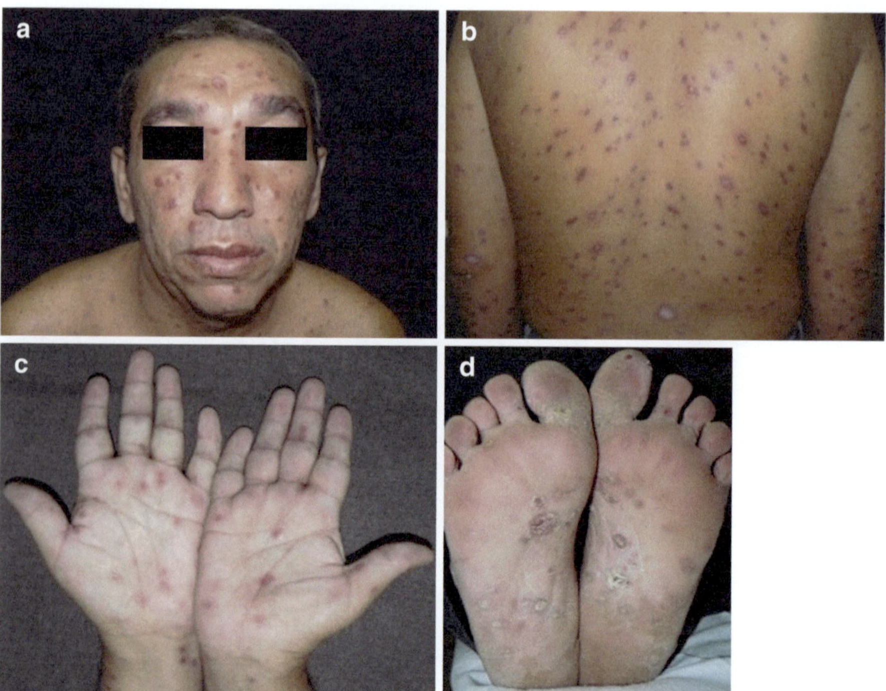

Fig. 16 Secondary Syphilis. Numerous small, oval, erythematous papules (syphilitic roseola) on the face (**a**), trunk (**b**), and the palms (**c**) and soles (**d**)

3.2 Lobomycosis or Jorge Lobo's Disease

Caused by the *Lacazia loboi* fungus, this mycosis is restricted to the Amazon region. It affects the skin and subcutaneous tissue. Nodules and plaques with frankly keloid-like nodules and plaques are present all over the body, with a greater predilection for exposed areas. The lesions are asymptomatic and follow a chronic course. The diagnosis is made by histopathological examination and identification of the fungus in the lesion. It may affect the auricular pavilion, as does the virchowian form of HD (VHD), but unilateral involvement is more common in Jorge Lobo's disease while bilateral involvement is more common in VHD.

3.3 Kaposi's Sarcoma

This is a proliferative tumor of vascular endothelial cells. Both macular lesions, nodules and plaques of angiomatous appearance may be found, with coloration ranging from erythematous-violaceous to brownish (Fig. 17).

Fig. 17 Kaposi's sarcoma

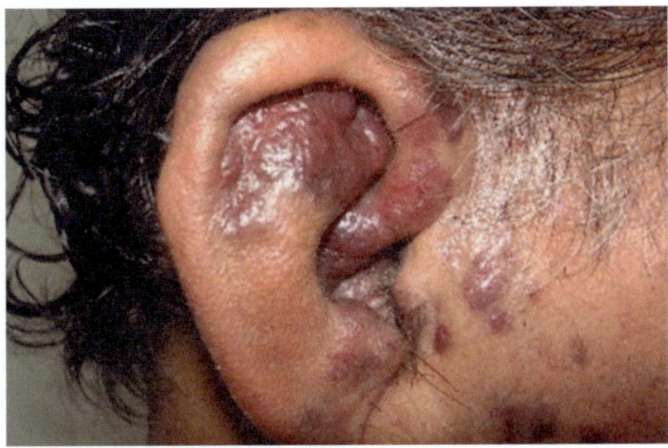

3.4 Diffuse Cutaneous Leishmaniasis

A disease caused by *Leishmania amazonensis* or *Leishmania aethiopica*, it constitutes the anergic pole of infection, presenting as a generalized nodular eruption with symmetrical distribution (Fig. 18). Diagnosis is made by identifying amastigotes within macrophages obtained by biopsy or smear of skin lesions.

3.5 Neurofibromatosis

This is a genodermatosis where nodular and tumoral lesions appear in childhood or later. The skin lesions vary in size and are asymptomatic (Fig. 19a, b).

3.6 Mycosis Fungoides

This is a malignant proliferation of T lymphocytes (cutaneous lymphoma), producing infiltrated macules and plaques of varying sizes, shapes, and colors (Fig. 20a–c). As the disease develops, nodules may appear in previously uninfiltrated areas. Sensitivities are preserved. Diagnosis is confirmed by histopathology of the skin.

3.7 Plaque Parapsoriasis

A skin disease caused by the proliferation of T-lymphocytes. It presents initially as macules evolving to yellowish-erythematous slightly desquamative plaques (Fig. 21). The diagnosis is confirmed by histopathological findings.

Fig. 18 Diffuse cutaneous leishmaniasis

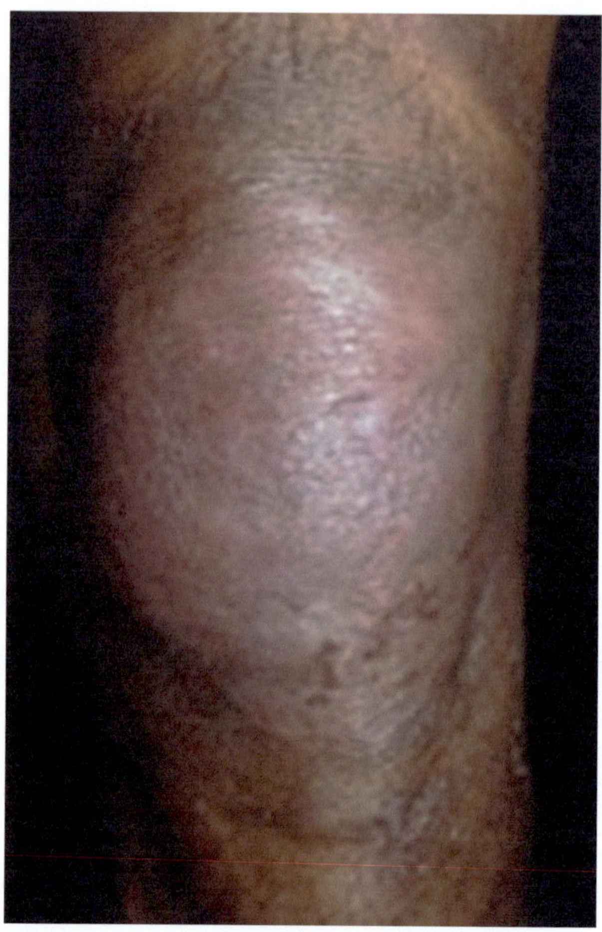

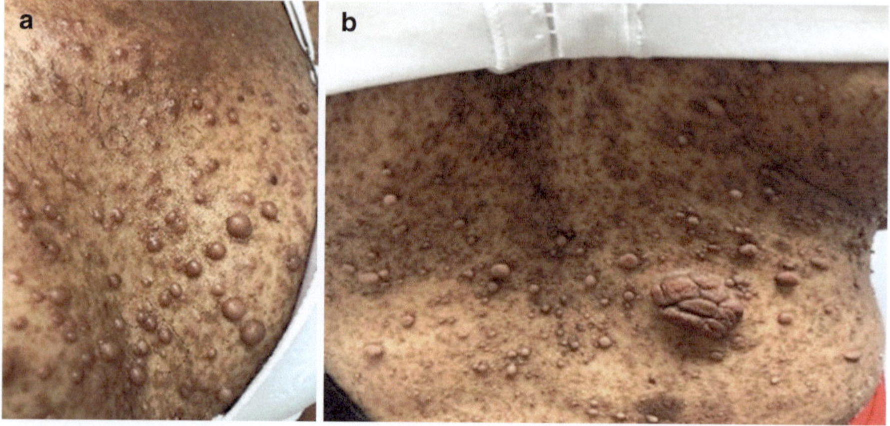

Fig. 19 Neutofibomatosis. Papules, nodules and tumours of skin colour (**a**, **b**)

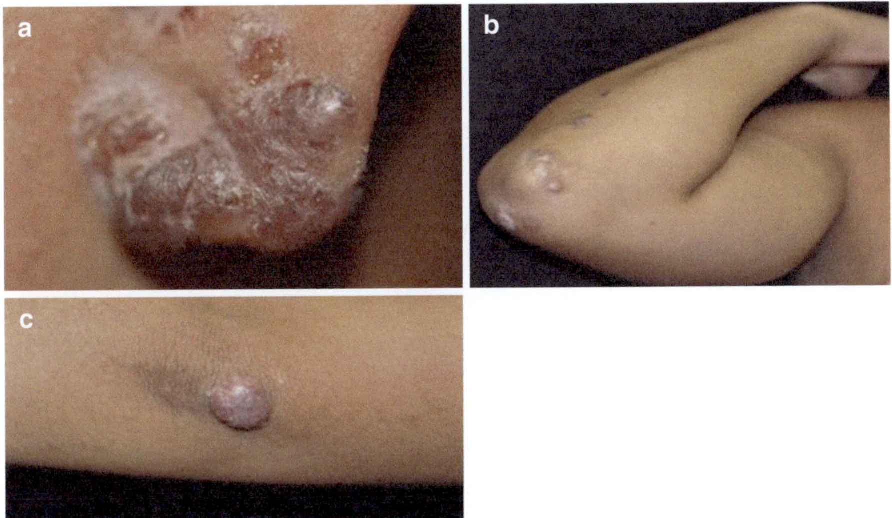

Fig. 20 Mycosis fungoides. Papules, nodules and erythematous plaques (**a–c**)

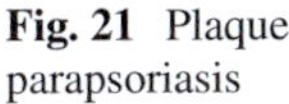

Fig. 21 Plaque parapsoriasis

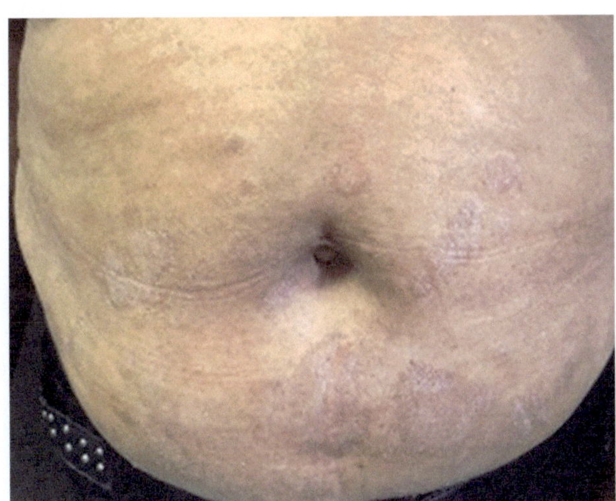

3.8 *Actinic Reticuloid*

A disease caused by persistent and severe photosensitivity. It presents with infiltration, erythema, edema, and thickening of the skin of the face, neck, and hands. Sensitivities are preserved. The diagnosis is confirmed by histopathological findings.

3.9 Symmetrical Drug-Related Intertriginous and Flexural Exanthema (SDRIFE)

SDRIFE or "Baboon syndrome" is characterized by symmetrical exanthema in the gluteal, intergluteal, and inguinal region and at least one intertriginous area (Fig. 22). It begins hours or up to 2 days after exposure to the causal agent. The most commonly implicated medications are beta-lactams, particularly amoxicillin, sulphamides, anti-inflammatory drugs, barbiturates, tetracyclines, and carbamazepine.

3.10 Erythema Elevatum Diutinum

This occurs between 30 and 60 years of age in both sexes. It is characterized initially by macules or purpuric plaques on the extensor surfaces of the extremities and evolves with the formation of nodules that simulate keloids, HD, or fibrous tumors (Fig. 23). It may be associated with tumors in solid organs, lympho-hematic, inflammatory, or autoimmune diseases.

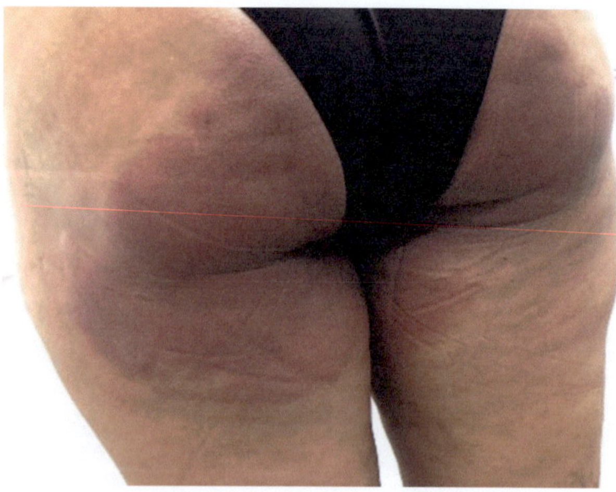

Fig. 22 Symmetrical drug-related intertriginous and flexural exanthema (SDRIFE)

Fig. 23 Erythema
elevatum diutinum

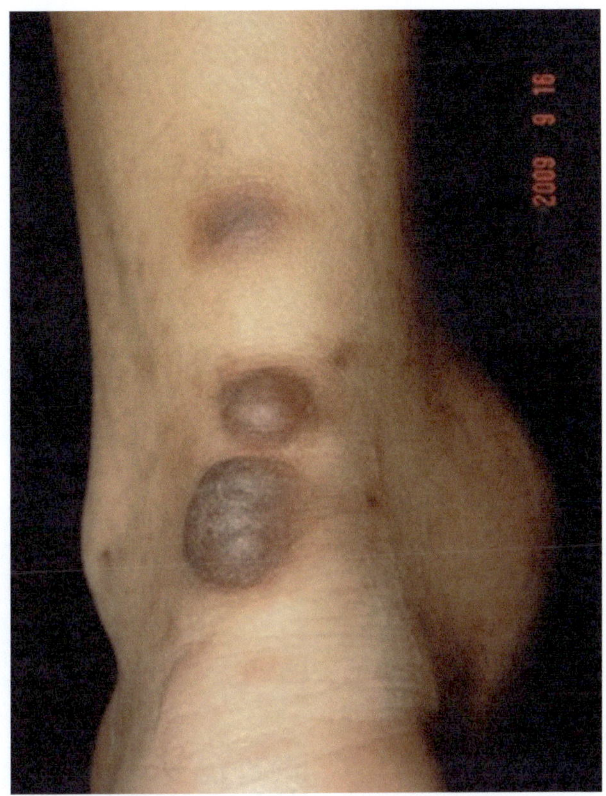

4   Differential Diagnosis of Reactions in Hansen's Disease

4.1   *Plaque Psoriasis*

This is a chronic inflammatory desquamative disease which can affect the skin and joints. It is characterized by well-defined, erythematous-descaling plaque lesions, generally affecting the scalp, elbows, knees, and the sacral region (Fig. 24). Psoriasis is recurrent and can be physically or socially disabling. Plaque psoriasis is a differential diagnosis with borderline forms of HD and Type 1 reactions.

4.2   *Erythema Multiforme*

An acute and recurrent skin condition that is considered to be a hypersensitivity reaction to infections or drugs [11]. The clinical picture may be preceded or accompanied by fever, malaise, arthralgia, and myalgia. It presents as a polymorphous eruption of macules, papules, and characteristic "target" lesions (pale center) that

Fig. 24 Plaque psoriasis

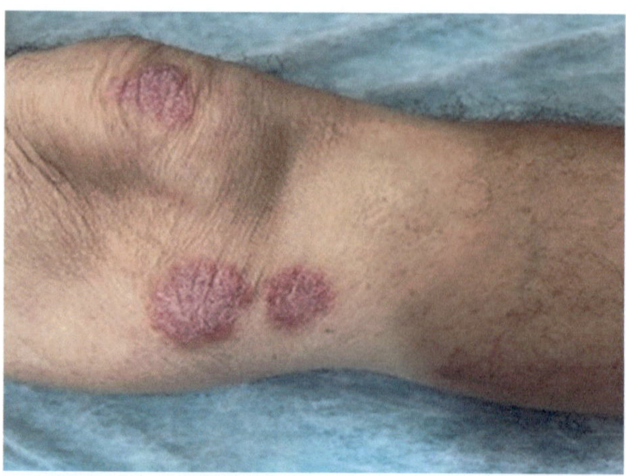

Fig. 25 Erythema multiforme

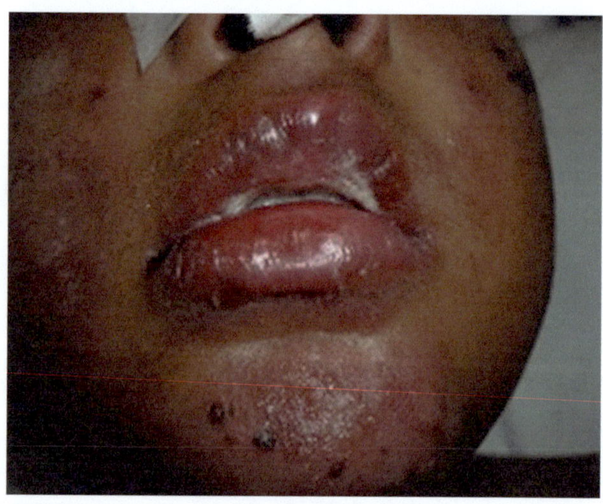

are distributed symmetrically with propensity for the distal extremities, and which may evolve to ulcerated lesions (Fig. 25). When the picture is more intense, generalized, and affecting mucous membranes, with vesicles and blisters, the possibility of Stevens-Johnson Syndrome or Toxic Epidermal Necrolysis must be considered. Differential diagnosis with Type 2 reactions of HD [11].

4.3 Erythema Nodosum (Non Leprosum)

The erythema nodosum is defined and characterized by erythematous lesions that are more palpable than visible and may be caused by infections, as in the reaction pictures of infection by *M. tuberculosis*, in pharyngitis caused by *Streptococcus*, or caused by medication, among other causes. It can also occur in autoimmune diseases such as systemic lupus erythematosus (SLE).

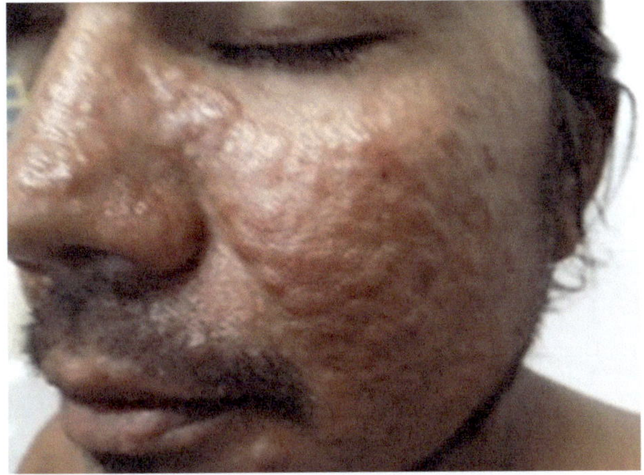

Fig. 26 Post-kala-azar dermal leishmaniasis

4.4   Post Kala-Azar Dermal Leishmaniasis (PKDL)

After treatment, visceral leishmaniasis (VL) may present clinically as macules, plaques, or nodular lesions (Fig. 26), usually beginning on the face and spreading to the neck and extremities. It also affects the small cutaneous nerves. Although rare, co-infections of HD and VL have been reported [12].

4.5   Sweet's Syndrome

This is an acute febrile neutrophilic dermatosis presenting with papules that tend to group into painful erythematous and erythematous-violaceous plaques. The intense edema of the lesions gives a characteristic appearance of the syndrome called pseudo-vesiculation. In some cases, the lesions resemble those of erythema multiforme and should be differentiated from Type 2 reactions whose cutaneous picture is indistinguishable from erythema multiforme. The presence of bacilli on histopathological examination confirms the diagnosis [13].

References

1. Rodney IJ, Kindred C, Angra K, et al. Hypopigmented mycosis fungoides: a retrospective clinicohistopathologic study. J Eur Acad Dermatol Venereol. 2017;31:808–14. https://doi.org/10.1111/jdv.13843.
2. George R, George A, Kumar TS. Update on management of morphea (localized scleroderma) in children. Indian Dermatol Online J. 2020;11:135–45. https://doi.org/10.4103/idoj.IDOJ_284_19.
3. Chamli A, Souissi A. Lichen sclerosus. In: Stat pearls. Treasure Island (FL): Stat Pearls Publishing; 2022.
4. Wang J, Khachemoune A. Granuloma annulare: a focused review of therapeutic options. Am J Clin Dermatol. 2018;19:333–44. https://doi.org/10.1007/s40257-017-0334-5.

5. Kovitwanichkanont T, Chong AH. Superficial fungal infections. Aust J Gen Pract. 2019;48:706–11. https://doi.org/10.31128/AJGP-05-19-4930.

6. Avelleira JCR, Lupi O, Caterino-de-Araujo A, de Los Santos-Fortuna E. Seroprevalence of HHV-8 infection in the pediatric population of two university hospitals in Rio de Janeiro, Brazil. Int J Dermatol. 2006;45:381–3. https://doi.org/10.1111/j.1365-4632.2006.02523.x.

7. Jaka-Moreno A, López-Núñez M, López-Pestaña A, Tuneu-Valls A. Lupus vulgaris caused by mycobacterium bovis. Actas Dermosifiliogr. 2012;103:251–3. https://doi.org/10.1016/j.ad.2011.03.031.

8. Condé K, Guelngar CO, Mohamed A, et al. Lupus pernio in chronic sarcoidosis. Cureus. 2021;13:e18331. https://doi.org/10.7759/cureus.18331.

9. Sève P, Pacheco Y, Durupt F, et al. Sarcoidosis: a clinical overview from symptoms to diagnosis. Cell. 2021;10(4):76. https://doi.org/10.3390/cells10040766.

10. Usatine RP, Riojas M. Diagnosis and management of contact dermatitis. Am Fam Physician. 2010;82:249–55.

11. Lamoreux MR, Sternbach MR, Hsu WT. Erythema multiforme. Am Fam Physician. 2006;74:1883–8.

12. Trindade MAB, da Cruz Silva LL, LMA B, et al. Post-kala-azar dermal leishmaniasis and leprosy: case report and literature review. BMC Infect Dis. 2015;15:543. https://doi.org/10.1186/s12879-015-1260-x.

13. Chiaratti FC, Daxbacher ELR, Neumann ABF, Jeunon T. Type 2 leprosy reaction with Sweet's syndrome-like presentation. An Bras Dermatol. 2016;91:345–9. https://doi.org/10.1590/abd1806-4841.20164111.

Differential Diagnoses of the Neurological Manifestations of Hansen's Disease

Patrícia D. Deps, Francisco Marcos B. Cunha, and José Antônio Garbino

Clinical suspicion of Hansen's disease should be raised in patients presenting with sensory alterations including paraesthesia, tingling, burning, and/or sensory deficit corresponding to the area of a thickened nerve, associated or not with motor and/or autonomic deficits, and with or without Hansen's disease skin lesions [1].

In a Brazilian Hansen's disease reference centre study involving 481 patients, Hansen's disease was confirmed in 320 (66.5%) cases, and differential diagnoses in the other 161 patients included: (a) metabolic and deficiency diseases—diabetes mellitus, hypothyroidism, uraemia, secondary amyloidosis, alcoholic neuropathy; (b) hereditary neuropathies—Charcot-Marie-Tooth I and II (Fig. 1), congenital insensitivity to pain, compression susceptibility neuropathy, neurofibromatosis type I; (c) inflammatory and immune-mediated diseases—vasculitis, systemic lupus erythematosus, panarteritis nodosa, chronic inflammatory demyelinating polyneuropathy, monoclonal gammopathy; (d) traumatic and compressive spinal and spinal cord diseases—radiculopathies, cervical syringomyelia, sequelae of transverse myelitis, neurogenic thoracic outlet syndrome; (e) motor neuron disease; (f) effects of drug toxicity—isoniazid, chloroquine, and antiretrovirals; (g) other non-neurological diseases—palmar tendinopathy, camptodactyly (Fig. 2) and osteoarthropathies [2].

P. D. Deps
Universidade Federal do Espírito Santo, Vitória, Brazil
e-mail: patricia.deps@ufes.br

F. M. B. Cunha
Universidade Federal do Cariri, Juazeiro do Norte, Ceara, Brazil
e-mail: marcos.cunha@ufca.edu.br

J. A. Garbino (✉)
Instituto Lauro de Souza Lima, Bauru, Brazil

P. D. Deps (ed.), *Hansen's Disease*, https://doi.org/10.1007/978-3-031-30893-2_21

"""

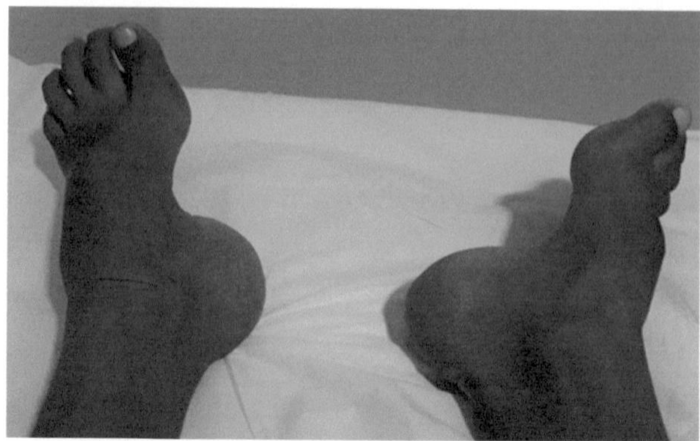

Fig. 1 Charcot-Marie-Tooth I and II Disease

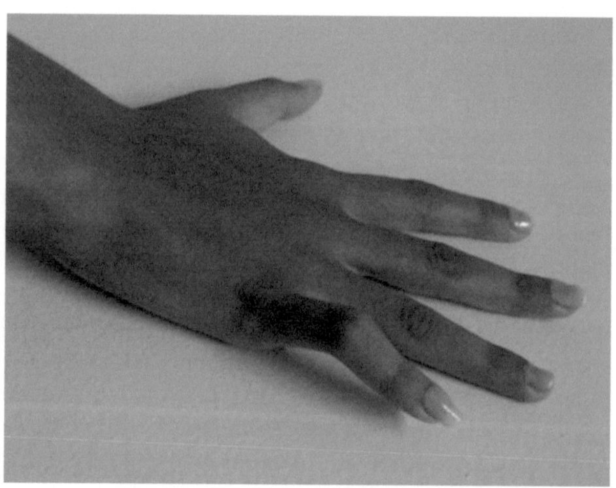

Fig. 2 Camptodactyly

Investigation of peripheral neuropathies begins with the anamnesis, research of personal and family antecedents, and a physical-neurological examination. Complementary examinations should include: general laboratory examinations, skin smears, clinical investigations of sensibility and motor examination, electro-neurophysiological evaluation, imaging examinations, and skin pathology. Biopsy of the affected nerve may be needed if skin smear and PCR are inconclusive.

1 Differential Diagnoses in Primary Neural Hansen's Disease and Peripheral Neuropathies

Primary neural Hansen's disease (PNHD) is characterised by the clinical and laboratory absence of skin involvement, at least at the outset, when abnormalities are restricted to the peripheral nervous system [3]. It is also referred to as the 'pure neuritic' or 'pure neural' form of Hansen's disease (see chapter "Neurological Manifestations of Hansen's Disease").

The prevalence of PNHD may be overestimated when identification of skin lesions in suspected cases is not correctly performed because of inadequate skin smears or poorly conducted skin biopsy [4, 5]. Conversely, patients presenting with nerve lesions of various aetiologies may be misdiagnosed as PNHD because of failure to perform a dermatological examination. In a Brazilian study using nerve biopsy on 162 patients with suspected PNHD, this diagnosis was confirmed in 34 cases (21%) [6].

Mononeuropathies and multiple mononeuropathies are the most plausible differential diagnoses for Hansen's disease neuropathy (HDN) (Table 1).

Table 1 Clinical conditions that mimic focal and multiple mononeuropathies

Peripheral and central neurological disorders					
Peripheral Neuropathies				Plexopathies	Genetically determined or developmental myelopathies
Focal mononeuropathies	Multiple mononeuropathies	Distal and symmetric polyneuropathies	Polyradiculoneuropathies		
THD	BTHD, BBHD, BVHD, AND VHD	VHD	BVHD, VHD	THD, BBHD	BTHD, BBHD
Ulnar Tunnel Syndrome, Carpal Tunnel Syndrome (CTS), Fibular Entrapment at Retro-fibular Tunnel (cross Leg Syndrome), Tibial at Posterior Tarsal Tunnel (TTS)	Vasculitic neuropathies	Nutritional deficiencies, vasculitic neuropathies	Lewis-Summer Syndrome or Multifocal Acquired Demyelinating Sensory and Motor Neuropathies (MADSAM)	Acute brachial plexus neuritis or neuralgic amyotrophy (Parsonage-Turner syndrome)	Syringomyelia
Paresthetica Meralgia, superficial radial Paresthetica Neuralgia (Cheiralgia Paresthetica)	Collagenosis neuropathies (systemic erythematous lupus, Sjögren syndrome)	Diabetes mellitus	Chronic Inflammatory Demyelinating Polyradiculoneuropathy (CIDP)—atypical presentation	Thoracic Outlet Syndrome (neurogenic TOS)	Hirayama disease (monomelic amyotrophy)
AIDS	AIDS, hepatitis B, and C, and HIV infection/AIDS	AIDS	AIDS		
Nerve tumour	Multifocal motor neuropathy with conduction block	Systemic erythematosus lupus			

Tardy ulnar nerve palsy	Hereditary Neuropathy with Pressure Palsy (HNPP)	Hereditary neuropathies: Familial Amyloid Polyneuropathy (FAP), Acute Intermittent Porphyria			
		Arsenic, lead, mercury, and thallium poisoning			
		ddC, ddI, d4T, isoniazid, dapsone, metronidazole, and chemotherapy drugs			

HD Hansen's disease, *THD* Tuberculoid form of HD, *BT* Borderline Tuberculoid form of HD, *BBHD* Borberline Borderline form of HD, *BVHD* Borderline Virchowian form of HD, *VHD* Virchowian form of HD

2 Mononeuropathies

The mononeuropathies with the greatest similarities to HDN, especially the paucibacillary forms, are ulnar tunnel syndrome, 'Saturday night' radial paralysis in the arm spiral groove and 'crossed leg' fibular syndrome in the retrofibular tunnel [7–9]. The latter two may be confused with the neural form of tuberculoid Hansen's disease, but their acute nature and spontaneous improvement help differentiate them from HDN. Nerve tumours present difficulties in differentiation them from nerve abscesses of the tuberculoid forms of Hansen's disease [10].

3 Multiple Mononeuropathies

Multiple mononeuropathies can occur as a result of vasculitis, arteritis, collagen diseases, systemic lupus erythematosus, and Sjögren's syndrome (sensory or sensory and axonal motor neuropathies), and infectious diseases such as hepatitis B and C (axonal) and HIV (axonal or myelinated) [11] (Table 1).

Multifocal motor neuropathy may be confused with HDN, but the fact that it preserves sensory fibres is a clear differentiator. Lewis-Sumner syndrome or MADSAM (multifocal acquired demyelinating sensory and motor neuropathy) is an inflammatory neuropathy with sensory involvement that can be more confusing. Polyradicular involvement, i.e. in nerves proximally, assists in differential diagnosis.

Hereditary neuropathy with susceptibility to pressure presents as asymmetrical neuropathy with focal accentuation at sites of compression, involving the same nerves as HDN; anamnesis may reveal its hereditary character. Evolution occurs in outbreaks at compression sites, predominantly myelinic, with total or partial improvement [12].

4 Plexopathies

4.1 Acute Brachial Plexus Neuritis, Brachial Neuralgic Amyotrophy, or Parsonage-Turner Syndrome

This is an inflammatory neuropathy of probable immune-mediated cause often preceded by viral upper airway infections. Pain is sudden onset, intense and acute, localised in the scapular girdle, generally unilateral, followed by weakness and/or muscular atrophy, with partial anaesthesia of the limb (Figs. 3 and 4). It has a myelinic and asymmetric character, like Hansen's disease, but involvement of the scapular waist is not frequent in Hansen's disease [13].

Fig. 3 Compressive syndrome of the posterior interosseous nerve in the left hand. The patient is unable to make the 'OK' sign

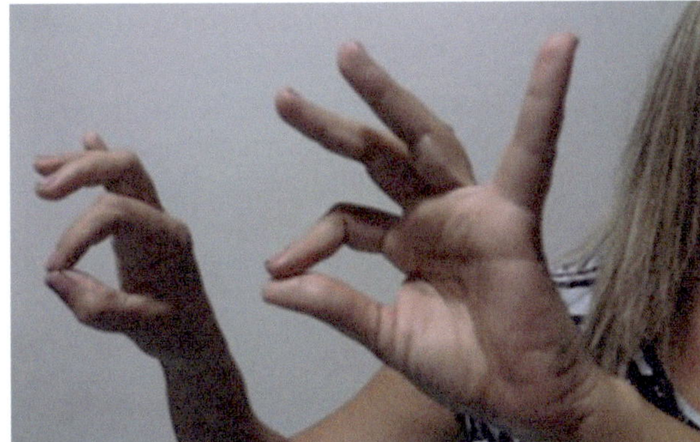

Fig. 4 Brachial Neuralgic Amyotrophy or Parsonage-Turner Syndrome. Posterolateral view: shows amyotrophy of the levator scapulae, supraspinatus, and infraspinatus muscles. The patient will have difficulty abducting the shoulder

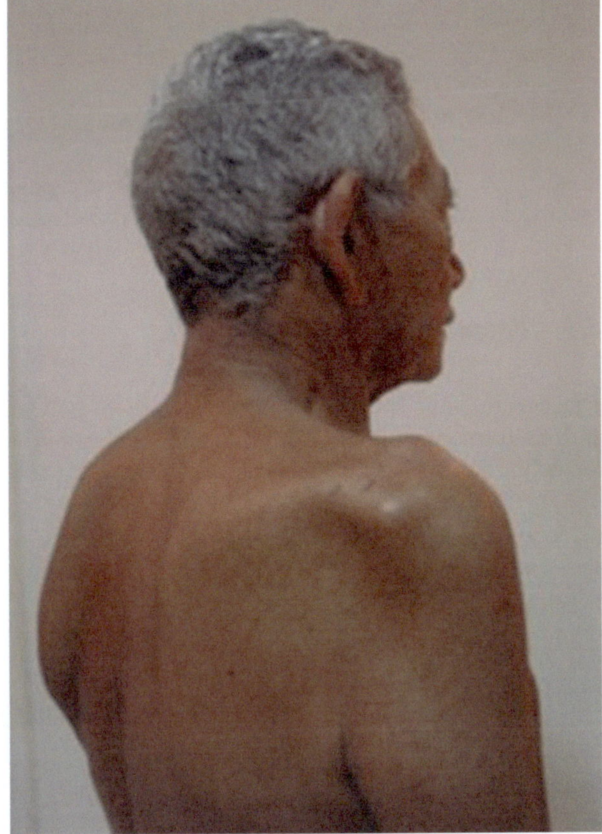

4.2   Neurogenic Thoracic Outlet Syndrome (NTOS)

NTOS mimics HDN because it affects the Lower Trunk of the Brachial Plexus, roots C8 andT1. Motor impairment predominating in the median nerve (C8, T1) and sensory impairment in the ulnar nerve (C8) is characteristic of NTS [14]. The vessels may suffer compression in the thoracic outlet which can be demonstrated by decreased radial pulse when performing the Adson's manoeuvre [5].

5   Polyneuropathies

Distal polyneuropathies resemble multibacillary forms of Hansen's disease with multiple confluent mononeuropathy [3]. They are defined by presenting diffuse peripheral nerve involvement and bilateral, symmetrical, and length-dependent distribution, that is, compromising nerve fibres more distally, lower limbs first, than proximally (Fig. 5).

The most relevant polyneuropathies in the differential diagnosis of HDN are related to diabetes mellitus, acquired immunodeficiency syndrome, systemic lupus erythematosus, familial amyloid polyneuropathy, poisoning by arsenic and other metals, genetic neuropathies, and neuropathy related to alcoholism [15, 16].

5.1   Polyneuropathy of Diabetes

Diabetes mellitus is the most common cause of polyneuropathy and can present in various forms including multiple mononeuropathy. In Hansen's disease endemic areas, these diseases coexist. Although it also affects the motor nerves, diabetic

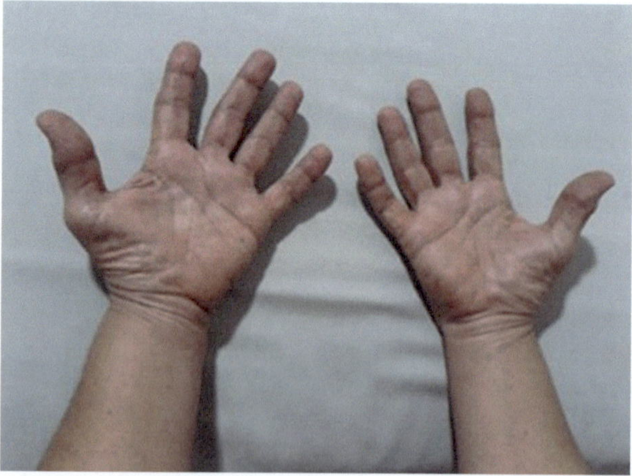

Fig. 5 Carpal tunnel syndrome. Atrophy in the thenar region

polyneuropathy is symmetric, length-dependent, and predominantly sensory. The patient complains of burning pain, paraesthesia, and hyperaesthesia, and allodynia is frequent in the lower extremities, making contact with bedsheets difficult at night. It may progress with decreased tactile, thermal, pain and vibratory sensibility, dysautonomia and complete abolition of deep reflexes. Clinically, diabetic polyneuropathy differs from HDN because it is length-dependent, i.e. it compromises long fibres more intensely, predominating in the lower limbs, and the motor deficit is symmetrical and diffuse, being initially sub-clinical [17–19].

5.2 Polyneuropathy of Systemic Lupus Erythematosus

This polyneuropathy appears as a sensory or motor disorder of the peripheral nerves, of variable duration, characterised by symmetric symptoms and distal distribution. In general, it is related to disease activity. It may affect 60% of patients with late-onset disease [20, 21].

5.3 Polyneuropathy of HIV/AIDS

The mechanisms of nerve damage include the direct action of the virus, immunological alterations, use of antiretroviral drugs, and opportunistic infections. HIV neuropathy presents in multiple forms including: demyelinating inflammatory polyneuropathy; symmetrical distal sensory-motor polyneuropathy; mononeuropathies and multiple mononeuropathies; progressive polyradiculopathies; ganglioneuropathies and autonomic neuropathies; drug toxicity neuropathies caused by ddC (zalcitabine), ddI (didanosine), d4T (stavudine), isoniazid, and metronidazole; ascending neuromuscular weakness associated with metabolic acidosis and secondary to side effects of antiretroviral drugs, especially d4T [22].

5.4 Inflammatory Demyelinating Polyradiculoneuropathies

Guillain-Barré syndrome (GBS) is an acute extensive demyelinating polyradiculoneuropathy, sensory and motor, symmetrical and extensive, with onset within 2 weeks, progressing from distal to proximal [23]. Although also a demyelinating disease, these clinical features easily differentiate GBS from Hansen's disease. However, chronic inflammatory demyelinating polyradiculoneuropathy (CIDP) may present in a typical or atypical form, with only half of patients expressing the typical phenotype exhibiting symmetrical sensory and motor symptoms over a period of 8 weeks or more. It may progress in alternating outbreaks with periods of stabilisation or remission. The atypical phenotype may present predominantly focal, sensory, motor, distal, or asymmetric symptoms. As a chronic demyelinating inflammatory neuropathy, this atypical form may be confused with Hansen's disease [24]. Cerebrospinal fluid (CSF) examination is mandatory for the diagnosis of these polyradiculoneuropathies [25].

6 Hereditary Neuropathies

6.1 Familial Amyloid Polyneuropathy (FAP) 1 and 3

These are autosomal dominant disorders which occur in the age group 30–40 years. The neuropathy progresses with sensorial and motor symptoms with predominant involvement of fine fibres, resulting initially in loss of pain sensitivity and dysautonomy and progressively affecting large fibres. Clinical features of FAP are: family history of neuropathy and/or cardiomyopathy, neuropathic pain, orthostatic hypotension, diarrhoea, constipation or alternating bowel rhythm, dysphagia, and severe weight loss [26].

Sequencing of the TTR (transthyretin) gene should be requested to determine the genetic form of FAP because the TTR V30M (Val30Met mutation) form progresses more slowly (10–15 years) than the non-V30M form [26].

6.2 Acute Intermittent Porphyria (AIP)

AIP is typically of autosomal dominant inheritance, with incomplete penetrance, but occasionally autosomal recessive. Rare before puberty, it results from failure of heme synthesis with accumulation of porphyrins and their precursors. The neuropathy is predominantly motor due to axonal degeneration. Of acute or subacute onset, with asthenia of the proximal muscles, more frequent in the arms than in the legs, it may be asymmetric and focal and can involve cranial and sensory nerves. Neuropathy will occur rarely without abdominal symptoms—colicky pain, nausea, vomiting, and constipation.

7 Genetically Determined or Developmental Myelopathies

7.1 Syringomyelia

In syringomyelia, there is formation of a cavity in the central canal of the medulla, with expansion of this canal, of the medullary substance and of the cerebral trunk resulting from alterations in CSF circulation. It may be caused by Chiari's malformation, tumoral growth in the marrow, infections, trauma, or have no identified cause (idiopathic) (Figs. 6, 7 and 8). It affects more the cervical and high thoracic spinal cord, generating asymmetric segmental weakness and atrophy of the hands and arms. There is a lesion of the fibres which form the lateral spinothalamic tracts. Thermal and pain sensitivity is lost, while tactile sensitivity is preserved ('hypoesthesia of suspended distribution'). As the involvement is preganglionic, sensory conduction is preserved despite the clinical sensory loss, which differentiates syringomyelia from HDN.

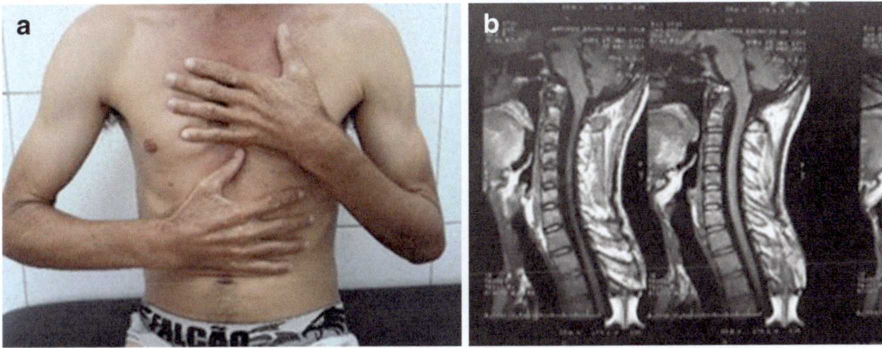

Fig. 6 Chiari's syndrome. (**a**) Amyotrophy of the first interosseous space. (**b**) Magnetic resonance imaging of the cervical spine showing invagination of the brainstem and cerebellum by the foramen magnum

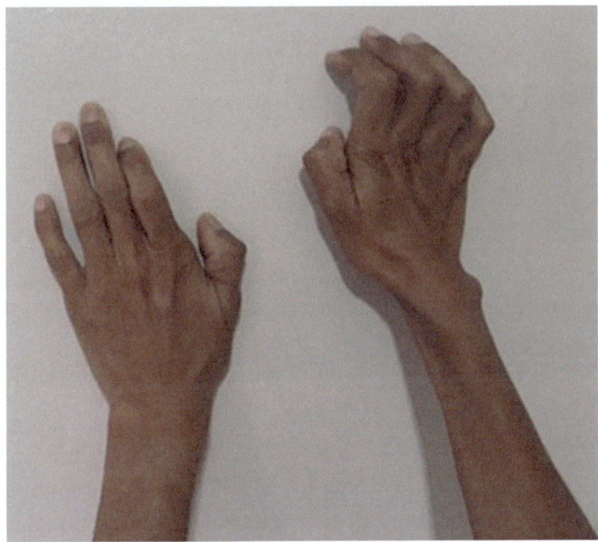

Fig. 7 Syringomyelia. Atrophy of the interosseous muscles of the hands. Right hand with radial-median-ulnar claw and in the left-hand radial claw

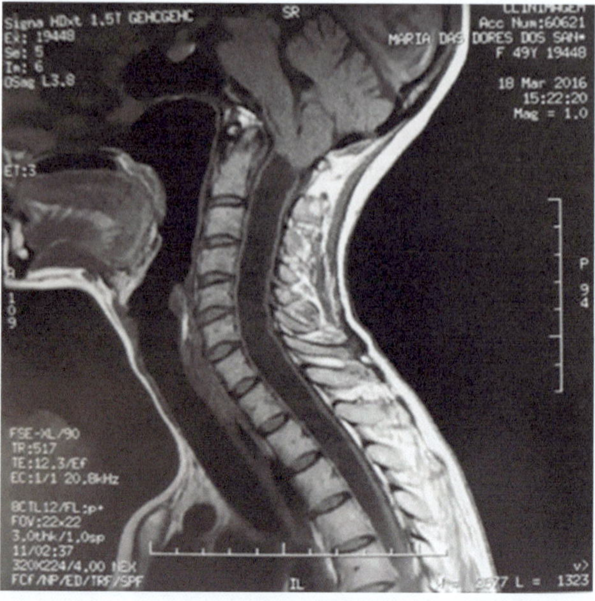

Fig. 8 Syringomyelia. MRI sagittal view—shows an enlargement of the spinal canal in the cervical and thoracic region

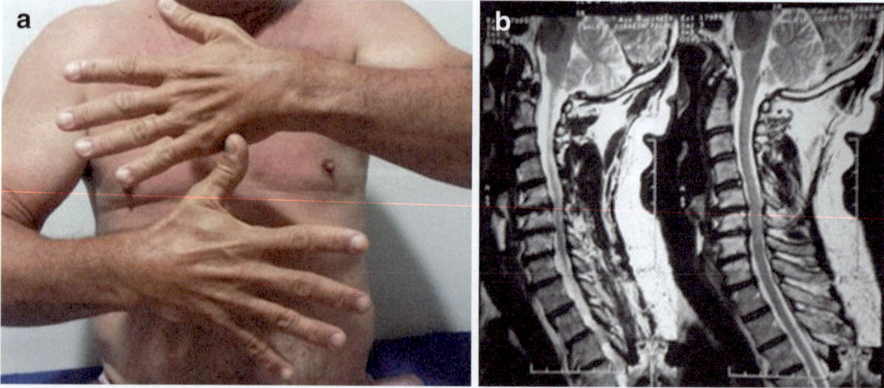

Fig. 9 (**a**) Cervical radiculopathy. Atrophy of the wrist and hand muscles. (**b**) MRI (sagittal view): cervicoarthrosis, the rectification of the spine, and narrow cervical spinal canal

7.2 *Myelopathy with Monomelic Amyotrophy or Hirayama Disease*

Hirayama disease is most prevalent in Asia, in young men. There are few reports from the Americas [27]. In this disease, there is hypodevelopment of the spinal dura mater, a posterior dural 'detachment' in the cervical and upper thoracic region during neck flexion movements. It leads to focal and asymmetric compression and ischaemia of the motor neurons in the anterior horn of the spinal cord, causing paralysis without loss of sensation (Figs. 9a, 10a and 10b). These clinical findings

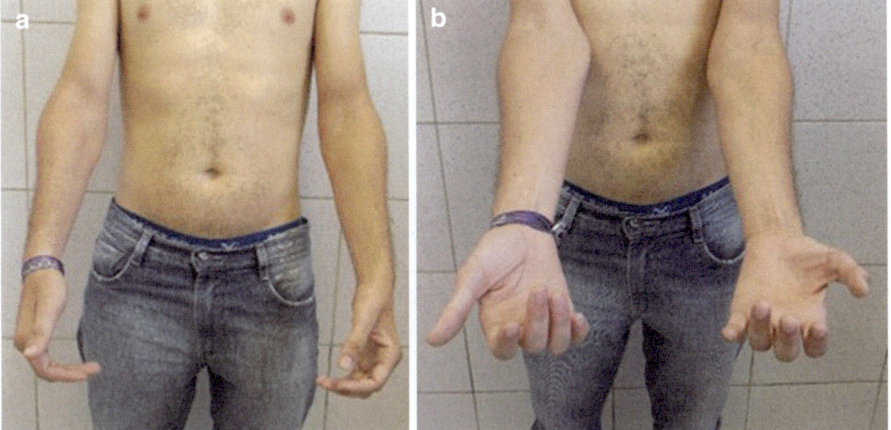

Fig. 10 Distal juvenile muscular atrophy of the upper limb or Hirayama's disease. (**a**) Atrophy of the forearm and hand and palmar interosseous muscles. (**a, b**) Hands showing atrophy of the left thenar and hypothenar regions with clawing of the 2nd to 5th fingers

differentiate this disease from HDN and syringomyelia, which always present sensory loss. MRI studies of the cervical spine in flexion may show the posterior venous plexus intensely engorged compared to the neutral position (Fig. 9b) [27].

8 Toxicity-Related Peripheral Neuropathies

8.1 Drugs

Chemotherapy-induced peripheral neuropathy presents as sensory-predominant and length-dependent polyneuropathy with a 'gloves and socks' distribution [28, 29]. The chemotherapeutic drugs most commonly implicated are oxaliplatin, cisplatin, paclitaxel, bortezomib, vincristine, combination of cisplatin and paclitaxel [30].

8.2 Heavy Metals

The increase in environmental contamination by heavy metals means that reports of their toxic effects on human health, including peripheral neuropathies are becoming more common. The metals most frequently reported as causing peripheral neuropathies are as follows:

(a) Inorganic mercury can cause peripheral nervous system disorders, as long as 30 years after exposure [31]. Ingestion of organic mercury in contaminated

foodstuffs such as fish affects the dorsal root and trigeminal ganglion, causing proximal sensory polyneuropathy and ganglionopathy [32].
(b) Lead poisoning causes asymmetric sensory and motor neuropathies similar to the neuropathy of Hansen's disease, including paralysis of the extensors of the hands and fingers and dorsiflexors of the dropped foot [33–35].
(c) Inorganic arsenic poisoning manifests as sensory neuropathy with neuropathic pain and symmetrical distal polyneuropathy, progressing to severe polyradiculoneuropathy similar to Guillain-Barré Syndrome [36].
(d) Use of thallium as a component of pesticides and rodenticides has been banned in several countries. Thallium poisoning is characterised by alopecia (1–2 weeks' onset) and peripheral neuropathy similar to inorganic arsenic poisoning [33, 37] (Figs. 7, 8, and 10).

References

1. Pfaltzgraff RE, Ramu G. Clinical leprosy. In: Hastings RC, editor. Leprosy. 2nd ed. Edinburgh: NY: Churchill Livingstone; 1994.
2. Pereira Leite Neto M, Bezerra da Cunha FM, e Silva CGL, et al. Clinical neurological profile of patients with leprosy in Fortaleza, Ceará, Brazil. Int Arch Med. 2015;8. https://doi.org/10.3823/1817.
3. Garbino JA, Marques W Jr, Barreto JA, et al. Primary neural leprosy: systematic review. Arq Neuropsiquiatr. 2013;71:397–404. https://doi.org/10.1590/0004-282X20130046.
4. Singh G, Dash K, Grover S, Sangolli P. Skin patches heralding relapse in a treated case of neuritic leprosy. Lepr Rev. 1998;69:400–1.
5. Garbino JA, Cury Filho M. Uma suspeita de mononeuropatia do nervo ulnar e o diagnóstico diferencial com síndrome do desfiladeiro torácico. Hansen Int. 2010;35:67–8.
6. Garbino JA. O paciente com suspeita de hanseníase primariamente neural. Hansen Int. 2007;32:203–6.
7. de Freitas MRG, Nascimento OJM, de Freitas MR, Hahn MD. Isolated superficial peroneal nerve lesion in pure neural leprosy: case report. Arq Neuropsiquiatr. 2004;62:535–9. https://doi.org/10.1590/s0004-282x2004000300030.
8. Garbino JA, Ura S, de Faria Fernandes Belone A, et al. Clinical and diagnostic aspects of the primarily neural leprosy. Hansen Int. 2004;29:130–6.
9. Theuvenet WJ, Finlay K, Roche P, et al. Neuritis of the lateral femoral cutaneous nerve in leprosy. Int J Lepr Other Mycobact Dis. 1993;61:592–6.
10. de Almeida JEM, Kirchner DR, Cury Filho M, et al. Peripheral nerve tumor, a differential diagnosis with primary neural leprosy: five case reports. Hansen Int. 2021;43:2367.
11. Höke A, Cornblath DR. Peripheral neuropathies in human immunodeficiency virus infection. Suppl Clin Neurophysiol. 2004;57:195–210. https://doi.org/10.1016/s1567-424x(09)70358-7.
12. Marques MAM, Antônio VL, Sarno EN, et al. Binding of α2-laminins by pathogenic and non-pathogenic mycobacteria and adherence to Schwann cells. J Med Microbiol. 2001;50:23–8. https://doi.org/10.1099/0022-1317-50-1-23.
13. Rachid A, Bem RS, Lacerda DC, Seitenfus JL. Parsonage-turner syndrome in HIV seropositive patient. Rev Bras Reumatol. 2005;45:39–42. https://doi.org/10.1590/S0482-50042005000100008.

14. Colli BO, Carlotti CG, Assirati JA, Marques W. Neurogenic thoracic outlet syndromes: a comparison of true and nonspecific syndromes after surgical treatment. Surg Neurol. 2006;65:262–71. Discussion 271-272. https://doi.org/10.1016/j.surneu.2005.06.037.

15. Chopra K, Tiwari V. Alcoholic neuropathy: possible mechanisms and future treatment possibilities: clinical management of alcoholic neuropathy. Br J Clin Pharmacol. 2012;73:348–62. https://doi.org/10.1111/j.1365-2125.2011.04111.x.

16. Rosewell A, Clark G, Mabong P, et al. Concurrent outbreaks of cholera and peripheral neuropathy associated with high mortality among persons internally displaced by a volcanic eruption. PLoS One. 2013;8:e72566. https://doi.org/10.1371/journal.pone.0072566.

17. Moreira RO, Castro AP, Papelbaum M, et al. Tradução para o português e avaliação da confiabilidade de uma escala para diagnóstico da polineuropatia distal diabética. Arq Bras Endocrinol Metabol. 2005;49:944–50. https://doi.org/10.1590/S0004-27302005000600014.

18. Martin CL, Albers J, Herman WH, et al. Neuropathy among the diabetes control and complications trial cohort 8 years after trial completion. Diabetes Care. 2006;29:340–4. https://doi.org/10.2337/diacare.29.02.06.dc05-1549.

19. Zaupa C, Zanoni JN. Diabetes Mellitus–Aspectos Gerais e Neuropatia Diabética. Arq Ciênc Saúde UNIPAR. 2000;4:19–25. https://doi.org/10.25110/arqsaude.v4i1.2000.1005.

20. Almeida RT, de Arruda Campos LM, Aikawa NE, et al. Polineuropatia periférica em pacientes com lúpus eritematoso sistêmico juvenil. Rev Bras Reumatol. 2009;49:362–74. https://doi.org/10.1590/S0482-50042009000400004.

21. Staub HL. Vasculites imunológicas—diagnóstico e diagnóstico diferencial. Temas Reumatol Clínica. 2008;9:72–6.

22. Chad DA, Hedley-Whyte ET. Case records of the Massachusetts General Hospital. Weekly clinicopathological exercises. Case 1-2004. A 49-year-old woman with asymmetric painful neuropathy. N Engl J Med. 2004;350:166–76. https://doi.org/10.1056/NEJMcpc030034.

23. Dyck PJ, Thomas PK. Peripheral neuropathy. 4th ed. Philadelphia: Saunders; 2005.

24. Robles MAM, Baldisserotto CM, Garbino JA. Neuropatia da hanseníase versus CIDP: Caso clínico de paciente com hanseníase do Instituto Lauro de Souza Lima. Hansen Int. 2011;36:64–5.

25. Hahn AF, Hartung HP, Dyck PJ. Chronic inflammatory demyelinating polyradiculoneuropathy. In: Dyck PJ, Thomas PK, editors. Peripheral neuropathy. 4th ed. Amsterdam: Elsevier; 2005. p. 2992.

26. Pinto MV, Dyck PJB, Liewluck T. Neuromuscular amyloidosis: unmasking the master of disguise. Muscle Nerve. 2021;64:23. https://doi.org/10.1002/mus.27150.

27. Bogoni M, de Almeida Teixeira BC, Cioni M. Rare occurrence of Hirayama disease in Brazil. Arq Neuropsiquiatr. 2019;77:370–1. https://doi.org/10.1590/0004-282X20190036.

28. Grisold W, Cavaletti G, Windebank AJ. Peripheral neuropathies from chemotherapeutics and targeted agents: diagnosis, treatment, and prevention. Neuro-Oncology. 2012;14 Suppl 4:iv45–54. https://doi.org/10.1093/neuonc/nos203.

29. Kandula T, Farrar MA, Cohn RJ, et al. Chemotherapy-induced peripheral neuropathy in long-term survivors of childhood cancer: clinical, neurophysiological, functional, and patient-reported outcomes. JAMA Neurol. 2018;75:980–8. https://doi.org/10.1001/jamaneurol.2018.0963.

30. Colvin LA. Chemotherapy-induced peripheral neuropathy: where are we now? Pain. 2019;160:S1–S10. https://doi.org/10.1097/j.pain.0000000000001540.

31. Letz R, Gerr F, Cragle D, et al. Residual neurologic deficits 30 years after occupational exposure to elemental mercury. Neurotoxicology. 2000;21:459–74.

32. Jackson AC. Chronic neurological disease due to methylmercury poisoning. Can J Neurol Sci. 2018;45:620–3. https://doi.org/10.1017/cjn.2018.323.

33. Jang DH, Hoffman RS. Heavy metal chelation in neurotoxic exposures. Neurol Clin. 2011;29:607–22. https://doi.org/10.1016/j.ncl.2011.05.002.

34. Staff NP, Windebank AJ. Peripheral neuropathy due to vitamin deficiency, toxins, and medications. Continuum (Minneap Minn). 2014;20:1293–306. https://doi.org/10.1212/01. CON.0000455880.06675.5a.
35. Windebank AJ. Metal neuropathy. In: Dyck PJ, Thomas PK, editors. Peripheral neuropathy. 4th ed. Philadelphia: Saunders; 2005.
36. Ratnaike RN. Acute and chronic arsenic toxicity. Postgrad Med J. 2003;79:391–6. https://doi. org/10.1136/pmj.79.933.391.
37. Zhao G, Ding M, Zhang B, et al. Clinical manifestations and management of acute thallium poisoning. Eur Neurol. 2008;60:292–7. https://doi.org/10.1159/000157883.

Immune and Chemoprophylaxis in Hansen's Disease

Marcos Cesar Florian

The prevalence of Hansen's disease in the world has decreased over the past decades after the introduction of multidrug therapy (MDT) in the 1980s, but the detection of new cases remains high with a slight decline of about 2% per year [1]. There are numerous cases that are still undiagnosed, therefore unrecorded, leading to an underestimation of the occurrence of the disease in some countries [2]. Because it is a chronic disease with great clinical variability and with possible neurological involvement as the initial signs and symptoms, there is the possibility of many late diagnoses, contributing to the occurrence of physical disabilities and to the maintenance of transmission in endemic countries and regions [3]. The understanding and comprehension about Hansen's disease, its signs and symptoms, as well as the general perception of Hansen's disease among the population are still low in many endemic areas [4]. All these factors also contribute to the difficulty in controlling the disease.

Some strategies to combat Hansen's disease have been developed over the years:

- Early diagnosis through spontaneous demand, active demand through campaigns, active search for new cases and training of health teams.
- Therapeutic with multidrug therapy (MDT) recommended by the World Health Organization (WHO).
- Close examination of household and social contacts of people affected by Hansen's disease.

Thus, in addition to these control proposals, which seem insufficient to reduce the number of cases more decisively, other strategies need to be sought [5]. Immunoprophylaxis and/or chemoprophylaxis, including the use of "post-exposure prophylaxis" (PEP), are included in these proposals. PEP can be

M. C. Florian (✉)
Department of Dermatology, Federal University of São Paulo, São Paulo, Brazil
e-mail: mcflorian@unifesp.br

P. D. Deps (ed.), *Hansen's Disease*, https://doi.org/10.1007/978-3-031-30893-2_22

administered among contacts of Hansen's disease patients, which include household contact, neighbor contact, and social contact [1]. PEP is a term used for chemoprophylaxis and/or immunoprophylaxis and has been studied in randomized clinical trials and observational studies since the 1960s in some endemic areas of the world [6]. The first clinical trials used dapsone and acedapsone. However, with the advent of dapsone resistance, its use in population-based chemoprophylaxis intervention studies has been discontinued. Rifampin, mainly as a single dose, [6, 7] but also in combination with other drugs, has been evaluated as a chemoprophylaxis option.

1 Immunoprophylaxis

Immunoprophylaxis is a mode of prevention in which the host uses its immune system to fight an infectious process. It can be passive, such as the administration of antiviral serum and breastfeeding, or active, such as vaccines.

The BCG (bacillus Calmette-Guérin) vaccine, which is produced with attenuated *Mycobacterium bovis*, was developed for the prevention of tuberculosis, especially its severe forms, and is part of the immunization scheme for children. It is routinely given to newborns in many parts of the world. In Brazil, in addition to being applied right at birth, it is also applied again to the examined contacts. When it comes to Hansen's disease immunoprophylaxis, the BCG vaccine is the most relevant since it confers a partial boost of immune response to *Mycobacterium leprae*. BCG vaccination in childhood reduces by about 50% the chance of contracting *M. leprae* in a high-risk population, such as contacts of patients newly diagnosed with Hansen's disease [8]. Its effectiveness against Hansen's disease seems to be significantly higher among contacts than in the general population: 68% versus 53% [9].

2 Chemoprophylaxis

Chemoprophylaxis is based on the administration of one or more drugs to stop *Mycobacterium leprae* infection in people who have had contact with Hansen's disease—affected individuals who are transmitters, or to reduce the chance that someone who has already been infected will develop Hansen's disease. Therefore, chemoprophylaxis is primarily aimed at reducing the transmission of the bacillus, especially among contacts.

Contacts living in the same household as people with Hansen's disease are about ten times more likely to be detected as having undiagnosed Hansen's disease than the general population, regardless of age, disease classification, and genetic distance [9, 10]. Thus, contacts should be one of the main focuses for applying plans for monitoring and controlling the disease.

In the 1960s and 1970s, clinical trials using dapsone and acedapsone as chemo-prophylactics were conducted in children's schools in Uganda and in endemic villages in India. An overall reduction of Hansen's disease of 40% among contacts where dapsone was administered and 51% among contacts where acedapsone was administered has been demonstrated [4].

The disadvantages of dapsone as a chemoprophylactic agent are the development of resistance to this drug and lack of patient compliance due to the need for long-term administration. New drugs were considered, including rifampin.

Rifampin, a bactericidal drug against *M. leprae* and one of drugs of the multidrug therapy, has been used in chemoprophylaxis studies, either as the sole drug (COLEP study, Project PEP-Hans) or together with other drugs (ROM: rifampin, ofloxacin, minocyclin. PEP++: rifampin and clarithromycin in three doses) [4, 11] or with immunoprophylaxis.

- Some points in favor of using single-dose rifampicin post-exposure prophylaxis (PEP-SDR):

  - A beneficial and effective effect in reducing *M. leprae* infection in the first 2 years after administration of PEP with a single dose of rifampicin in contacts of persons with Hansen's disease [10].
  - Allow greater adherence to treatment since it is very common for people with Hansen's disease to live long distances from the places where medication and treatment are distributed. This situation often makes it unfeasible to receive the treatment because the worker has difficulty in attending the health service due to his or her work routine [10].
  - Low cost.
  - The possibility of being implemented in Family Health Strategies allowing easy access to the person with Hansen's disease, as well as their contacts for the administration of PEP, facilitating the work of health professionals in the treatment and epidemiological control of Hansen's disease [10];
  - No need of a second dose of medication [10].
  - Low risk of side effects and resistance to rifampicin used as a single dose PEP [10, 12].
  - The possibility of a reduction in the number of new cases in the first 2 years after chemoprophylaxis [10].

- Some unfavorable points for the use of post-exposure prophylaxis of one dose of rifampicin (PEP-SDR):

  - The goal of contacts who need to receive PEP to achieve a significant reduction in the incidence of Hansen's disease must be achieved with difficulty since there are many cases still undiagnosed, therefore with their contacts also undetected [10, 13].
  - The risk of resistance to rifampicin used as a single-dose PEP is considered low, but it is not zero.
  - Lack of information or inadequate information can lead to rejection of rifampicin use as PEP by contacts.

- The risk of developing Hansen's disease, even in people who are carriers of the bacillus, tends to decrease naturally in all contacts, even those who have not received PEP [10].
- The different results in the studies depend on the type of study and the observation time [14].

There are clinical trials looking at the efficacy of combining BCG with rifampicin, including using the combination of BCG vaccine with heat-inactivated *M. leprae* [6]. Chemoprophylaxis with rifampicin had an overall protective effect of approximately 60% and, when combined with prior immunization with BCG vaccine, could reach 80%, and this effect was demonstrated within 2 years of the intervention [15]. It is unclear whether this combination of BCG immunoprophylaxis with single-dose rifampin chemoprophylaxis would have a lasting additional protective effect in preventing Hansen's disease [15, 16].

The different chemoprophylaxis and/or immunoprophylaxis schemes target especially the contacts [5].

The contact settings are:

- Household contact: contact living in the same dwelling or sharing the same kitchen with an index case. This includes family members but also domestic staff or aids or co-workers or others sharing the same accommodation. A family member living elsewhere should not be considered as a household contact.
- Neighbor contact: a person living in the neighborhood of an index case, typically defined as an adjacent household or living within 100 m [17]. Because of geographic proximity, these persons have a higher probability of being exposed and/or infected.
- Social contact: other persons having prolonged contact with an index case and who are not classified as household or neighbor contact. These may include friends, persons sharing workplace (e.g., factory workers, office colleagues) or school (students and teachers) or leisure venue (e.g., sports club) [1].

The World Health Organization (WHO) puts as one of the current strategic pillars "tracing household contacts along with 25–50 neighbors and social contacts of each patient, accompanied by the offer of a single dose of rifampicin as preventive chemotherapy." [18–21].

With the current information, endemic countries should evaluate whether to adopt chemoprophylaxis (and what regimen) in their national programs based on the pros and cons of this intervention modality [22, 23]. In countries where PEP-SDR is adopted, it will be reviewed in terms of coverage of contacts provided with SDR and number of new cases detected during chemoprophylaxis activities [20, 24].

References

1. WHO. Leprosy/Hansen disease: contact tracing and post-exposure prophylaxis: technical guidance. New Delhi: World Health Organization, Regional Office for South-East Asia; 2020. https://www.who.int/publications/i/item/9789290228073

2. Burki TK. Leprosy and the rhetoric of elimination. BMJ. 2013;347:f6142.
3. Barth-Jaeggi T, Steinmann P, Mieras L, van Brakel W, Richardus JH, Tiwari A, Bratschi M, Cavaliero A, Vander Plaetse B, Mirza F, Aerts A, LPEP study group. Leprosy post-exposure prophylaxis (LPEP) programme: study protocol for evaluating the feasibility and impact on case detection rates of contact tracing and single dose rifampicin. BMJ Open. 2016;6:e013633.
4. Van't Noordende AT, Lisam S, Ruthindartri P, Sadiq A, Singh V, Arifin M, van Brakel WH, Korfage IJ. The role of perceptions and knowledge of leprosy in the elimination of leprosy: a baseline study in Fatehpur district, northern India. PLoS Negl Trop Dis. 2019;13:e0007302.
5. Taal AT, Blok DJ, van Brakel WH, de Vlas SJ, Richardus JH. Number of people requiring post-exposure prophylaxis to end leprosy: a modeling study. PLoS Negl Trop Dis. 2021;15:e0009146.
6. Richardus JH, Oskam L. Protecting people against leprosy: chemoprophylaxis and immunoprophylaxis. Clin Dermatol. 2015;33:19–25.
7. Smith CM, Smith WC. Chemoprophylaxis is effective in the prevention of leprosy in endemic countries: a systematic review and meta-analysis. MILEP2 study group. Mucosal Immunology of Leprosy. J Infect. 2000;41:137–42.
8. Schuring RP, Richardus JH, Pahan D, Oskam L. Protective effect of the combination BCG vaccination and rifampicin prophylaxis in leprosy prevention. Vaccine. 2009;27:7125–8.
9. Moet FJ, Pahan D, Oskam L, Richardus JH. Effectiveness of single dose rifampicin in preventing leprosy in close contacts of patients with newly diagnosed leprosy: cluster randomised controlled trial. BMJ. 2008;336:761–4.
10. Cunha SS, Bierrenbach AL, Barreto VH. Chemoprophylaxis to control leprosy and the perspective of its implementation in Brazil: a primer for non-epidemiologists. Rev Inst Med Trop São Paulo. 2015;57:481–7.
11. NHR Brasil (2022) Programa PEP++. NHR Brasil. https://www.nhrbrasil.org.br/publicacoes.htlm. Accessed 28 Apr 2022 [in Portuguese].
12. Mieras L, Anthony R, van Brakel W, Bratschi MW, van den Broek J, Cambau E, Cavaliero A, Kasang C, Perera G, Reichman L, Richardus JH, Saunderson P, Steinmann P, Yew WW. Negligible risk of inducing resistance in mycobacterium tuberculosis with single-dose rifampicin as post-exposure prophylaxis for leprosy. Infect Dis Poverty. 2016;5:46.
13. Ortuno-Gutierrez N, Baco A, Braet S, Younoussa A, Mzembaba A, Salim Z, Amidy M, Grillone S, de Jong BC, Richardus JH, Hasker E. Clustering of leprosy beyond the household level in a highly endemic setting on the Comoros, an observational study. BMC Infect Dis. 2019;19:501.
14. Dos Santos DS, Duppre NC, Sarno EN, Pinheiro RO, Sales AM, Nery JADC, Moraes MO, Camacho LAB. Chemoprophylaxis of leprosy with rifampicin in contacts of multibacillary patients: study protocol for a randomized controlled trial. Trials. 2018;19:244.
15. Richardus RA, Alam K, Pahan D, Feenstra SG, Geluk A, Richardus JH. The combined effect of chemoprophylaxis with single dose rifampicin and immunoprophylaxis with BCG to prevent leprosy in contacts of newly diagnosed leprosy cases: a cluster randomized controlled trial (MALTALEP study). BMC Infect Dis. 2013;13:456.
16. Moet FJ, Pahan D, Schuring RP, Oskam L, Richardus JH. Physical distance, genetic relationship, age, and leprosy classification are independent risk factors for leprosy in contacts of patients with leprosy. J Infect Dis. 2006;193:346–53.
17. Bakker MI, Hatta M, Kwenang A, Van Benthem BH, Van Beers SM, Klatser PR, Oskam L. Prevention of leprosy using rifampicin as chemoprophylaxis. Am J Trop Med Hyg. 2005;72:443–8.
18. WHO. Guidelines for the diagnosis, treatment and prevention of leprosy. 2017.
19. WHO. Towards zero leprosy. Global leprosy (Hansen's disease) strategy 2021–2030. New Delhi: World Health Organization, Regional Office for South-East Asia; 2017.
20. WHO. Task force on definitions, criteria and indicators for interruption of transmission and elimination of leprosy. New Delhi: World Health Organization, Regional Office for South-East Asia; 2021.
21. Schoenmakers A, Mieras L, Budiawan T, van Brakel WH. The state of affairs in post-exposure leprosy prevention: a descriptive meta-analysis on immuno- and chemo-prophylaxis. Res Rep Trop Med. 2020;11:97–117.

22. Lockwood DN, De Barros B, Walker SL. Single-dose rifampicin and BCG to prevent leprosy. Int J Infect Dis. 2020;92:269–70.
23. Richardus JH, Tiwari A, Barth-Jaeggi T, Arif MA, Banstola NL, Baskota R, Blaney D, Blok DJ, Bonenberger M, Budiawan T, Cavaliero A, Gani Z, Greter H, Ignotti E, Kamara DV, Kasang C, Manglani PR, Mieras L, Njako BF, Pakasi T, Pandey BD, Saunderson P, Singh R, Smith WCS, Stäheli R, Suriyarachchi ND, Tin Maung A, Shwe T, van Berkel J, van Brakel WH, Vander Plaetse B, Virmond M, Wijesinghe MSD, Aerts A, Steinmann P. Leprosy post-exposure prophylaxis with single-dose rifampicin (LPEP): an international feasibility programme. Lancet Glob Health. 2021;9:e81–90.
24. Palit A, Kar HK. Prevention of transmission of leprosy: The current scenario. Indian J Dermatol Venereol Leprol. 2020;86:115–23.

Psychosocial Aspects of Hansen's Disease

Anna T. van 't Noordende, Suresh Dhondge, and Wim H. van Brakel

1 Hansen's Disease and Stigma

Persons affected by Hansen's disease often have to deal both with physical effects, such as damage to the skin, nerves, and eyes, and psychosocial aspects of the disease. An important factor, if not the most important, in producing and sustaining a negative psychosocial effect on persons affected is stigma. Stigma against Hansen's disease dates back to many centuries ago [1]. Stigma refers to "a social process, experienced or anticipated, characterised by exclusion, rejection, blame or devaluation that results from experience, perception or reasonable anticipation of an adverse social judgment about a person or group" [2].

Persons affected by Hansen's disease may be stigmatised because of the visible impairments associated with their condition, fear of transmission, a lack of knowledge about Hansen's disease and cultural and religious perceptions about the disease, for example, about the cause or mode of transmission [3–5]. Inequalities between people in age, gender, and socioeconomic status can also contribute to and increase experiences of stigma [6]. For example, women have been found to experience more Hansen's disease-related stigma than men [7]. Stigma can occur in the family, community, and at the health centre and people can also internalise stigma [8].

A. T. van 't Noordende (✉) · W. H. van Brakel
NLR, Amsterdam, The Netherlands

Department of Public Health, Erasmus MC, University Medical Center Rotterdam, Rotterdam, The Netherlands
e-mail: w.vanbrakel@nlrinternational.org

S. Dhondge
The Leprosy Mission Trust India, New Delhi, India
e-mail: Suresh.dhondge@leprosymission.in

Both impairments caused by Hansen's disease and stigma can affect mobility and lead to participation restrictions, such as restrictions in work, education, and participation in community life, and problems in interpersonal interactions and relationships, including marriage [9]. Stigma can also undermine the availability of social support and psychological resources and may prevent people from seeking help [8, 10]. Impairments and stigma may also negatively affect mental wellbeing and quality of life [11]. Hansen's disease has been associated with depressive and anxiety disorders, suicide (attempts), and negative feelings such as fear, sadness, shame, and low self-esteem [11]. Family members of persons affected, and health workers sometimes experience stigma by association [11].

2 Hansen's Disease Often Has a Psychosocial Impact

Being diagnosed with a major disease is often a turning point in an individual's life [12]. People may experience anger, vulnerability, sadness, shame, loss of control, fear about the prognosis of the disease and of discrimination, and concerns about the future. For some people, it may be a relief to find out their disease status because it provides clarity. Before and after diagnosis, people may seek to conceal their condition because of fear of what other people may think or do. Especially when Hansen's disease is visible, this may be difficult [9]. While concealment may avoid negative attitudes from others, it may also lead to feelings of stress, anxiety, and depression [13, 14]. Some people may decide to disclose their condition. This makes them vulnerable to social stigma and mental distress but may also lead to care and social support [13, 15].

Following diagnosis, persons affected by Hansen's disease go through a process of psychosocial adaptation and adjustment to their new situation. There is great variation in how people adjust to their disease. This depends on personal and environmental factors, but also on the manifestation and severity of the disease [16, 17]. Hansen's disease is curable, but medication has to be taken daily for 6–12 months, depending on the classification of the disease [18]. This requires adjustment to people's daily routine. Side effects of treatment are common and may include red urine, darkening and dryness of the skin, itchiness, and feeling weak [19]. These side effects may be a reason for people to stop taking their treatment [19]. In addition, changes in appearance, because of side effects or because of Hansen's disease-related impairments, may cause a loss of self-esteem and fear of disclosure [20].

Hansen's disease-related impairments may hamper people's daily functioning, such as their ability to perform certain tasks, and their social participation. When people are for example no longer able to work and contribute to the family, this may threaten their (social) identity, and may negatively impact their wellbeing and self-esteem [21]. In addition, physical impairments may require people to change their behaviour and lifestyle to prevent impairments from progressing [22, 23]. People may need to use protective footwear and gloves, be careful when using a hot stove and regularly practise self-care. Self-management routines sometimes need to be practised life-long [23]. The need to keep up with self-management may cause stress, and it can be difficult to accept that some impairments may never go away. It can be difficult to explain to persons affected, their family members and community that the person is cured of Hansen's disease, yet still continuous to have visible signs and disabilities. Even after treatment, people may fear the recurrence of their disease.

Both persons affected by Hansen's disease and their family members are confronted with (negative) perceptions of others [8]. Hansen's disease can also have psychosocial effects on family members. Family members may experience mental distress, discrimination, and restrictions in social participation, and they may lose family income. In addition, providing care can affect the psychosocial health of family members [24].

3   Adapting to a Life with Hansen's Disease

For most people, medical treatment for Hansen's disease is available, but access to mental health care is often either very difficult or not considered a need for persons affected. There is a lack of mental health care for those who are living in the general community. Grassroot health workers are providing medical care, but there is no attention for mental health care. Even health workers who are trained in mental health care do not have enough time to implement it in a systematic manner. Grassroot health workers are overburdened, as they are taking care of all diseases of community members, so the mental wellbeing of persons affected by Hansen's disease is not given any priority.

Due to lack of awareness and social stigma many persons affected by Hansen's disease delay going for treatment, which may result in permanent, visible impairments. These visible impairments can cause stigma and discrimination, loss of self-esteem and hope. Many try to hide their disease or isolate themselves. Quite a few develop depression and even suicidal tendencies [25, 26]. The disease may also cause them to lose their faith and reduce spiritual activities, while others find comfort and hope in their faith and spiritual practices like prayer [8]. Professional and social support from health workers, family members, friends, and colleagues plays a vital role in the mental wellbeing of persons affected by Hansen's disease. Experiences of from many persons affected show that those who received such support were able to overcome the disease, as well as stigma and discrimination, and become role models for others or even champions for the cause [27]. Family support is crucial for learning to live with the consequences of Hansen's disease and family counselling has been found to be helpful in improving acceptance of the person with the disease. This in turn will also help to reduce the stigma in the community (personal communication, Suresh Dhondge).

> **Box 1: Personal Story of the Second Author, Who Has Had Hansen's Disease Himself**
>
> "When I was diagnosed with Hansen's disease it was very shocking for me. Due to side effects of the leprosy medicines I had to drop out of college. After that I started working on a farm. Working on the farm was comfortable for me, as there was nobody to ask me anything about my disease or about visible signs of the disease and its treatment. I was spending more time on the farm and returned home after sunset so nobody would notice my disease. I even chose routes that were less crowded. When I was admitted in the leprosy hospital at Pune, I became habituated to watch television and Bollywood movies, to reduce my stress. My faith in God was gone. However, I used to read books which helped me to restart my education and completed a bachelor of law and three master degrees (arts, business administration, and social work). I felt so confident after that. With time I regained my faith. I found employment with a leprosy organisation (the Leprosy Mission Trust India), first as a student and later as a Programme Officer. This was also when I met my wife, Mangala, who also has had Hansen's disease. I work at TLMTI for over 20 years now, am often invited as a speaker at religious events, and have three healthy daughters!"

4 Interventions to Address Psychosocial Issues

A special focus is needed on mental wellbeing of persons affected by Hansen's disease, given the profound impact the disease can have on mental wellbeing. General mental health services often have very limited coverage in countries and areas where Hansen's disease is endemic. Usually only few mental health professionals are available, such as psychiatrists and psychologists and they tend to practise in urban areas. Specialist Hansen's disease centres often have a counsellor or psychologist on the staff, but while their work is very important, their remit is often limited to working with hospital in- and outpatients [28, 29]. Mental health programmes therefore focus on task shifting regarding diagnosis and management of mental health conditions to other cadres of health workers, such as nurses in peripheral health centres, and even peers and community groups and volunteers. Lusli and colleagues showed that peer counselling was effective in reducing the psychosocial impact of Hansen's disease in a trial in Indonesia [30]. They developed the so-called Rights-based counselling module that included factual information about the condition, training on how to use human rights and coping skills. Peer counsellors conducted on average five weekly sessions, comprising individual, family, and group sessions. This work has now been used to develop an NTD-adapted version of the Psychological First Aid tool developed by WHO, called the Basic

Psychological Support for persons affected by NTDs (BPS-N) (publication to be submitted). The BPS-N approach is intended for use by peer supporters with personal experience of either Hansen's disease or other NTDs, such as lymphatic filariasis.

Somar and colleagues conducted a systematic review on the impact of Hansen's disease on the mental wellbeing of affected persons and their family members, including interventions to address this. Very few intervention studies were found [11]. Several interventions were shown to be effective in reducing depression and/or anxiety among persons affected. In one study in Brazil, therapeutic workshops were conducted during which affected persons were able to share experiences, socialise, and collectively work on problems encountered. Several studies used forms of cognitive behavioural therapy (CBT) and showed that this was able to reduce depression rates. One study in Taiwan showed that reminiscence group therapy (RGT) significantly lowered depression scores among elderly persons affected by Hansen's disease. A few studies demonstrated psychological benefits of combining either surgical or medical interventions and psychological treatment. Available approaches to improving the social and mental wellbeing of persons affected by Hansen's disease have been detailed in Guide 2 'How to reduce the impact of stigma' of the ILEP/NNN Guides on Stigma and Mental Wellbeing.[1] These approaches focus on the strategies to adapt, described in section three, and include psychosocial (family) support and counselling, peer and group support, role models and champions, and promoting resilience. More research is needed to develop and test simple, low-cost, and scalable approaches to the prevention and treatment of mental health problems due to Hansen's disease or other NTDs.

There are very effective tools to help persons affected to adapt to life with Hansen's disease. One is to provide a platform and opportunities for their participation and inclusion at various forums. There are many role models who used such opportunities and now working for the cause. If persons affected by Hansen's disease will get opportunities in the same way as other human beings, they will be able to show the importance of their contributions to the society. Various skills development and vocational training programmes have been shown to be effective in enhancing their skills to promote social and economic growth [30, 31]. The successful placements of persons affected by Hansen's disease in reputed companies by NGOs who are running Vocational Training Centres are good examples of this [32].

---

[1] https://www.infontd.org/toolkits/stigma-guides/guide-2-how-reduce-impact-stigma

References

1. Rao PS. Study on differences and similarities in the concept and origin of leprosy stigma in relation to other health-related stigma. Indian J Lepr. 2010;82:117–21.
2. Weiss MG, Ramakrishna J, Somma D. Health-related stigma: rethinking concepts and interventions. Psychol Health Med. 2006;11:277–87.
3. Adhikari B, Kaehler N, Raut S, Marahatta SB, Ggyanwali K. Risk factors of stigma related to leprosy-a systematic review. J Manmohan Mem Inst Health Sci. 2013;1:3–11.
4. Sermrittirong S, van Brakel W. Stigma in leprosy: concepts, causes and determinants. Lepr Rev. 2014;85:36–47.
5. van't Noordende AT, Lisam S, Ruthindartri P, Sadiq A, Singh V, Arifin M, et al. Leprosy perceptions and knowledge in endemic districts in India and Indonesia: differences and commonalities. PLoS Negl Trop Dis. 2021;15:e0009031.
6. Heijnders ML. The dynamics of stigma in leprosy. Int J Lepr Other Mycobact Dis. 2004;72:437–47.
7. Varkevisser CM, Lever P, Alubo O, Burathoki K, Idawani C, Moreira TMA, et al. Gender and leprosy: case studies in Indonesia, Nigeria, Nepal and Brazil. Lepr Rev. 2009;80:65.
8. van't Noordende AT, da Silva Pereira ZB, Kuipers P. Key sources of strength and resilience for persons receiving services for Hansen's disease (leprosy) in Porto Velho, Brazil: what can we learn for service development? Int Health. 2021;13(6):527–35.
9. van Brakel WH. Measuring leprosy stigma-a preliminary review of the leprosy literature. Int J Lepr Other Mycobact Dis. 2003;71:190.
10. Engelbrektsson UB, Subedi M. Stigma and leprosy presentations, Nepal. Lepr Rev. 2018;89:1–8.
11. Somar P, Waltz M, van Brakel W. The impact of leprosy on the mental wellbeing of leprosy-affected persons and their family members–a systematic review. Glob Ment Health. 2020;7:7. https://doi.org/10.1017/gmh.2020.3.
12. Moos RH, Schaefer JA. The crisis of physical illness. In: Moos RH, editor. Coping with physical illness. Boston, MA: Springer; 1984. p. 3–25.
13. Peters RMH, Hofker ME, van Brakel WH, Zweekhorst MBM, Seda FSSE, Irwanto I, et al. Narratives around concealment and agency for stigma reduction: a study of women affected by leprosy in Cirebon District, Indonesia. Disabil CBR Inclusive Dev. 2014;25:5–21. https://doi.org/10.5463/DCID.v25i4.389.
14. Rai SS, Irwanto I, Peters RM, Syurina EV, Putri AI, Mikhakhanova A, et al. Qualitative exploration of experiences and consequences of health-related stigma among Indonesians with HIV, leprosy, schizophrenia and diabetes. Kesmas. 2020;15:7–16.
15. Adhikari B, Kaehler N, Raut S, Gyanwali K, Chapman RS. Stigma in leprosy: a qualitative study of leprosy affected patients at green pastures hospital, western region of Nepal. J Health Res. 2013;27:295–300.
16. Stanton AL, Revenson TA. Adjustment to chronic disease: progress and promise in research. Oxford University Press; 2012.
17. Zhang X, Wang A, Shi T, Zhang J, Xu H, Wang D, et al. The psychosocial adaptation of patients with skin disease: a scoping review. BMC Public Health. 2019;19:1–15.
18. Suzuki K, Akama T, Kawashima A, Yoshihara A, Yotsu RR, Ishii N. Current status of leprosy: epidemiology, basic science and clinical perspectives. J Dermatol. 2012;39:121–9.
19. Deps PD, Nasser S, Guerra P, Simon M, Birshner RDC, Rodrigues LC. Adverse effects from multi-drug therapy in leprosy: a Brazilian study. Lepr Rev. 2007;78:216–22.
20. Ebenso B, Fashona A, Ayuba M, Idah M, Adeyemi G, S-Fada S. Impact of socio-economic rehabilitation on leprosy stigma in Northern Nigeria: findings of a retrospective study. Asia Pac Disabil Rehabil J. 2007;18:98–119.
21. Major B, O'Brien LT. The social psychology of stigma. Annu Rev Psychol. 2005;56:393–421. https://doi.org/10.1146/annurev.psych.56.091103.070137.

22. Barlow J, Wright C, Sheasby J, Turner A, Hainsworth J. Self-management approaches for people with chronic conditions: a review. Patient Educ Couns. 2002;48:177–87.
23. Barrett R. Self-mortification and the stigma of leprosy in northern India. Med Anthropol Q. 2005;19:216–30.
24. van't Noordende AT, Aycheh MW, Schippers A. The impact of leprosy, podoconiosis and lymphatic filariasis on family quality of life: a qualitative study in northwest Ethiopia. PLoS Negl Trop Dis. 2020;14:e0008173.
25. van Dorst MMAR, van Netten WJ, Waltz MM, Pandey BD, Choudhary R, van Brakel WH. Depression and mental wellbeing in people affected by leprosy in southern Nepal. Glob Health Action. 2020;13:1815275. https://doi.org/10.1080/16549716.2020.1815275.
26. Govindasamy K, Jacob I, Solomon RM, Darlong J. Burden of depression and anxiety among leprosy affected and associated factors—a cross sectional study from India. PLoS Negl Trop Dis. 2021;15:e0009030.
27. Cross H, Choudhary R. STEP: an intervention to address the issue of stigma related to leprosy in Southern Nepal. Lepr Rev. 2005;76:316–24.
28. Floyd-Richard M, Gurung S. Stigma reduction through group counselling of person s affected by leprosy ± a pilot study. Lepr Rev. 2000;71:499–504.
29. Stevelink SAM, van Brakel WH, Augustine V. Stigma and social participation in Southern India: differences and commonalities among persons affected by leprosy and persons living with HIV/AIDS. Psychol Health Med. 2011;16:695–707.
30. Lusli M, Peters R, van Brakel W, Zweekhorst M, Iancu S, Bunders J, et al. The impact of a rights-based counselling intervention to reduce stigma in people affected by leprosy in Indonesia. PLoS Negl Trop Dis. 2016;10:e0005088.
31. Ebenso B, Ayuba M. "Money is the vehicle of interaction": insight into social integration of people affected by leprosy in northern Nigeria. Lepr Rev. 2010;81:99.
32. The Leprosy Mission Trust India. The livelihood focus. Beating the marginalisation due to leprosy 2020. https://www.leprosymission.in/what-we-do/institutions-and-projects/vocaitonal-training-centres/. Accessed 15 Feb 2022.

Peripheral Nerve by Ultrasound in Hansen's Disease

Glauber Voltan ⓘ

Ultrasonography (US) can be used as a complementary diagnostic method in Hansen's Disease (HD) by identifying neuropathy. HD is the only condition in which assessment of neural hypertrophy is central to the diagnosis [1], and it is proposed by the World Health Organization as one of the three criteria for case definition of the disease [2]. The simplified neurological physical examination, including palpation of the peripheral nerves, aids in the diagnosis of neural thickening and neuritis but is subjective even for well-trained professionals [3]. HD is a neural disease with or without cutaneous manifestations [4–10] (Fig. 1). On the other hand, cases of peripheral neuropathy accompanied by neural thickening, with or without cutaneous manifestations, should lead the clinician to suspect the diagnosis of HD.

Supplementary Information The online version contains supplementary material available at https://doi.org/10.1007/978-3-031-30893-2_24.

G. Voltan (✉)
Faculdade de Medicina de Ribeirão Preto da Universidade de São Paulo, Ribeirão Preto, Brazil

Instituto Humanizare—Clínica de Médica de Especialistas, Juina, Mato Grosso, Brazil

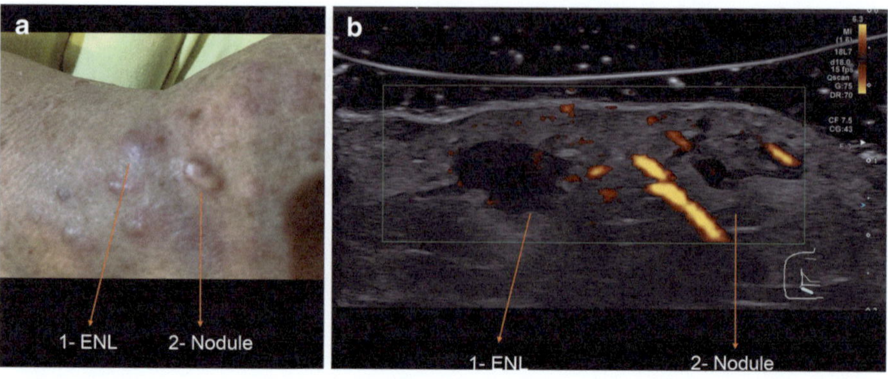

Fig. 1 Nodule and erythema nodosum of Hansen's disease, clinical image real photo (**a**) ultrasound image (**b**)

1   High-Resolution Ultrasound

High-resolution ultrasound (HRUS) two-dimensional and Doppler modes make it possible to assess the entire extent of superficial and deep peripheral nerves; assess and quantify the cross-sectional area (CSA) and the diameter of the epineurium and perineurium in various neural segments; characterize fascicular patterns and echogenicity; identify the presence or absence of endoneurial or perineural vascularization [11].

HRUS in two-dimensional and Doppler modes make it possible to:

- Assess the full extent of superficial and deep peripheral nerves.
- Gauging and quantifying the cross-sectional area (CSA) and diameter of the epineurium and perineurium in various neural segments.
- Characterize fascicular patterns and echogenicity.
- Identify the presence or absence of endoneurial or perineural vascularization [11].

HRUS is able to identify a greater number of altered nerves and a greater extent of alterations, even in areas inaccessible to palpation or when the clinical examination of peripheral nerve palpation leaves the examiner in doubt as to whether or not there is thickening. Being accurate and objective may help bring new parameters for the diagnosis of HD and the early recognition of neuritis, especially in the reaction phases of the disease [12–14]. Comparing HRUS with electrophysiological study, it is concluded that they are complementary methods. And, HRUS is more cost-effective compared to MRI [15, 16].

2   Anatomical Aspects of Peripheral Nerves

Peripheral nerves are made up of axons held together by a thin endoneuro (inner layer), grouped into fascicles covered by the perineural and reunited into the nerve, which is surrounded by the epineural (outer layer) (Fig. 2). The echo graphic images show the nerves as hypoechoic structures with a fine fascicular pattern. In the longitudinal axis, it appears as hypoechoic tubular structures interspersed by hyperechoic lines and externally lined by a hyperechoic line (cord or rope pattern) (Fig. 3a). On the transverse axis, it appears rounded or oval, with multiple rounded hypoechoic images (neural fascicles) inside, located on a hyperechoic background (epineurium + perineurium), an appearance described as a "honeycomb" or connective fascicular (Fig. 3b) [17–19].

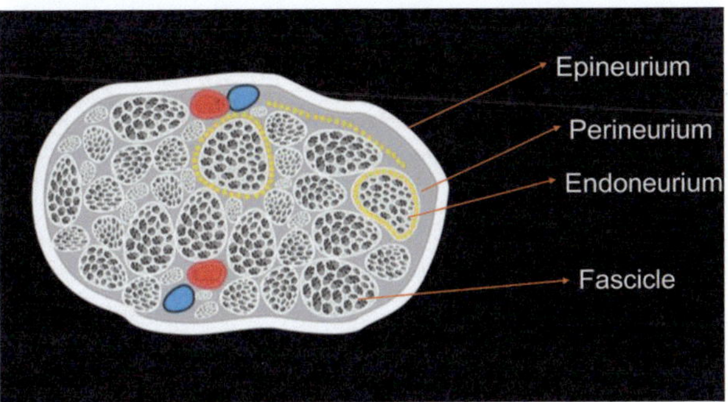

Fig. 2 Schematic drawing of the cross-sectional area of a peripheral nerve image seen by a high-resolution ultrasound image

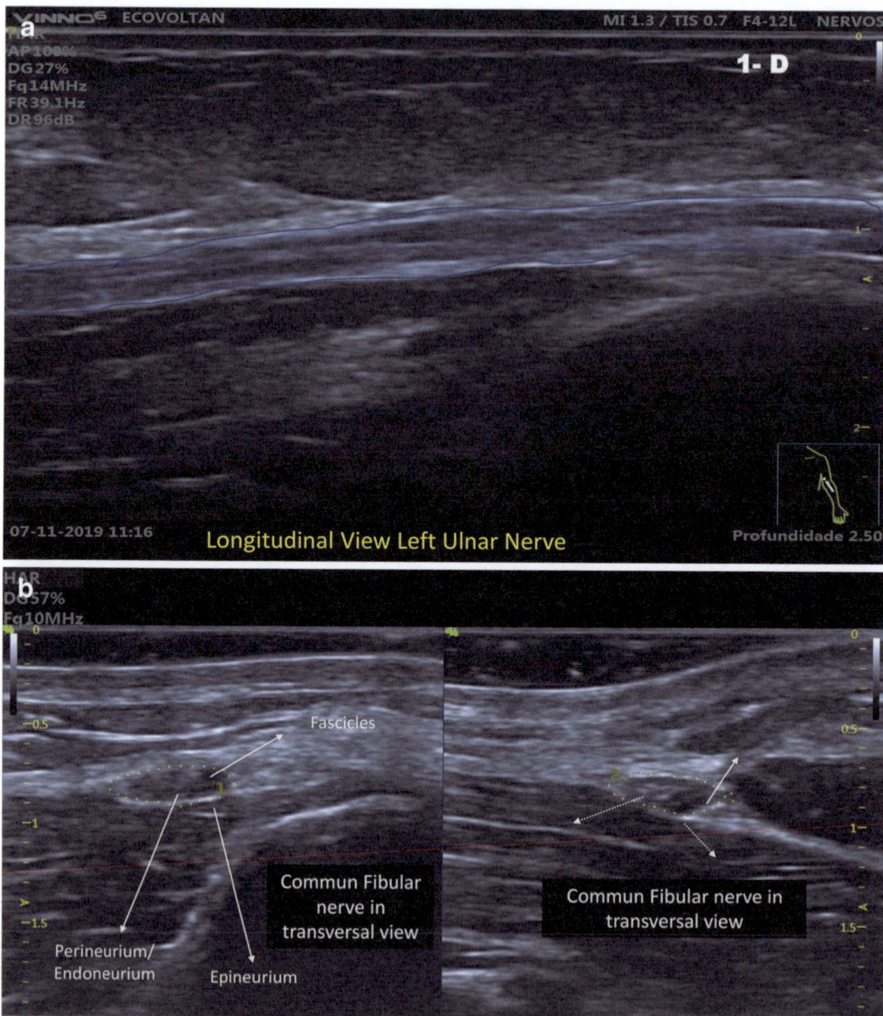

Fig. 3 Ultrasound image of normal left ulnar nerve in longitudinal view (**a**); Ultrasound image of normal common fibular nerve in transversal view, on the left side at head fibula and on the right side proximal of head fibular (**b**)

3 Morphologic Aspects of Hansen's Disease (HD) Neuropathy Seen by High-Resolution USG

USG of the peripheral nerves should verify the CSA, analyze the presence or absence of Doppler, and be done bilaterally. This method has high sensitivity and accuracy to diagnose, localize, and evaluate peripheral nerve thickening when compared with clinical neurological examination and other imaging methods. In general, it is performed on the following nerves: median in the carpal and forearm tunnels; ulnar in the cubital and proximal tunnels, common fibular in the fibular head and proximal, tibial in the popliteal fossa and/or tarsal tunnel; sural in the leg and ankle; and radial in the radial groove of the arm (Groove).

In HD, we observe greater thickening of the neural trunks represented by increased CSA, in addition to more morphological alterations of echogenicity, fascicular pattern, perineurium, and vascularization in the peripheral nerves. The findings of the ulnar nerve with more severe thickening above the medial epicondyle, the median nerve proximal to the carpal tunnel, the common fibular nerve at the fibular head, and the tibial nerve at the medial malleolus are noteworthy; these points should be in the routine ultrasound evaluation [9, 12].

In addition to the parameters of the absolute values of the CSA measurements, other authors [9, 14], suggest the asymmetry index [Δ CSA = (> CSA right or left)—(< CSA right or left)] in the evaluation of HD neuropathy, demonstrating that the asymmetry index between the right and left peripheral nerves has high sensitivity and specificity in differentiating between nerves from healthy individuals and nerves from HD patients. It is concluded that asymmetry of peripheral nerve thickening is a characteristic of HD patients, regardless of their classification in multibacillary or paucibacillary.

Focal thickening of the ulnar nerve starts at the ulnar sulcus and reaches its maximum 4 cm above the medial epicondyle [14, 20], and this characteristic finding may help mainly in the diagnosis of primary or pure neural HD (PNH), in which skin lesions are absent, and also in differentiating HD from other neuropathies in which diffuse nerve enlargement may occur (Fig. 4).

The absence of neural thickening or other peripheral nerve changes does not exclude a diagnosis of HD because the lesion may be in the neural ramus and not in the nerve trunks. On the other hand, the identification of neural thickening does not confirm the diagnosis of Hansen's Disease, and a thorough investigation of the clinical, bacteriological, and electrophysiological aspects of the disease is required.

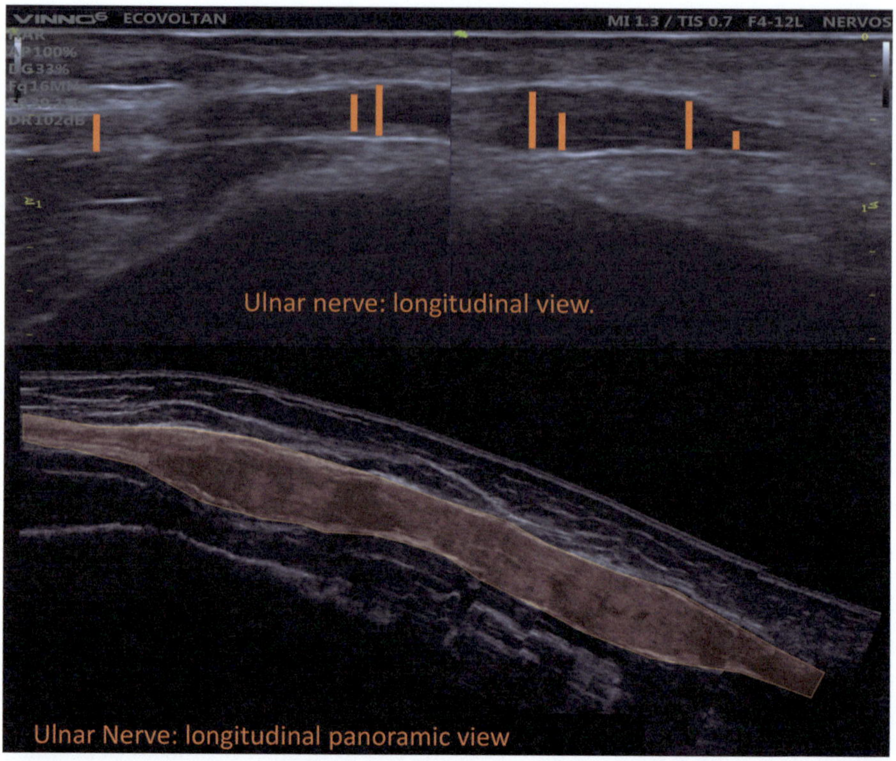

Fig. 4 Fusiform or focal thickening of pathological ulnar nerve, on the upside dual ultrasound image and on the downside panoramic view of the ultrasound image

References

1. Donaghy M. Enlarged peripheral nerves. Pract Neurol. 1994;2003:40–5. https://doi.org/10.1046/j.1474-7766.2003.00121.x.
2. WHO. Guidelines for the diagnosis, treatment and prevention of leprosy. 2017; 1: 87.
3. Van Brakel WH, Saunderson P, Shetty V, et al. International workshop on neuropathology in leprosy–consensus report. Lepr Rev. 2007;78(4):416–33.
4. Alemu Belachew W, Naafs B. Position statement: leprosy: diagnosis, treatment and follow-up. J Eur Acad Dermatology Venereol. 2019;33(7):1205–13. https://doi.org/10.1111/jdv.15569.
5. Scollard D. Mechanisms of nerve injury in leprosy: an overview neuropathy in leprosy acute and chronic neuritis reactions and neuritis in leprosy: clinician's perspective reactions and neuritis in leprosy: basic science perspective. 2008.
6. Garbino JA, Marques W, Barreto JA, et al. Primary neural leprosy: systematic review. Hanseníase neural primária: Revisão sistemática. Arq Neuropsiquiatr. 2013;71(6):397–404. https://doi.org/10.1590/0004-282X20130046.
7. Filho FB, De Paula NA, Leite MN, et al. Evidence of hidden leprosy in a supposedly low endemic area of Brazil. Mem Inst Oswaldo Cruz. 2017;112(12):822–8. https://doi.org/10.1590/0074-02760170173.

8. Lugão HB, MAC F, Marques W Jr, Foss NT, Nogueira-Barbosa MH. Ultrasonography of leprosy neuropathy: a longitudinal prospective study. PLoS Negl Trop Dis. 2016;10(11):e0005111. https://doi.org/10.1371/journal.pntd.0005111.

9. Frade MC, et al. New sonographic measures of peripheral nerves: a tool for diagnosis of peripheric nerve involvement in leprosy. Hansen Int. 2013;36(1):71. https://doi.org/10.1590/s0074-02762013000300001.

10. Lancet Neurology. Leprosy as a neurological disease. Lancet Neurol. 2009;8(3):217. https://doi.org/10.1016/S1474-4422(09)70026-2.

11. Peer S, Gruber H. Atlas of peripheral nerve ultrasound: with anatomic and MRI correlation. New York: Springer; 2013. https://doi.org/10.1007/978-3-642-25594-6.

12. Jain S, Visser LH, Praveen TLN, et al. High-resolution sonography: a new technique to detect nerve damage in leprosy. PLoS Negl Trop Dis. 2009;3(8):1–7. https://doi.org/10.1371/journal.pntd.0000498.

13. Gupta S, Bhatt S, Bhargava SK, Singal A, Bhargava S. High resolution sonographic examination: a newer technique to study ulnar nerve neuropathy in leprosy. Lepr Rev. 2016;87(4):464–75.

14. Lugão HB, Nogueira-Barbosa MH, Marques W, Foss NT, Frade MAC. Asymmetric nerve enlargement: a characteristic of leprosy neuropathy demonstrated by ultrasonography. PLoS Negl Trop Dis. 2015;9(12):1–11. https://doi.org/10.1371/journal.pntd.0004276.

15. Elias J, Nogueira-Barbosa MH, Feltrin LT, et al. Role of ulnar nerve sonography in leprosy neuropathy with electrophysiologic correlation. J Ultrasound Med. 2009;28(9):1201–9. https://doi.org/10.7863/jum.2009.28.9.1201.

16. Martinoli C, Derchi LE, Bertolotto M, et al. US and MR imaging of peripheral nerves in leprosy. Skelet Radiol. 2000;29(3):142–50. https://doi.org/10.1007/s002560050584.

17. Kowalska B, Sudoł-Szopińska I. Normal and sonographic anatomy of selected peripheral nerves. Part III: peripheral nerves of the lower limb. J Ultrason. 2012;12(49):148–63. https://doi.org/10.15557/jou.2012.0003.

18. Martinoli C, Bianchi S, Derchi LE. Ultrasonography of peripheral nerves. Semin Ultrasound CT MRI. 2000;21(3):205–13. https://doi.org/10.1016/S0887-2171(00)90043-X.

19. Wortsman X, Jemec G. Dermatologic ultrasound with clinical and histologic correlations. New York: Springer; 2013. https://doi.org/10.1007/978-1-4614-7184-4.

20. Bathala L, Krishnam VN, Kumar HK, et al. Extensive sonographic ulnar nerve enlargement above the medial epicondyle is a characteristic sign in Hansen's neuropathy. PLoS Negl Trop Dis. 2017;11(7):1–10. https://doi.org/10.1371/journal.pntd.0005766.

Electroneuromyography in Hansen's Disease

Ana Lucila Moreira

1 Introduction

Electroneuromyography is an ancillary test for peripheral nerve function investigation and comprises nerve conduction studies (that may include specific evaluations for diagnosis of small nerve fiber involvement) and needle electromyography. There are several techniques for performing nerve conduction studies, but basically, they record nerve and muscle responses to electrical stimulation of nerves. All tests are planned according to the clinical manifestation of the patient, and ideally should include at least upper and lower limb assessment.

Neuropathy in these patients has different characteristics considering the spectrum of the disease and can occur even without skin lesions [1, 2]. Early recognition is important to reduce the risks of permanent deficits.

Neurophysiological diagnosis is useful for: (1) defining the pattern and severity of peripheral nerve involvement [2]; (2) indicating the need for surgical treatment strategies [3]; (3) follow-up during treatment (including for monitoring nerve damage secondary to drugs) [1]; and (4) differentiate worsening or new neuropathies during type-1 and type-2 reactions.

2 Patterns of Peripheral Nerve Involvement in Hansen's Disease

Nerve damage in Hansen's disease can be as small as single nerve involvement, but as large as generalized peripheral nerve disease, including autonomic compromise.

A. L. Moreira (✉)
CENEC, Campinas, SP, Brazil

P. D. Deps (ed.), *Hansen's Disease*, https://doi.org/10.1007/978-3-031-30893-2_25

Some nerves are predominantly affected in specific locations, such as: (1) the ulnar in the distal arm and elbow, and the dorsal cutaneous branch of the ulnar in the distal forearm; (2) the median in the wrist; (3) the superficial radial in the distal forearm and hand; (4) peroneal nerve above the fibular head; and (5) tibial nerve above the ankle. Pure sensory nerves such as sural, posterior auricular, and supraorbital nerves can also be injured, some of those requiring special techniques for investigation, and it may be necessary to extend nerve conduction studies to detect involvement of nerves such as the facial and phrenic nerves [1]. And a major challenge for the clinical neurophysiologist is to suggest Hansen's disease in the case of an isolated mononeuropathy, which can sometimes mimic a common nerve entrapment [4], in a patient referred without specific suspicion.

The most common pattern linked to Hansen's disease diagnosis is the mononeuritis multiplex, with multiple sensory, motor, or mixed neuropathies occurring in an asymmetric, non-length-dependent pattern [2, 5]. However, as the disease progresses, the neuropathy can take on a confluent character, and it is very difficult to differentiate it from a polyneuropathy [4].

The cardinal feature of Hansen's disease nerve lesion is demyelination, and the abnormalities can be localized or diffuse [5]. They can be documented by latency prolongation, and segmental or generalized velocity reduction in the nerve portions that can be assessed by conduction nerve study [1]. Segmented studies with attention to the vulnerable sites are necessary to properly identify focal lesions: there may be temporal dispersion, and when there is weakness, there is a chance to detect conduction block (Fig. 1) [1]. And in sites where there is conduction block, it is very likely to find morphological changes of the nerve by ultrasound.

Axonal damage can occur as the disease progresses [6], and the patterns of axonal injury are reduced amplitude or even absence of responses in conduction studies, but reduced conduction velocity can also occur due to loss of fast conducting fibers. Axonal and demyelinating lesions can coexist, and demyelinating lesions can cause distal abnormalities that mimic axonal damage; besides, if there is an absence of responses, it is not possible to define whether the lesion is axonal or demyelinating.

Late responses such as F waves or the H reflex may be altered even early in the disease when other findings in conduction studies may not be present [1]. Similarly, autonomic studies such as the cutaneous sympathetic response and the study of R-R interval variability (Ewing tests) may be altered in isolation or accompany the neuropathies already described [1].

Needle recordings can show reduced recruitment secondary to focal demyelination, and when there is motor axonal loss, active denervation findings (positive sharp waves and fibrillation potentials) and those related to recent or long-term reinnervation (polyphasic and unstable units, stable units with larger duration of potentials which can have larger amplitudes, with increased frequency and progressive recruitment reduction) become present and are related to the territory of the affected nerve or nerves [6]. Therefore, the findings can suggest whether the injury is recent or chronic [1, 6], and whether there has been reinnervation; and considering recent injuries, it is important to emphasize that acute lesions may take at least 3 weeks to be detected in needle examination. Furthermore, it is important to plan the needle

Sensory Nerve Conduction Study

Site	Lat.1	Lat.2	Amp.	Area	Segment	Distance	Interval	NCV
Median	**Left**							
Wrist-3rd finger	2.7ms	3.6ms	5.6uV	0.4uVms	Wrist-3rd finger	140mm	2.7ms	52.6m/s
Wrist-2nd finger	2.5ms	3.3ms	7.3uV	0.2uVms	Wrist-2nd finger	140mm	2.5ms	56.0m/s
Median	**Right**							
Wrist-3rd finger	3.8ms	4.7ms	9.3uV	0.5uVms	Wrist-3rd finger	140mm	3.8ms	36.8m/s
Wrist-2nd finger	3.3ms	4.1ms	9.3uV	0.2uVms	Wrist-2nd finger	140mm	3.3ms	42.7m/s
Ulnar	**Left**							
Wrist-5th finger	2.5ms	3.2ms	18.6uV	0.8uVms	Wrist-5th finger	140mm	2.5ms	55.1m/s
Ulnar	**Right**							
Wrist-5th finger	2.6ms	3.2ms	14.2uV	0.3uVms	Wrist-5th finger	140mm	2.6ms	54.7m/s
Radial	**Left**							
Wrist-dorsum	2.2ms	2.7ms	11.9uV	0.6uVms	Wrist-dorsum	130mm	2.2ms	59.6m/s
Radial	**Right**							
Wrist-dorsum	2.0ms	2.6ms	12.2uV	0.4uVms	Wrist-dorsum	130mm	2.0ms	64.4m/s

Motor Nerve Conduction Study

Site	Lat.	Dur.	Amp.	Area	Segment	Distance	Interval	NCV
Median	**Left**							
Wrist	3.0ms	5.4ms	9.7mV	16.3mVms	Wrist		3.0ms	
Above elbow	9.0ms	4.4ms	5.2mV	7.1mVms	Wrist - elbow	250mm	6.0ms	41.5m/s
Lumbrical II	3.1ms	4.8ms	1.1mV	1.9mVms	Lumbr II – interosseous II		0.3ms	
Interosseous II	2.8ms	4.6ms	9.9mV	16.3mVms				
Median	**Right**							
punho	4.3ms	4.9ms	10.4mV	19.3mVms	Wrist		4.3ms	
Wrist	8.7ms	5.0ms	9.8mV	19.4mVms	Wrist - elbow	215mm	4.4ms	49.1m/s
Above elbow	1.8ms	4.9ms	11.2mV	21.7mVms	Wrist - palm	60mm	2.6ms	23.4m/s
Lumbrical II	4.0ms	4.2ms	2.7mV	4.2mVms	Lumbr II – interosseous II		0.9ms	
Interosseous II	3.1ms	4.1ms	6.3mV	9.4mVms				

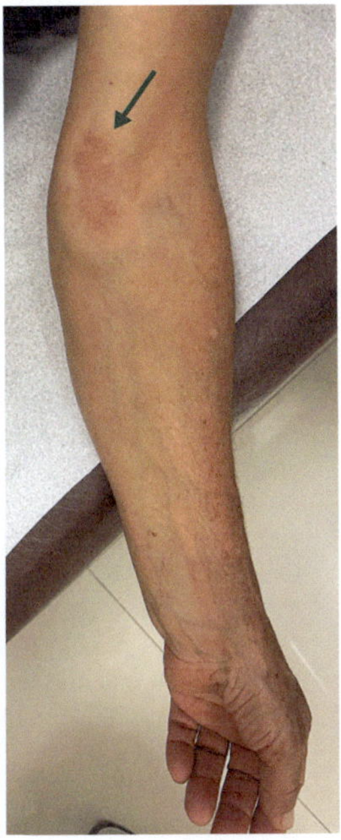

Fig. 1 A 64-year-old female patient with burning hands and symptoms of carpal tunnel syndrome on the right hand. Sensory conduction studies (on top) showed reduced amplitudes for median nerves and superficial radial nerves (suggesting polyneuropathy), and delayed latencies with reduced conduction velocities only for right median. Motor conduction studies (bottom) confirmed the right median nerve compromise in the carpal tunnel (entrapment neuropathy), with prolonged distal latency (4.3 ms) and reduced velocity in the wrist-palm segment (23 m/s). And showed a conduction block in proximal median nerve, with a marked reduction in amplitude in proximal stimulation compared to distal stimulation (a 53% amplitude drop from 9.7 mV to 5.2 mV) and conduction velocity slowing (41.5 m/s) in the location where there was a hyperemic lesion in the proximal forearm (picture on the right). *ms* milliseconds, *mV* millivolts, *m/s* meters/second

study according to the clinical manifestations and the findings of the nerve conduction studies, and differentiation from pre-existing pathologies can be difficult depending on the extent, nerve territory, and duration of symptoms.

Finally, silent neuropathy can be detected in electroneuromyography without skin lesions, neurologic symptoms, or nerve enlargement [1, 5]. For that reason, electroneuromyography should be considered in all patients in the scenario of Hansen's disease diagnosis.

3 Conclusion

Electroneuromyography is important for diagnosis, follow-up, and prognostic evaluation in Hansen's disease, and abnormalities can be detected even in silent neuropathies, without skin lesions, neurologic symptoms, or nerve enlargement.

Considering the complexity of the neurophysiological study described above, it is recommended that the professional performing the examination to be qualified in clinical neurophysiology and have a previous experience in the diagnosis and follow-up of this disease.

References

1. Srinivasan J, Ooi WW. Leprosy and the peripheral nervous system: basic and clinical aspects. Muscle Nerve. 2004;30:393–409.
2. Shukla B, Verma R, Kumar V, et al. Pathological, ultrasonographic, and electrophysiological characterization of clinically diagnosed cases of pure neuritic leprosy. J Peripher Nerv Syst. 2020;25:191–203.
3. Brasil-Neto JP. Electrophysiologic studies in leprosy. Arq Neuropsiquiatr. 1992;50(3):313–8.
4. DeFaria CR, Silva IM. Electromyographic diagnosis of leprosy. Arq Neuropsiquiatr. 1990;48(4):403–13.
5. Jardim MR, Chimelli L, Faria SC, et al. Clinical, electroneuromyographic and morphological studies of pure neural leprosy in a Brazilian referral Centre. Lepr Rev. 2004;75(3):242–53.
6. Garbino JA, Heise CO, Marques W Jr. Assessing nerves in leprosy. Clin Dermatol. 2016;34(1):51–8.

Treatment of Hansen's Disease

Marcos Cesar Florian and Patrícia D. Deps

1   A Short History of Treatments

The treatment of Hansen's disease, including drug approaches, is a challenge and one of the crucial points in controlling the endemic. Information regarding conduct in earlier times is scarce.

The history of Hansen's disease includes several empirical attempts at curative treatment. The first attempt at treatment was introduced by Mouat in 1854, who used "Chaulmoogra oil" extracted from the seeds of trees of the genus *Hydnocarpus*, in the Asian region [1, 2]. In the first decades of the twentieth century, it was widely used with low therapeutic response, especially in patients in the virchowian pole of the disease [3]. In the 1930s, medications against streptococcal infections began to be used, among them sulfonamides. In 1941, Guy Faget and collaborators used sodium glycosulfone (Promin®) to treat patients in Carville, USA, beginning the era of sulfones for the treatment of Hansen's disease [4]. Sulfones had been known since 1833 and were used as artificial tannins and insecticides until the appearance of DDT (dichlorodiphenyltrichloroethane). Diamino-diphenyl-sulfone (DDS) was synthesized by Fromm and Whittmann in Germany in 1908 [5], and sulfonamides were synthesized that same year. In the absence of toxicological and safety studies, the use of analogous doses of the two drugs led to adverse side effects and treatments using these drugs were unfeasible for many years.

M. C. Florian
Universidade Federal de São Paulo, São Paulo, Brazil
e-mail: mcflorian@unifesp.br

P. D. Deps (✉)
Universidade Federal do Espírito Santo, Vitória, Brazil
e-mail: patricia.deps@ufes.br

P. D. Deps (ed.), *Hansen's Disease*, https://doi.org/10.1007/978-3-031-30893-2_26

Following Faget et al. [4], Hansen's disease experts in several regions of the world—Cochrane and collaborators in India [6], Lowe in Nigeria [7], Floch in French Guiana [8]—confirmed the drug's activity at low doses given orally. This brought about a profound change in the treatment of the disease which, until then had been based mainly on isolation and segregation of patients.

In 1960, Shepard was able to multiply *M. leprae* in the plantar cushion of mice [9], allowing proof of sulfone activity and experimentation with new drugs. Only a few years later, clinical suspicion of sulfone resistance was demonstrated by the same method [10].

The emergence of secondary resistance to sulfones in several countries led the World Health Organization (WHO) to recommend, in 1976, a two-drug treatment regimen instead of the sulfone monotherapy [11]. Rifampicin, a drug with high bactericidal activity that had been used for the first time in 1963 by Opromolla, was combined with dapsone [12].

In the 1970s, besides dapsone, several drugs were used in various combinations: acedapsone, rifampicin, clofazimine, prothionamide/ethionamide, isoniazid, thiacetazone, thiambutosine, and long-acting sulfonamides.

The main objective of this recommendation—to prevent the emergence of primary dapsone resistance—began to fail as early as 1977, when Pearson described sulfone resistance in five treatment-naïve patients [13]. This led to a new recommendation, in 1981, that the standard treatment should include a third drug, clofazimine, a riminophenazine dye derived from aniline, first synthesized in 1954.

2 WHO Multidrug Therapy (MDT/WHO)

In 1981, the WHO organized an expert meeting in Geneva (Switzerland) and recommended the adoption of MDT/WHO. The combination of three antimicrobial drugs for the treatment of Hansen's disease represents the most significant advance in the fight against the disease [14].

Following the roll-out of MDT/WHO, the number of registered (prevalent) cases decreased dramatically, mainly due to the effectiveness and shorter duration of MDT. However, new case detection rates have remained stubbornly high in endemic countries, and elimination of the disease remains a major public health challenge.

Prompt treatment of new patients is essential to reducing endemicity, and early MDT treatment is effective in preventing disease progression, breaking the epidemiological chain of transmission, avoiding resistance to monotherapy, and preventing or minimizing the onset of physical disability and the psychosocial consequences of Hansen's disease [14, 15].

In addition to the initiation of MDT, the comprehensive management of the individual diagnosed with Hansen's disease includes evaluation of the patient to monitor the progression of skin lesions and his nerve involvement, checking and monitoring for the onset of reactions and neuritis. This assessment should be performed during monthly administration of treatment (supervised doses) plus whenever necessary. Patients should also receive guidance on self-care techniques and prevention of disabilities [16].

MDT is effective, but multidrug-resistant strains have started to occur in the last two decades, reaching 2% among new cases and 5% among relapsed cases that had been adequately treated [17]. In such cases, MDT can be extended for an additional 12 months, or specific substitute regimens can be used, but these treatment decisions should be evaluated in conjunction with a Hansen's disease reference service [16].

MDT/WHO comprises rifampicin (RMP), dapsone (DDS), and clofazimine (CFZ) given according to a regimen determined by the operational classification of Hansen's disease [16]. In adult and paediatric cases where there is intolerance to one or more of the component drugs, a substitute regimen is indicated usually with referral to a disabilities reference service [16].

MDT is administered in supervised doses monthly (28-day) at a health unit, plus daily self-administered doses at home. The patient is discharged as cured after receiving at least the full number of doses in the recommended regimen and according to the findings of dermato-neurological examination [16].

For the treatment of children under 15 years of age, weight is the most important indicator. Children weighing more than 50 kg receive the adult dose; from 30 to 50 kg, use the MDT/WHO children's blister packs (brown/blue); for children under 30 kg, dose adjustments must be made [16].

Standard MDT is not contraindicated during pregnancy and breastfeeding. Similarly, in cases of patients with COVID-19 or HIV co-infection (or on HIV/AIDS treatment), the MDT/WHO regimen according to Hansen's disease operational classification is maintained.

3 MDT/WHO Regimens for Paucibacillary (PB) and Multibacillary (MB) Hansen's Disease

PB patients receive a 6-month MDT/PB regimen (6 monthly doses supervised over up to 9 months). MB patients a 12-month MDT/MB regimen (12 monthly doses supervised over up to 18 months) [15]. For patients who still have multiple skin lesions at the end of MDT, an additional 12 doses of MDT may be required. Table 1 shows the dosages of clofazimine, dapsone, and rifampicin for adults and children.

4 Treatment Insufficiency

Treatment insufficiency is evident in those patients who, at the end of the standard treatment, need to continue MDT. Patients incorrectly classified as PB may complete 12 doses of MDT-MB/WHO. Patients classified as MB should receive 12

Table 1 Recommended treatment regimens [16]

Age group	Drug	Dosage and frequency[a]	Duration	
			MB	PB
Adult[a]	Rifampicin	600 mg once a month	12 months	6 months
	Clofazimine	300 mg once a month and 50 mg daily		
	Dapsone	100 mg daily		
Children (10–14 years)[a]	Rifampicin	450 mg once a month	12 months	6 months
	Clofazimine	150 mg once a month, 50 mg on alternate days		
	Dapsone	50 mg daily		
Children < 10 years old or < 40Kg[a]	Rifampicin	10 mg/kg once a month	12 months	6 months
	Clofazimine	100 mg once a month, 50 mg twice weekly		
	Dapsone	2 mg/kg daily		

Note: The treatment for children with body weight below 40 kg requires single formulation medications since no MDT blister packs are available
[a]At patient's monthly clinic appointment, the daily dose on that day can be supervised.

additional doses if, after being treated with a 12-dose regimen, they still show signs of clinical activity and/or have well-defined intact bacilli on dermal scrapings and/ or by histopathological examination of the skin and, if serological tests are available, have elevated levels of anti-PGL-1 antibodies (IgM). Treatment insufficiency with standard MDT-MB/WHO is thought to occur due to sub-optimal bioavailability, drug interactions, and/or absorption failure.

5 Treatment Failure

Treatment failure is when an MB patient has received 24 doses of MDT/MB due to treatment insufficiency but still shows signs of clinical activity and/or has well-defined intact bacilli on dermal scrapings and/or by histopathological examination of the skin and, if serological tests are available, have elevated levels of anti-PGL-1 antibodies (IgM). In such cases, tests to assess drug resistance may be performed and treatment continued using a combination of three or four drugs, substituting the drug identified in the resistance test if appropriate. Hansen's disease reactions after discharge from MDT in principle do not mean treatment failure and may occur due to antigenic persistence of non-viable bacilli. However, situations of persistent and/or sub-intrant Hansen's disease reactions after MDT discharge should be carefully evaluated for possible treatment failure or relapse, and in such cases should be retreated and evaluated for drug resistance [18].

6 Treatment of Drug-Resistant Hansen's Disease

As chemotherapy for Hansen's disease has been used more than 70 years and MDT is a treatment that has been used since the 1980s, surveillance, monitoring, and knowledge of the actual rates of bacterial resistance in Hansen's disease in different parts of the world are of fundamental importance [19]. Rates vary in reports, and it is important to know their magnitude in each country and region. Molecular techniques are used to detect the level of drug resistance [20]. Although MDT is considered effective, drug resistance rates to one or more drugs at or above 8% are also reported [17, 21, 22]. The WHO guidelines for rifampicin-resistant patients recommend using at least two of the second-line drugs (clarithromycin, minocycline, or a quinolone) with daily clofazimine for 6 months, followed by clofazimine plus one of these drugs for a further 18 months (Table 2) [16]. When there is resistance to ofloxacin, quinolones should not be considered (Table 3).

Clarithromycin is part of the therapeutic arsenal for Hansen's disease. This drug is important to replace rifampicin and dapsone, especially for children and pregnant women contraindicated for minocycline and quinolones, and for patients diagnosed with therapeutic failure.

Table 2 Recommended treatment regimens for Rifampicin intolerance and/or resistance [16]

First 6 months (daily)	Next 18 months (daily)
Ofloxacin 400 mg[a] + Minocycline 100 mg + Clofazimine 50 mg	Ofloxacin 400 mg[a] OR Minocycline 100 mg + Clofazimine 50 mg
Ofloxacin 400 mg[a] + Clarithromycin 500 mg + Clofazimine 50 mg	Ofloxacin 400 mg[a] + Clofazimine 50 mg

[a] *Ofloxacin 400 mg can be replaced by levofloxacin 500 mg OR moxifloxacin 400 mg*

Table 3 Recommended treatment regime for Rifampicin intolerance and/or resistance and ofloxacin resistance [16]

First 6 months (daily)	Next 18 months (daily)
Clarithromycin 500 mg + Minocycline 100 mg + Clofazimine 50 mg	Clarithromycin 500 mg OR Minocycline 100 mg + Clofazimine 50 mg

7 Substitute Regimens

If any of the MDT/WHO component drugs are not tolerated or if drug resistance is detected, substitute regimens should be considered. Patients should be evaluated in a referral centre and ofloxacin, minocycline), and/or clarithromycin should be used, as described below.

- *Dapsone intolerance and/or resistance*
  Discontinue use of dapsone and replace it with ofloxacin 400 mg OR minocycline 100 mg daily. The duration of treatment remains the same as for standard MDT/WHO.
- *Clofazimine intolerance*
  Discontinue use of clofazimine and replace it with ofloxacin 400 mg OR minocycline 100 mg daily. The duration of treatment remains the same as for standard MDT/WHO.
- *Dapsone intolerance and/or resistance and Clofazimine intolerance*
  Discontinue use of dapsone and clofazimine and replace them with ofloxacin 400 mg AND minocycline 100 mg daily. The duration of treatment remains the same as for standard MDT/WHO.
- *Rifampicin intolerance and/or resistance* (with or without Dapsone intolerance and/or resistance)
  Use one of the regimens in Table 2 for 24 months for either PB or MB patients. Maintain monthly patient clinical consultations.
- *Rifampicin intolerance and/or resistance AND ofloxacin resistance* (with or without Dapsone intolerance and/or resistance)
  Use the regimen in Table 3 for 24 months for either PB or MB patients. Maintain monthly patient clinical consultations.

8 Treatment of Hansen's Disease Reactions

All possible urgent care and attention should be given to patients experiencing suspected reaction episodes, and correct treatment given according to the type of reaction [23]. This requires comprehensive knowledge of reactional states in Hansen's disease. A thorough neurological examination should be carried out and treatment should be started within the first 24 h, typically on an out-patient basis by a doctor. In some cases, hospitalization may be necessary. Other interventions such as surgical drainage of abscesses and decompression of nerves may be required [24].

8.1 Treatment of Type 1 Reactions

A corticosteroid (prednisone/prednisolone) is the elective treatment for type 1 Hansen's disease reactions. The recommended starting dose is 1 mg/kg/day, maintained until regression of the reaction, then slowly reduced at fixed intervals, guided by clinical evaluation [13]. Factors in prolonged use of oral corticosteroid therapy should be considered and monitored: weight, fasting glycemia, blood pressure, ocular alterations, and proceed with prophylactic treatment for strongyloidiasis and osteoporosis [23].

In cases of neuritis, the affected limb should be immobilized. If the patient is on MDT/WHO treatment, this should be continued except in special cases as judged by the medical team.

To avoid physical disability, the patient should always be regularly monitored for affected peripheral nerve function through a simplified neurological assessment with attention paid to the degree of disability. Neuritis can be early detected and best followed by ultrasound, if available [25].

In cases of recalcitrant Hansen's disease reactions with severe neuritis that do not improve with long-term use of high-dose oral corticosteroids, intravenous pulse therapy with corticosteroids is indicated [26]. This type of treatment must be carried out in reference centres, with or without hospitalization. For the first pulse, intravenous methylprednisolone at a dose of 1 g/day for three consecutive days is used. Subsequent pulses are administered (single doses of 1 g of IV methylprednisolone) at 15- or 30-day intervals. Discontinuation of pulse therapy and replacement with a lower dose of oral prednisone is indicated by clinical improvement [16]. When necessary, other strategies for control neuritis can be used using immunosuppressive drugs, such as cyclosporin A and other drugs (see also Chap. 10) [27].

8.2 Treatment of Type 2 Reactions (Erythema Nodosum Leprosum, ENL)

Thalidomide (alpha-N-pthali-midoglutarimide) is recommended as first-line treatment [23, 28–30]. However, the use of corticosteroids is mandatory when there is associated neural involvement, reactive hands and feet, neuritis, iritis, iridocyclitis, orchitis, nephritis, and/or necrotic ENL [23].

Thalidomide is used in adults at a dose of 100–400 mg/day, according to the involvement and severity of the condition. The main contraindications are pregnancy or the possibility of pregnancy. It can only be prescribed to women of childbearing age who use at least two effective methods of contraception (at least one barrier method), according to the health rules of each country. In these cases, the drug can be considered, but only where improvements due to thalidomide cannot be achieved by other means. High-sensitivity pregnancy tests should be done before the start of thalidomide use and regularly during treatment. Men taking thalidomide must use a condom during sexual intercourse with women of childbearing age, even if vasectomized.

If thalidomide is contraindicated, pentoxifylline at a dose of 400 mg 8/8 h can be used with or without prednisone at a dose of 1 mg/kg/day or dexamethasone at an equivalent dose (0.15 mg/kg/day). General caution should be observed when using systemic corticosteroid therapy, and when using corticosteroids together with thalidomide, acetyl salicylic acid should be prescribed at a dose of 100 mg/day to prevent thromboembolism. The doses of thalidomide and corticosteroids should be reduced slowly according to the therapeutic response. MDT/WHO treatment should be maintained, and limbs affected by neuritis should be immobilized if necessary.

Betamethasone [31], pentoxifylline [32], clofazimine [33, 34], acetyl salicylic acid [35], chloroquine [35], indomethacin [35, 36], levamisole [37], and other drugs have been tried in the treatment of ENL, as has clofazimine at a dose of 300 mg/day although with few reports on its efficacy (see also Chap. 10).

Especially in cases of reaction (type 1 or 2) with little improvement with treatments, the possibility of comorbidities should be considered, such as concomitant infections including orodental bacterial foci, hormonal changes, emotional stress, anxiety disorders, and diabetes [23].

8.3   Treatment of Severe Nerve Pain

For chronic neuropathic pain, antidepressants such as amitriptyline hydrochloride at a dose of 25–300 mg/day or nortriptyline hydrochloride at a dose of 10–150 mg/day can be considered. Other possible therapeutic agents include neuroleptics, such as chlorpromazine at a dose of 25–200 mg/day: anticonvulsants, such as carbamazepine at a dose of 200–3000 mg/day and gabapentin at 900–2400 mg/day [23].

Botulin toxin has been used for recalcitrant chronic neuropathic pain, and its use can be evaluated in these situations in the Hansen's disease [38]. Uncontrolled neural pain should be evaluated by a reference service for possible surgical decompression.

8.4   Treatment of Reactions in Children

In type 1 and type 2 reactions and neuritis, corticosteroids are the drugs of choice in doses that can range from 0.5–1.0 mg/kg/day. There are no studies on the safety of thalidomide in the treatment of type 2 reactions in children under 12 years of age.

9   Adverse Effects of Components of Multidrug Therapy

The frequency of side effects caused by MDT varies widely, ranging from 0.6% to 45% of patients treated in Brazil, for example. Although not serious or preventing continuation of treatment, the most observed side effect is a change in skin pigmentation which occurs in most patients who take clofazimine [15, 39–41].

9.1   Dapsone

Diamino-diphenyl-sulfone (DDS) is a bacteriostatic drug, and its mode of action is to compete with paraminobenzoic acid for an enzyme, dihydropteroate synthetase, thereby preventing the formation of folic acid by mycobacteria. Despite being considered a safe drug at the dosage used for MDT [39], it is the component that causes the most serious side effects.

The main side effect is allergic reaction, ranging from pruritic rashes to exfoliative dermatitis [41]. Researchers have described not uncommon dapsone-related side effects, including haemolytic anaemia, methaemoglobinaemia, jaundice, psychotic reactions, and dapsone syndrome [15, 39–43]. The hepatic alterations, when they occur, are more frequent in the first 3 months of treatment, usually manifesting with increased bilirubin and transaminases, with or without jaundice [15].

9.2   Rifampicin

Rifampicin has potent bactericidal action against *M. leprae* acting by inhibiting DNA-dependent RNA polymerase [12]. Few side effects have been reported with monthly administration [14]. However, there are reports of effects including skin rashes, thrombocytopenic purpura, hepatitis, influenza syndrome, haemolytic anaemia, shock, respiratory failure, and acute renal failure [15, 39–41, 43, 44].

9.3   Clofazimine

Clofazimine is a riminophenazine dye with bacteriostatic and anti-inflammatory properties whose mechanism of action is not well understood. It is well tolerated but can cause side effects including hyperpigmentation of the skin, conjunctiva and body fluids, integumentary and eye dryness, gastrointestinal symptoms, abdominal pain, nausea, vomiting, diarrhoea, anorexia, weight loss, and bowel obstruction. A more serious side effect is small bowel syndrome, characterized by persistent diarrhoea, weight loss, and abdominal pain [45, 46].

A rare side effect of MDT is haemophagocytic lymphohistiocytosis (HLH) [47], an abnormal (overactive) immune system response characterized by fever, splenomegaly, pancytopenia, marked hyperferritinaemia, hypertriglyceridaemia, and histiocytic haemophagocytosis in the bone marrow. It can occur during Hansen's disease treatment because MDT does not reach the bone marrow, which serves as a niche for *M. leprae*. HLH may be confused with dapsone syndrome and type 2 Hansen's disease reaction, which means that bone marrow evaluation is essential for correct diagnosis and management [48].

References

1. Mouat FJ. Notes on native remedies no. 1: the chaulmoogra. Indian Ann Med Sci. 1854;1:646–52.
2. McCoy GW. Chaulmoogra oil in the treatment of leprosy. Public Health Rep. 1942;57:1727–33. https://doi.org/10.2307/4584277.
3. Skinsnes OK. Origin of chaulmoogra oil-another version. Int J Lepr Other Mycobact Dis. 1972;40:172–3.
4. Faget GH, Pogge RC, Johansen FA, et al. The Promin treatment of leprosy. A progress report. Public Health Rep. 1943;58:1729–41.
5. Fromm E, Wittmann J. Derivate desp-Nitrothiophenols. Ber Dtsch Chem Ges. 1908;41:2264–73. https://doi.org/10.1002/cber.190804102131.
6. Cochrane RG, Ramanujam K, Paul H, Russell D. Two-and-a-half years' experimental work on the Sulphone Group of Drugs. Lepr Rev. 1949;20:4–64.
7. Lowe J. Treatment of leprosy with diamino-diphenyl sulphone by mouth. Lancet. 1950;1:145–50. https://doi.org/10.1016/s0140-6736(50)90257-1.
8. Floch HA. Sulfone-resistance of Mycobacterium leprae–monotherapy with diaminodiphenyl-sulfone–the value of triple-drug combinations. Int J Lepr Other Mycobact Dis. 1986;54:122–5.
9. Shepard CC. The experimental disease that follows the injection of human leprosy bacilli int foot-pads of mice. J Exp Med. 1960;112:445–54. https://doi.org/10.1084/jem.112.3.445.
10. Gillis TP, Williams DL. Dapsone resistance in mycobacterium leprae. Lepr Rev. 2000;71(Suppl):S91–5.
11. World Health Organization. WHO expert committee on leprosy. Fifth report. Geneva: WHO; 1977.
12. Opromolla DVA. First results of the use of rifamycin SV in the treatment of lepromatous leprosy. In: Transactions of the VIIIth International congress of leprology, vol. 2; 1963. p. 346–55.
13. Pearson JM, Haile GS, Rees RJ. Primary dapsone-resistant leprosy. Lepr Rev. 1977;48:129–32. https://doi.org/10.5935/0305-7518.19770016.
14. Sansarricq H, UNDP/World Bank/WHO special programme for research and training in tropical diseases. Multidrug therapy against leprosy: development and implementation over the past 25 years. Geneva: World Health Organization; 2004.
15. Deps PD, Nasser S, Guerra P, et al. Adverse effects from multi-drug therapy in leprosy: a Brazilian study. Lepr Rev. 2007;78:216–22.
16. World Health Organization. Guidelines for the diagnosis, treatment and prevention of leprosy. Geneva: World Health Organization; 2018.
17. Cambau E, Saunderson P, Matsuoka M, et al. Antimicrobial resistance in leprosy: results of the first prospective open survey conducted by a WHO surveillance network for the period 2009-15. Clin Microbiol Infect. 2018;24:1305–10. https://doi.org/10.1016/j.cmi.2018.02.022.

18. Lastoria JC, Almeida TSC, Putinatti MSMA, Padovani CR. Effectiveness of the retreatment of patients with multibacillary leprosy and episodes of erythema nodosum leprosum and/or persistent neuritis: a single-center experience. An Bras Dermatol. 2018;93:181–4.

19. Aubry A, Rosa PS, Chauffour A, et al. Drug resistance in leprosy: as update following 70 years of chemotherapy. Infect Dis Now. 2022;52:243–51.

20. Matsuoka M. Drug resistance in leprosy. Jpn J Infect Dis. 2010;63:1–7.

21. Maymone MBC, Venkatesh S, Laughter M, et al. Leprosy: treatment and management of complications. J Am Acad Dermatol. 2020;83:17–30.

22. Rosa PS, D'Espindula HRS, Melo ACL, et al. Emergence and transmission of drug–/ multidrug-resistant *Mycobacterium leprae* in a former leprosy colony in the Brazilian Amazon. Clin Infect Dis. 2020;70:2054–61.

23. World Health Organization. Leprosy/Hansen disease: management of reactions and prevention of disabilities. Geneva: World Health Organization; 2020.

24. Lugão HB, Frade MAC, Mazzer N, et al. Leprosy with ulnar nerve abscess: ultrasound findings in a child. Skelet Radiol. 2017;46:137–40. https://doi.org/10.1007/s00256-016-2517-1.

25. Spitz CN, Mogami R, Pitta IJR, et al. Ultrasonography as a diagnostic tool for neural pain in leprosy. PLoS Negl Trop Dis. 2022;16(4):e0010393.

26. Lu P-H, Lin J-Y, Tsai Y-L, Kuan Y-Z. Corticosteroid pulse therapy for leprosy complicated by a severe type 1 reaction. Chang Gung Med J. 2008;31:201–6.

27. Jesus JB, Sena CBC, Macchi BM, do Nascimento JLM. Cyclosporin a as an alternative Neuroimmune strategy to control neurites and recover neuronal tissues in leprosy. Neuroimmunomodulation. 2022;29(1):15–20.

28. Pearson JM, Vedagiri M. Treatment of moderately severe erythema nodosum leprosum with thalidomide–a double-blind controlled trial. Lepr Rev. 1969;40:111–6. https://doi.org/10.5935/0305-7518.19690022.

29. Sheskin J, Convit J. Results of a double blind study of the influence of thalidomide on the lepra reaction. Int J Lepr Other Mycobact Dis. 1969;37:135–46.

30. Waters MF. An internally-controlled double blind trial of thalidomide in severe erythema nodosum leprosum. Lepr Rev. 1971;42:26–42. https://doi.org/10.5935/0305-7518.19710004.

31. Girdhar A, Chakma JK, Girdhar BK. Pulsed corticosteroid therapy in patients with chronic recurrent ENL: a pilot study. Indian J Lepr. 2002;74:233–6.

32. Sales AM, de Matos HJ, Nery JA, et al. Double-blind trial of the efficacy of pentoxifylline vs thalidomide for the treatment of type II reaction in leprosy. Braz J Med Biol Res. 2007;40:243–8. https://doi.org/10.1590/s0100-879x2007000200011.

33. Helmy HS, Pearson JM, Waters MF. Treatment of moderately severe erythema nodosum leprosum with clofazimine–a controlled trial. Lepr Rev. 1971;42:167–77. https://doi.org/10.5935/0305-7518.19710020.

34. Iyer CG, Languillon J, Ramanujam K, et al. WHO co-ordinated short-term double-blind trial with thalidomide in the treatment of acute lepra reactions in male lepromatous patients. Bull World Health Organ. 1971;45:719–32.

35. Karat AB, Thomas G, Rao PS. Indomethacin in the management of erythema nodosum leprosum–a double-blind controlled trial. Lepr Rev. 1969;40:153–8. https://doi.org/10.5935/0305-7518.19690027.

36. Ing TH. Indomethacin in the treatment of erythema nodosum leprosum, in comparison with prednisolone. Singap Med J. 1969;10:66–70.

37. Arora SK, Singh G, Sen PC. Effect of levamisole therapy on lepromin reaction in lepromatous leprosy cases. Int J Lepr Other Mycobact Dis. 1985;53:113–4.

38. Sousa EJS, Sousa GC, Baia VF, et al. Botulinum toxin type A in chronic neuropathic pain in refractory leprosy. Arq Neuropsiquiatr. 2019;77(5):346–51.

39. Brasil MT, Opromolla DV, Marzliak ML, Nogueira W. Results of a surveillance system for adverse effects in leprosy's WHO/MDT. Int J Lepr Other Mycobact Dis. 1996;64:97–104.

40. Cunha Mda G, Schettini AP, Pereira ES, et al. Regarding Brasil, et al.'s adverse effects in leprosy's WHO/MDT and paramedic's role in leprosy control program. Int J Lepr Other Mycobact Dis. 1997;65:257–9.
41. Goulart IMB, Arbex GL, Carneiro MH, et al. Adverse effects of multidrug therapy in leprosy patients: a five-year survey at a health Center of the Federal University of Uberlândia. Rev Soc Bras Med Trop. 2002;35:453–60. https://doi.org/10.1590/s0037-86822002000500005.
42. White C. Sociocultural considerations in the treatment of leprosy in Rio de Janeiro, Brazil. Lepr Rev. 2002;73:356–65.
43. Hilder R, Lockwood D. The adverse drug effects of dapsone therapy in leprosy: a systematic review. Leprosy. 2020;91:232–43. https://doi.org/10.47276/lr.91.3.232.
44. Girling DJ. Adverse reactions to rifampicin in antituberculosis regimens. J Antimicrob Chemother. 1977;3:115–32. https://doi.org/10.1093/jac/3.2.115.
45. Jopling WH. Side-effects of antileprosy drugs in common use. Lepr Rev. 1985;56:61–70.
46. Rastogi P, Chhabria BA, Sreedharanunni S, et al. Leprosy and bone marrow involvement. QJM. 2017;110:189–90. https://doi.org/10.1093/qjmed/hcw204.
47. Saidi W, Gammoudi R, Korbi M, et al. Hemophagocytic lymphohistiocytosis: an unusual complication of leprosy. Int J Dermatol. 2015;54:1054–9. https://doi.org/10.1111/ijd.12792.
48. Somanath P, Vijay KC. Bone marrow evaluation in leprosy: clinical implications. Lepr Rev. 2016;87:122–3.

Index